Praise for Pumping Insulin

Knowledge is a very powerful tool in the management of diabetes. Pumping Insulin gives you all the knowledge you need to enjoy the health and lifestyle benefits of insulin pump therapy. You will find many of the pages in your copy dog-eared in no time! It's a great resource.

> — Melanie Hellstern
> Mother of a successful pumper
> Toronto, Ontario, Canada

I find myself stealing a few minutes throughout the day to get back to reading this book.

> — Judith Jones Ambrosini, Sea Girt, NJ
> Author and chef extraordinaire at the Diabetes Cyber Kitchen
> www.diabetesnet.com/cyber_kitchen/

Diabetes is NOT for dummies... this book will measurably raise your diabetes IQ and lower your A1c. **Pumping Insulin** distills extensive professional knowledge and personal experience of advanced diabetes care into bite-sized wisdom available no where else.

Don't leave injections without it !

> — Timothy Bailey, MD, FACE, FACP
> North County Endocrine, Escondido, CA

Wow! You managed to jam pack the 4th edition of **Pumping Insulin** Edition 4 with information, yet keep it user friendly for people like me. You've provided everyone with another "must have" resource that is current and comprehensible.

> — Barb Chafe, President, Insulin Pumpers Canada™
> Nova Scotia, Canada

A pumper's must-have bible. Read it and refer to it regularly to optimize your pump and blood sugar control.

> — Hope Warshaw, MMSc, RD, CDE, BC-ADM
> Co-author of **Complete Guide To Carb Counting**
> Alexandria, VA

John and Ruth's **Pumping Insulin** makes sense of an incredibly sophisticated science by transforming complex ideas into practical use. We recommend this comprehensive reference to all our families using an insulin pump.

> — Andrea Huber, RN, BSN, CDE, and
> Laura Adema Barba, RN, MS, NP, CDE
> Pediatric Insulin Pump Educators
> Children's Hospital, San Diego, CA

Insulin pump companies in the U.S.:

Animas Corporation	(877) 937-7867	www.animascorp.com
Disetronic Medical Systems, Inc.	(800) 280-7801	www.disetronic-usa.com
Insulet Corporation	(800) 591-3455	www.insulet.com
Medtronic Minimed, Inc.	(800) 646-4633	www.minimed.com
Smiths Medical MD, Inc	(800) 826-9703	www.cozmore.com

The latest pump information at our web site:

Current insulin pumps	www.diabetesnet.com/diabetes_technology/insulinpumps.php
Pump models & features	www.diabetesnet.com/diabetes_technology/insulin_pump_models.php
Infusions sets	www.diabetesnet.com/diabetes_technology/infusion_sets.php
Continuous monitors	www.diabetesnet.com/diabetes_technology/new_monitoring.php
The Insulin Wizard	www.diabetesnet.com/diabetes_tools/

Other web sites of interest in pumping or diabetes

Children With Diabetes	www.childrenwithdiabetes.com
Diabetes Health	www.diabeteshealth.com
Topix.net	www.topix.net/health/diabetes
American Diabetes Assoc.	www.diabetes.org
Insulin Pumpers Group	www.insulin-pumpers.org
Medline	www.ncbi.nlm.nih.gov/PubMed/
Clinical trials in diabetes	www.centerwatch.com/patient/studies/area4.html
Nutrition and carb data	www.medexplorer.com/nutrition/nutrition.dbm

Pumping INSULIN

Everything You Need For Success On A Smart Insulin Pump

by John Walsh, P.A., C.D.E., and Ruth Roberts, M.A.

Torrey Pines Press
San Diego

Torrey Pines Press
1030 West Upas Street
San Diego, California 92103-3821
1-619-497-0900

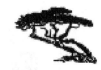

Library of Congress Cataloging in Publication Data
Walsh, John and Roberts, Ruth

Pumping Insulin:

Everything you need for success on a smart insulin pump, 4th edition
by John Walsh, P.A., C.D.E. and Ruth Roberts, M.A.

p. cm.
Includes bibliographical references.
Includes index.
1. Diabetes Popular Books
2. Diabetes Insulin
3. Diabetes Insulin-dependent diabetes
4. Diabetes Research
5. Insulin Therapeutic use
I. Title

Library of Congress Card Number: 00-190817
ISBN 1-884804-86-1 $23.95   Paperback

Printed in the United States of America

10 9 8 7 6 5 4 3 2

More Praise...

Pumping Insulin 4th Edition gives us new information on figuring safe basals, and carb and correction boluses, and how to adjust these for exercise and other life events. It shows us how to effectively use the new features in today's Super Insulin Pumps. You will find this a great addition to your diabetes library.

> — JoAnne Scott, RN, BSN, CDE
> Spokane, WA

This new edition of **Pumping Insulin** is a must read for both patients and physicians alike. An authoritative work for anyone who is contemplating insulin pump therapy or any physician who cares for patients who want to benefit from wearing an insulin pump.

> — Alan B. Schorr, DO, FAAIM, FACE,
> Langhorne, PA

Once again, John Walsh and Ruth Roberts have compiled the modern-day "bible" for intensive diabetes management. Pumping Insulin incorporates the latest technology and know-how to help people with diabetes (and their clinicians) get the most out of pump therapy.

> — Gary Scheiner MS, CDE
> President, Integrated Diabetes Services, Wynnewood, PA
> Author, **Think Like A Pancreas: A Practical Guide To Managing Diabetes With Insulin**

This is a smart book for the smart person with diabetes. It will build your knowledge of pumping and equip you with the tools you need to leverage this technology to achieve optimal well-being and health. Run, don't walk, to get your copy, and dig in! I'd recommend this book in a heartbeat.

> — Kelly Close
> Principal, Close Concerns (www.closeconcerns.com), and pumper
> San Francisco, CA

Pump users get the hang of basals and boluses in a couple of days. That's the easy part. To get the most out of all the smart features of your pump you need **Pumping Insulin** – the manual that should come with all insulin pumps. Walsh and Roberts share decades of experience, wisdom, and real-world lessons to improve your blood sugar control and health on a pump.

> — Jeff Hitchcock, Founder and President
> Children With Diabetes, Hamilton, OH
> www.childrenwithdiabetes.com – education and support for families with children with Type 1, both online and through conferences and events

The newest edition of **Pumping Insulin** truly gives the state of the art, up to date, review of practical information for any person with diabetes considering pump therapy, current pump users who want to fine tune their control, and professionals interested in insulin pumps. **Pumping Insulin** is easily the gold standard.

> —Steve Edelman, MD – Type 1 diabetes since age 15 and pumper
> Assoc. Professor of Medicine, Univ. of Cal., San Diego School of Medicine
> Founder of *Taking Control of Your Diabetes* – a seminar series that promotes education, motivation, and self-advocacy for people with diabetes

I have been in diabetes education for 20 years. **Pumping Insulin** is awesome! All patients, diabetes educators, and physicians will benefit from this new edition.

> — Pi Merzanis, RN, CDE
> North County Endocrine Medical Group, Escondido, CA

Walsh and Roberts have created the ultimate user's manual for those who refuse to take a back seat in life or in their diabetes care.

> — Bruce A. Perkins, MD, MPH
> Division of Endocrinology and Metabolism, University of Toronto, Toronto, Ontario, Canada

Pumping Insulin has been the standard reference for people who use an insulin pump and their providers for years. The fourth edition continues this outstanding tradition with information that is invaluable to pumpers.

> — Carol Wysham, MD
> Rockwood Clinic, Spokane, WA

This book truly guides health care providers as well as patients through the complex world of diabetes and pump therapy better than any other book out there. I recommend it to all my patients on a pump. New to pumping or pumping for years, the book has a lot to teach you about how to achieve better glucose control.

> — Ken Cathcart, DO, FACE
> Northside Internal Medicine, Spokane, WA

I advise all my pump patients to have a copy of this excellent book. I often ask them to work through the exercises that help them troubleshoot their basal rates, carb boluses and correction factors when control deteriorates.

> — Diane Krieger, MD
> Medical Director, South Miami Hospital Diabetes Care Center
> Miami, FL

About the Authors

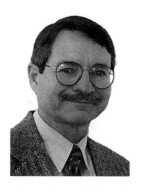

John Walsh, P.A., C.D.E., is a Physician Assistant and Diabetes Clinical Specialist who has provided clinical care to thousands of people with diabetes over the last 25 years in a wide variety of clinical settings, including private practice, HMO and university health science center. He has worn a pump for 23 years, and started and followed several hundred people on pumps.

Mr. Walsh is a popular presenter on a wide variety of diabetes topics to physicians, health professionals, diabetes educators, and people with diabetes, including the American Diabetes Association, Canadian Diabetes Association, International Diabetic Athletes Association (now DESA), Children With Diabetes, and pump support groups.

He serves as President of Diabetes Services, Inc. and is webmaster of www.diabetesnet.com, a highly trafficked source of diabetes information and online store. He has authored or coauthored hundreds of diabetes articles, as well as diabetes books and booklets. He is a consultant for medical corporations, and has developed many of the theories and assisted in the design of many of the dose-related features in today's and tomorrow's pumps and devices. He is considered an authority on pumps, devices, and intensive diabetes management, and sees patients at North County Endocrine Medical Group in Escondido, CA.

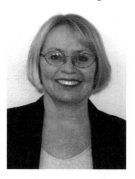

Ruth Roberts, M.A., is CEO of Diabetes Services, Inc, Diabetes Mall and Torrey Pines Press, and a widely-read medical writer and editor. She has served as a corporate training administrator, technical writer, and instructional designer for twenty years in San Diego. She has coauthored several books on diabetes, edited a weekly internet newsletter, "Diabetes This Week," and written numerous articles on diabetes.

She is a consultant for medical corporations and business start-ups specializing in diabetes products and services. She is a professional member of the American Diabetes Association and past board member of the International Diabetes Athletes Association, now DESA.

OTHER BOOKS BY JOHN WALSH, P.A., C.D.E. AND RUTH ROBERTS, M.A.:

Using Insulin, Torrey Pines Press, 2003

Pumping Insulin, 1st, 2nd, and 3rd edition, Torrey Pines Press, 2000, 1994, and 1989

STOP the Rollercoaster, Torrey Pines Press, 1996

Pocket Pancreas, Torrey Pines Press, 2000, 1998, 1995

Smart Charts, My Other CheckBook record book, Torrey Pines Press, 2000, 1995

Insulin Pump Therapy Handbook, 1990

Acknowledgments

Pumping Insulin is the product of years of personal and professional experience with diabetes and insulin pumps. During this time, major contributions have been made by our patients, colleagues, friends and fellow travelers.

Our heartfelt thanks go to the following individuals who graciously and critically reviewed and improved upon the fourth edition:

Nancy J. Bohanon, MD, FACP, FACE, San Francisco, CA, for her wise suggestions and insightful edits.

Gary Scheiner MS, CDE, President, Integrated Diabetes Services, Wynnewood, PA, for excellent advice and knowing when to use the brakes.

Helen Oswalt, proofreader and editor, par excellence, of San Diego, CA, who gets special thanks for all her revisions and encouragement.

John Rodosevich, Insulin Pumpers Support Group of San Diego, CA, for his generous support of pumpers over the last quarter century.

Carol Wysham, MD, of the Rockwood Clinic of Spokane, WA, for her thoughtful and dedicated care.

Timothy Bailey, MD, FACP, North County Endocrine, Escondido, CA, for his helpful advice and pushing the research envelope.

JoAnne Scott, RN, CDE of Spokane, WA, who helps her patients in very thoughtful ways only partly because of her own diabetes.

Daniel Einhorn, MD, FACP, FACE, Director of Sharp Healthcare Diabetes, Assoc. Clinical Professor of Medicine, U.C.S.D. School of Medicine, San Diego, CA, for his critical insights and many contributions to diabetes.

Steve V. Edelman, MD, Founder of *Taking Control of Your Diabetes*, Assoc. Professor of Medicine, U.C.S.D School of Medicine, San Diego, CA, for enlightening those with diabetes, their families and their health care providers.

Judith Jones Ambrosini, diabetes writer, Diabetes Cyber Kitchen (www.diabetesnet.com/cyber_kitchen/) and pump wearer, Sea Girt, NJ, for cooking up a storm with humor and mirth.

Bruce A. Perkins, MD, MPH, Division of Endocrinology and Metabolism, U. of Toronto, Toronto, Ontario, Canada, for his mighty contributions to exercise as an athlete with diabetes.

Ken Cathcart, DO, FACE, Northside Internal Medicine Clinic, Spokane, WA, for the excellent care he provides in diabetes.

Diane Krieger, MD, Medical Director, South Miami Hospital Diabetes Care Center, Miami, FL, who models patient care that people seek because of its results.

Alan B. Schorr, DO, FAAIM, FACE, in private practice in Langhorne, PA, for his excellent and insightful patient care.

Pi Merzanis, RN, CDE, diabetes educator at North County Endocrine Medical Group, Escondido, CA, whose patients love her because she know diabetes.

Jeff Hitchcock, Founder and President, Children With Diabetes (www.children-withdiabetes.com), Hamilton, OH, who expanded his love for his daughter with diabetes into improved care for children with diabetes worldwide.

Kelly Close, Principal, Close Concerns (www.closeconcerns.com), San Francisco, CA, who skillfully brings complex research concepts down to ground for others to see.

Andrea Huber, RN, BSN, CDE, and Laura Adema Barbara, RN, MS, NP, CDE, Pediatric Insulin Pump Educators, Children's Hospital, San Diego, CA, who make kids and families happy even with diabetes.

Melanie Hellstern, Toronto, Ontario, Canada, whose heart of gold is focused on better diabetes care for her son and others.

Hope Warshaw, MMSc, RD, CDE, BC-ADM, Alexandria, VA, who laughs with the best and writes like a dynamo.

Barb Chafe, President, Insulin Pumpers Canada™, Halifax, Nova Scotia, Canada, who has organized hundreds of Canadian families with members with diabetes into an effective voice for optimum care.

Our special thanks to Richard B. Morris, III, a graphics artist of San Diego, for the cover design, chapter headings, and all the wonderful tables, figures, text boxes and workspaces that present complex information in a clear, crisp way. Richard's hand is also at work at our website www.diabetesnet.com where he supplies technical expertise in design and communication. Visit his website at www.tingedesigns.com

We and everyone with diabetes are indebted to:

The American Diabetes Association, the Juvenile Diabetes Foundation, the National Institiute of Health, and other national agencies that generously support diabetes education and research.

All the health practitioners and the 1,441 volunteers with diabetes who participated in the Diabetes Control and Complications Trial which confirmed what early pumpers and pump proponents already assumed—that controlling blood sugars makes people healthier and reduces the complications of diabetes.

Table Of Contents

Tables

Text Boxes

Figures

Examples

Important Note

Pumping Insulin, 4th Edition, has been developed as a guide to use of a smart pump for diabetes control. Figures, charts, examples, tables, and tips provide basic as well as advanced information related to the use of an insulin pump. Insulin requirements and treatment protocols differ significantly from one person to the next. The information included in this book should be used only as a guide. It is not a substitute for the sound medical advice of your personal physician or health care team.

Specific treatment plans, insulin dosages, and other aspects of health care for a person with diabetes, must be based on individualized treatment protocols under the guidance of your physician or health care team. The information in this book is provided to enhance your understanding of diabetes and insulin pumps so that you can manage the daily challenges you face. It can never be relied upon as a sole source for your personal diabetes regimen.

While every reasonable precaution has been taken in the preparation of this information, the authors and publishers assume no responsibility for errors or omissions, nor for the uses made of the materials contained herein and the decisions based on such use. No warranties are made, expressed, or implied, with regard to the contents of this work or to its applicability to specific individuals. The authors and publishers shall not be liable for direct, indirect, special, incidental, or consequential damages arising out of the use of or inability to use the contents of this book.

Read This!

Never use this book on your own! Any suggestion made in this book for improving blood sugar control with an insulin pump should only be followed with the approval and under the guidance of your personal physician and health care team. We have provided the best information and tools available to make your insulin pump do its job of normalizing your blood sugars.

However, this book is not enough. We have worked with pumpers who have used this information together with the guidance of their physician, and they have excelled. We have also seen pumpers who get themselves into trouble by a selective use of this or other material, and by ignoring or not seeking excellent medical advice.

Always seek the advice and guidance of your physician and health care team. No book can ever help you as much as they will. They have the benefit of objectivity and experience gained from working with many other pumpers. Your own participation in the process of good control is essential, but never minimize the importance of good professional advice and support. Teams win where individuals fail, and teamwork takes trust and communication from everyone.

We wish all users of this book good health and great control with their pumps.

INTRODUCTION

If you're considering an insulin pump, beginning to use a pump, or already on a pump and have less control than you desire, the answers to your questions are here. This book gives the information and in-depth detail you need for success on a smart pump. It can help any prospective pumper, any current pumper, and anyone who assists pumpers.

Pumping Insulin is for:

- Everyone considering or beginning to use an insulin pump
- Existing pumpers who want to improve their control
- Physicians, nurses, dietitians, physician assistants, nurse practitioners, and others who follow people on pumps
- Everyone who wants to lower their glucose exposure and variability
- Everyone who wants to match insulin need with insulin delivery

Pumping Insulin tells you:

- What a pump is and how to set it up
- How to chart and analyze your blood sugar readings and other data
- How to count carbs
- How to regulate basal rates and boluses to improve your control
- How to manage and avoid low and high blood sugars
- How to minimize and solve pump problems
- How to get the most out of today's smart pumps
- How to feel better and live a healthier life
- When to seek help

This book explains how to improve control with a pump by mimicking the normal pancreas. Designed for those just starting and those who are already pumping, it contains information about new pump features, how to evaluate your control, how to set and test basal and bolus doses, and how to determine and use your personal carb and correction factors.

Included are step-by-step instructions for starting on a pump, how to test your pump settings, checklists to improve control, and specific examples of blood sugar management techniques, as well as advanced blood sugar charting methods, carbohydrate counting instructions, approaches to exercise and pregnancy, specific directions for children and teens on pumps, and information on how to avoid complications.

If you are preparing to start on a pump, read the first 13 chapters in **Pumping Insulin** before you start. These chapters explain how a pump works, how to switch from injected doses to a pump, and how to estimate and test your starting doses. Reading this make a startup easier and ensures a faster path to success.

Pump Terms

BASAL INSULIN OR BASAL RATE

A continuous 24-hour insulin delivery that matches background insulin need. Once correctly set, the blood sugar does not rise or fall when the pump user is not eating.

BASAL/BOLUS BALANCE

Basal insulin usually makes up half (40 to 60%) of the TDD with the rest as boluses.

BOB (BOLUS ON BOARD)

A pump feature that tells how much insulin from a recent bolus insulin is left to lower the blood sugar. Also called insulin on board, unused insulin, or active insulin.

BOLUS

A quick release of insulin from the pump to cover carbs or lower a high blood sugar.

BOLUS STACKING

Caused when frequent boluses overlap and causes a low blood sugar. Today's pumps prevent this by tracking BOB and Duration Of Insulin Action.

CARB BOLUS

A bolus delivered to match carbohydrates in an upcoming meal or snack.

CARB FACTOR

How many grams of carbohydrate one unit of insulin will cover.

CORRECTION BOLUS

A bolus delivered to bring a high blood sugar back to normal.

CORRECTION FACTOR

How many mg/dl (or mmol) one unit of insulin lowers the blood sugar. Used to correct highs.

DURATION OF INSULIN ACTION

A pump setting for how long a bolus of insulin lowers the blood sugar.

INFUSION SET

Delivers insulin from a reservoir to the body. Includes a hub, catheter (line), and insertion set. The insertion set is inserted through the skin. It may be a fine metal needle or a larger metal needle, which is removed to leave a small Teflon catheter under the skin.

INSULIN PUMP

A computerized device about the size of a beeper that is programmed to deliver basal insulin and carb or correction boluses. Rapid insulin is delivered from a reservoir through a plastic catheter to a Teflon or small metal needle inserted through the skin. Delivers doses as small as 0.025 unit. Programmed from information gained through frequent blood sugar monitoring.

TDD (TOTAL DAILY DOSE)

The total units of insulin a person uses in a day. Includes basal doses and bolus doses. It is used to determine the basal rate and carb and correction factors.

Benefits Of Pumping

The number of people using insulin pumps has grown rapidly since their introduction nearly 30 years ago. Much of this growth has come from pump wearers enthusiastically sharing the benefits they experience. When used well, an insulin pump allows the wearer to feel better, live more freely, and have fewer diabetes-related health problems.

The decision to go on a pump is often a turning point in a person's approach to diabetes care. Those who use pumps say things like, "For the first time in years, I can eat when I want to," or "I can really control my blood sugars now, and I feel better, too."

One enthusiastic pumper who started at the age of 70 says, "The insecurity is gone. I feel so much more hopeful and positive. According to my A1c, my control was good on injections, but I couldn't avoid overnight lows that created stress day after day. I now feel really in charge of my body again." An 11 year-old boy adds, "I can eat just like my friends if I count my carbs. Going on hikes this year at diabetes camp was easy."

This chapter explains

- Why people choose pumps
- Advantages of a smart pump over multiple injections
- Some drawbacks to pumping

Why Choose A Pump?

Keeping the blood sugar as close to normal as possible is your primary goal, whether you use conventional insulin therapy, multiple daily injections (MDI), or an insulin pump. Today's smart pumps, available since late 2002, have smart features which offer the best choice in insulin delivery. Most health professionals who have diabetes themselves prefer pumps because they know a pump offers the most convenient and effective way to mimic the pancreas. In 1998, when only 6% of people with Type 1 diabetes were using pumps, 60% of diabetes nurse educators and 52% of physicians who had Type 1 diabetes were wearing one.[1]

Dr. John Pickup published the first research report about insulin pumps in England in 1979.[2] Since then, the number of users has increased to over 325,000 worldwide. Most would never consider going back to injections. One review of 18 research studies that were conducted before 1991 with classic pumps looked at which therapy participants' preferred after they had used both a pump and multiple injections during crossover trials. Of the 520 participants, 62.5% chose to remain on a pump.[3]

Pump wearers become pump advocates because they can finally match their insulin need with the right amount given at the right time, thereby reducing stress and providing relief from unexpected emergencies. People with diabetes choose pumps for the reasons listed in Table 1.1, while health professionals recommend pumps for additional reasons listed in Table 1.2.

1.1 People With Diabetes Choose Pumps For

- A convenient and freer lifestyle
- Flexibility in when and how much to eat
- Improved blood sugar control
- Improved matching of insulin delivery to the body's variable needs
- Less hypoglycemia and hypoglycemia unawareness
- Prevention of long-term complications
- Assistance with calculations plus the data tracking required to achieve optimal control
- Reminders to bolus before meals and test afterwards
- Improved balancing of exercise with insulin
- Freedom to travel or perform shift work
- Membership in a health-conscious community
- Improved health and peace of mind

For people on multiple injections who may eat meals on a rigid schedule, require a snack every night before bed, wake up at 3 a.m. sweating profusely, face unexpected high morning readings, have returned to consciousness in an emergency room, or want to sleep late on the weekend, changing to a pump can offer a new confidence and a more enjoyable life. By allowing consistent, responsive, and precise insulin delivery, a pump can create more freedom and provide better health for the person who wears it.

Powered by common AAA or AA batteries, and using only a rapid insulin, an insulin pump creates a freer lifestyle with improved glucose readings. Pumps benefit people of all ages, from infants to those in their 80s and 90s. They have been shown to help people who have peripheral or autonomic neuropathy,[4,5] early kidney disease (microalbuminuria),[6,7] and retinopathy.[8] Pumps also benefit those who have Dawn Phenomenon, erratic control,[9,10] or insulin resistance.[11] Improved control on a pump may even reverse some health damage associated with complications.

Is A Pump Better Than Multiple Injections?

Other than the obvious benefits of fewer fingersticks per day, the ability to give insulin whenever spontaneous events arise, and quicker adjustments for changes in activity, a pump offers other benefits and conveniences:

Better Insulin Delivery

Whether provided by multiple injections or a pump, insulin delivery must mimic the way the body naturally works. In nondiabetic people, beta cells in the pancreas release precise amounts of insulin to cover two basic needs. Background insulin is released as a steady flow through the day to direct the release and uptake of glucose and fat as fuel. In addition the pancreas releases short bursts of insulin into the bloodstream to match the carbohydrate content of food eaten.

Multiple injections or a pump mimic the body by providing background insulin as basal insulin and carb boluses to cover carbohydrate. In addition correction boluses are taken to lower a high blood sugar, a state that does not occur in a nondiabetic person.

Insulin injections have four disadvantages: inconvenience, complexity, lack of precision, and variable daily activity. Success on injections is often limited to the lucky, those with a consistent lifestyle, those who retain some of their own internal insulin production, those blessed

1.2 Health Professionals Recommend Pumps For
• Sub-optimal glycemic control
• Dawn Phenomenon with elevated fasting blood sugars
• Frequent or severe hypoglycemia or hypoglycemia unawareness
• Nighttime hypoglycemia
• Postmeal hyperglycemia
• "Brittle" diabetes or high glucose variability, even with a good A1c
• Insulin requirement of less than 30 units a day
• Frequent travel
• Variable work schedule
• Intensive exercise or athletics
• Tracking insulin doses, carbs, glucose levels, and other information critical to control
• Reminders to carb bolus and test blood glucose
• Preventing, delaying, or reversing complications
• Improving control during growth and puberty in children and adolescents
• Managing gastroparesis with its erratic food absorption
• Lessening insulin resistance in Type 2 diabetes
• Preparing for conception or during pregnancy
• Frequent ketoacidosis
• Frequent hospitalizations for diabetes

with common sense, or those with a degree of obsessiveness in their personality.

Multiple daily injections or MDI involves three or more injections and at least four blood sugar tests a day. It allows a more flexible lifestyle with better control than one or two injections. A pump improves on this by providing a physiologic basal or background infusion of rapid insulin around the clock to keep the blood sugar level when no food is eaten. A bolus or quick release of insulin can be given whenever carbs are eaten. If a high blood sugar occurs, a correction bolus can immediately correct it.

A pump makes eating meals late or going all day without eating possible while maintaining great control. Because a pump excels at matching insulin to need, a person no longer has to experience the frequent highs or frightening lows characteristic of "brittle diabetes." High morning blood sugars cease to wreck the rest of the day, and exercise routines and eating can be varied without losing control.

More Convenience And Flexibility

MDI requires that an insulin bottle and syringe or an insulin pen be available for use whenever needed. Each injection must be taken in a timely fashion, whether at a restaurant or in a public restroom during times you are away from home.

Calculations can be cumbersome with MDI. Most people need a calculator to divide the grams of carb in a meal by their carb factor, and the dose becomes harder to calculate when they have to subtract a high reading from their target and divide this by a correction factor. Once the carb and correction doses are determined, an additional estimate must be made for how much rapid insulin is still active from recent injections.

> ### 1.3 Today's Smart Pumps Excel At Control
>
> Precise insulin delivery allows most pumpers to achieve blood sugars within their acceptable target range most of the time. If you use a smart pump and your blood sugar often goes too high or too low, your basal rates, carb factor, correction factor, or duration of insulin action can be changed to better fit your need.
>
> Never accept having high A1cs or experiencing erratic control if you use a smart pump. A smart pump should deliver excellent overall results. If it does not, modify your lifestyle and tweak your insulin settings until it does.

Dose calculations are much simpler with today's smart pumps. Your carb and correction factors are entered when you set up your pump. Then you enter how many carbs you will eat and your current blood sugar prior to each meal, and the pump will recommend an accurate bolus. The pump keeps track of bolus insulin on board (BOB) or active bolus insulin and adjusts carb and correction boluses to prevent insulin stacking caused by active insulin from recent boluses.

Most people prefer not to live a regulated life that is forced upon them by set doses of insulin, nor to have to take an injection every time their diet or life varies. Work hours vary, meetings and events occur randomly, meals are delayed or missed, and eating is often done on the run. On weekends, you may want to rise early or sleep late, and exercise more or less than usual and at different times of the day. Eating may change to accommodate larger family or holiday meals or late dining after a movie. As meals, activity, stress, and sleep change, so must insulin levels.

The best way to address the demands of daily life while maintaining diabetes control is to have a flexible and precise method to deliver insulin. People prefer a pump for the easy adjustment of bolus and basal doses it provides.

A pump delivers precise doses with greater flexibility than multiple injections.[12] With the variety of smart pumps now on the market, flexible insulin delivery has never been easier. "It's given me freedom for the first time. I never thought it would make this much difference," one young man responded to wearing a pump.

1.4 Normal Glucose Values

| | Normal glucose values measured in: | | |
	plasma	whole blood	interstitial fluid
before meals	110 mg/dl or less (6.1 mmol)	100 mg/dl or less (5.6 mmol)	90 mg/dl or less (5 mmol)
2 hrs after meals	140 mg/dl or less (7.8 mmol)	130 mg/dl or less (6.9 mmol)	120 mg/dl or less (6.3 mmol)

Plasma readings read by most glucose meters are similar to lab values. Whole blood readings are about 10% lower and interstitial values are about 20% lower than plasma values.

2006 Diabetes Services, Inc.

A German study looked at satisfaction scores among 77 people with Type 1 diabetes who switched from 1 or 2 injections a day to MDI and compared them to another group of 55 people who switched from MDI to an insulin pump. Those on 1 or 2 injections who switched to MDI reported greater satisfaction with MDI. The increase in satisfaction was even higher for the group who switched from MDI to insulin pump therapy.[13]

Pump wearers find that less effort is required for control with less impact from diabetes on their lives. Although the prevention of long-range problems is always a goal, most people find that the convenience and flexibility of a pump is a better personal motivator. They like the immediate sense of security and the better quality of life, along with the added benefit of knowing they are preventing future health problems through improved control.

Greater Precision

The precise insulin delivery of a pump better matches the demands of an active lifestyle than MDI. Basal insulin flow can be adjusted to keep the blood sugar in a normal range overnight or when meals are skipped. Settings that work well do not change until the wearer needs to change them, such as during long periods of exercise or activity. Exclusive use of rapid insulin allows both bolus doses and basal rates to be tailored quickly for spontaneous eating and exercise.

People who are sensitive to insulin and are on small doses especially benefit from the precision of a pump. Those who need less than 30 to 35 units a day love a pump where doses are delivered in increments as small as 0.025 (twenty five thousandths) of a unit. This precision, along with carefully calculated doses, can save them from the critical lows that often plagued them when using a syringe.

When a single unit of insulin lowers the glucose by 100 mg/dl (5.6 mmol) or more, even a small miscalculation spells disaster. A half unit or 50 mg/dl (2.8 mmol) is as close as a syringe or an insulin pen can get. It becomes understandable why the blood sugar often rises and falls on injections.

More Reliable Insulin Action

Insulin injections require that one or more doses of a long-acting insulin be given each day. These larger doses create a pool of insulin under the skin that causes its onset and peak action to vary considerably from day to day. In clinical studies of older insulins like Lente, NPH, and Ultralente, the amount of insulin that actually reached a person's bloodstream was shown to vary as much as 25% from one day to the next.[14] Unreliable dosing creates peaks and valleys that throw off control at unpredictable times.

1.5 Why Injected Insulin Action Varies
• Size of the insulin dose
• Where the injection is given
• Depth of the injection (IM vs SC)
• Exercise length and intensity
• Local heat or massage
• Outside temperature
• Mixing of different insulins
• Poor resuspension of cloudy insulins
• Smoking

Contrast this with newer long-acting insulins like Lantus (glargine) and Levemir (detemir) that display less peaking and have more consistent activity. Even so, variation in activity will still occur if the time of a daily injection varies as it may on weekdays versus weekends. In some users, Lantus has a slight peak and an action time shorter than 24 hours. Many diabetes clinics find that a third of their Lantus users require two injections a day to offset the variable action of the insulin and to accommodate lifestyle changes like sleeping in late on weekends. Also, when the action of a long-acting insulin is truly flat, it may not match a person's true basal insulin need.

Compared to using MDI with Lantus, pumps provide more stable glucose readings.[15] Basal delivery from a pump can be more easily matched to the variable background needs of those who have a Dawn Phenomenon, who change their waking or work hours, or who engage in strenuous exercise at different times. Over 75% of pumpers use more than two basal rates a day. Most use three, four, or five daily rates that can be adjusted every 30 minutes to match the body's need at different times of the day. In contrast to the variable action of a long-acting insulin, a pump uses a rapid-acting insulin delivered in small amounts throughout the day. This reduces variable insulin delivery from as much as 25% on injections to only 3% on a pump.[16]

Easier Problem Solving

If a glucose goes high or low on injections, it is difficult to determine whether the long-acting insulin is peaking erratically or the wrong dose of rapid insulin was given for a meal. On a pump, only one insulin is used for both basal and bolus doses. No long-acting insulin is in play to cause confusion from its variable action.

On a pump, the effects of basal rates and boluses are easier to separate and test so that problems can be clarified more easily. Basal delivery is tested and adjusted first. Then the pump user selects a carb factor that keeps the postmeal blood sugar from rising too high with a minimum of lows and highs before the next meal. If the carb count for a meal is inaccurate, the blood sugar two hours later will show an unwanted rise or fall. Because the basal rate has already been shown to be correct, the bolus for that particular meal has to be the problem.

If a blood sugar is high, a correction bolus will safely bring it back to a desired target range once an accurate correction factor or the number of points (mg/dl or mmol) your blood sugar drops per unit of insulin is put into your pump. The correction factor and bolus can be tested by whether they bring the blood sugar to your target range sometime between three hours, when much of the bolus activity has occurred, to as much as five to six hours later when the bolus activity has ended.

Less Hypoglycemia With A Lower A1c

The Diabetes Control and Complications Trial (DCCT) clearly showed that when people improve control they face a higher risk of hypoglycemia, shown in Fig. 1.6. The higher risk occurred regardless of whether the person used multiple injections or a pump. Luckily, the benefits of tighter blood sugar control greatly outweighed this extra risk for most people.

Severe hypoglycemia requiring the assistance of another person occurred three times as often in the intensive control group, or 62 events in 100 patient-years, compared to 19 events in 100 patient years in the conventionally treated group.[17] Some participants had several episodes of severe hypoglycemia, while others had none at all. Some of the 19 clinics involved in the DCCT improved glucose control in their pump patients with little increase in hypoglycemia. The skill of medical providers at various clinics appears to make a difference in whether tight control leads to hypoglycemia.

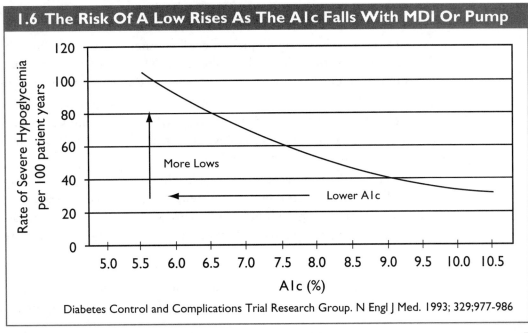

1.6 The Risk Of A Low Rises As The A1c Falls With MDI Or Pump

More Lows

Lower A1c

Diabetes Control and Complications Trial Research Group. N Engl J Med. 1993; 329;977-986

Several research studies have shown lower A1c values and less hypoglycemia with pumps, meaning that less time is spent in the low and high ranges.[18-22] As experience grows on a pump, low blood sugars generally become less frequent and less severe. In one study of 225 pumpers in Atlanta, the frequency of hypoglycemia during the first year of pump use was compared to the previous year on MDI. Severe episodes dropped from 138 events for every 100 years with MDI to 22 per 100 years in the first year of pump use. This lower rate persisted during the four years participants were on pumps.[23]

In 1998, the Disetronic pump company surveyed 6,890 pump users in the U.S. and Europe. Respondents had diabetes for an average of 21 years, with half having used a pump between 0 to 2 years and half for 3 to 15 years. In this large group, 62% reported that their hypoglycemia was less frequent, while 17% reported it was more frequent, and 21% said it was about the same compared to previously on injections.

Today's smart pumps and continuous monitors are more likely to prevent hypoglycemia through use of features listed in Table 1.7. Smart pumps have reminders to test after boluses, provide doses based on a meal's carb count and the current blood sugar, and adjust for any BOB (or bolus insulin on board – see pages 48-50). Tracking of active insulin allows a smart pump to determine exactly how many carbs are needed to prevent an upcoming low blood sugar once a blood sugar test is done, as shown in Text Box 5.5. Continuous monitors track blood sugar trends and sound an alarm before lows happen or when the blood sugar rises faster than expected, such as after a meal.

Less Hypoglycemia Unawareness

Hypoglycemia unawareness occurs when someone is not aware a low blood sugar is happening because their symptoms are reduced. Thinking becomes severely impaired before they notice any symptoms. This can be dangerous if no one is around to help. It is more common in anyone who has had diabetes for many years, whose insulin doses are excessive, or who is having frequent lows. Unawareness can be reversed by reducing the frequency of lows or avoiding them altogether. This allows counter-regulatory hormone levels to rise and produces stronger symptoms, so the person recognizes the low earlier.

An insulin pump allows the user more time to recognize symptoms and correct a low blood sugar.[24] Most episodes of hypoglycemia unawareness occur during sleep. A pump can be programmed to deliver nighttime basal rates so they match changing insulin need. This helps prevent nighttime lows.

Irl Hirsch, M.D. and Ruth Farkas-Hirsch, R.N. follow a large group of pumpers in Seattle. They say, "Hypoglycemia unawareness should be considered an important indication for an insulin pump.[25] Having fewer low blood sugar readings allows a person to experience stronger hypoglycemia symptoms.[26] See Chapter 17 for more information.

Fewer Morning Highs

"If I wake up high, my whole day is shot!" is a typical complaint from people with diabetes. Morning highs are difficult to bring down and often require several correction

1.7 Smart Pumps Help Prevent Hypoglycemia	
Cause For Lows	**How A Smart Pump Helps**
Excess bolus insulin	Protects against overbolusing with the premeal carb and correction factors programmed into the pump. When a glucose test is taken, a pump can reveal your bolus excess (carb deficit) using bolus tipping. (see Figure 5.5)
Insulin stacking	Avoided by taking into account the bolus on board (BOB) or active insulin from previous boluses when a new bolus is given.
Insulin absorption and carb need are increased with exercise.	Fast and precise insulin adjustments can be made, such as a temporary basal reduction, to reduce the risk of hypoglycemia during and after exercise.
Insulin absorption increased with heat absorption	Compared to large pools of long-acting insulin required with injections, pumps have only a small insulin pool under the skin. This reduces heat absorption during hot weather or when sitting in a sauna.
A bolus is taken but the meal is delayed or missed	Not solved by a smart pump. You must take responsibility here.

boluses, less food, or more exercise through the day to return the blood sugar to target. A precisely timed increase in the night basal rate lessens glucose production by the liver, improves uptake of glucose by muscle cells, and reduces excess fat release. This allows a person with Type 1 diabetes and a strong Dawn Phenomenon or someone with Type 2 and insulin resistance to wake up without a high blood sugar.

"I usually wake up with a normal blood sugar!" is a joy shared by many pumpers and makes a major difference in controlling the entire day's readings. Correcting a prior pattern of high morning blood sugar readings is done through simple basal adjustments. Easy programming allows a pumper to adjust basal rates to meet personal insulin need through the night.

Drawbacks To Pumping

Insulin pumps have many advantages, but they are also mechanical devices that depend on several components to work properly. Pumps use small computers to deliver sophisticated doses. Some can be started as a simple insulin delivery device and transformed into a device with all the advanced features that aid control, as discussed in Chapter 5. Like any device, a pump requires a conscientious user to go through a learning curve in order to make it work properly. A pump is not the answer for everyone. Consider the drawbacks of pumping before making your own decision.

Attachment And Acceptance

Attachment to a pump may seem inconvenient, annoying, or embarrassing to someone who has not worn one. Even though today's beeper-sized pumps weigh only a few ounces, being attached via a catheter and tubing to a small computerized device may seem intolerable. This common concern usually disappears quickly once a user is attached and begins to experience the advantages that a pump offers.

Once a person starts on a pump, they are usually surprised at its comfort and wearability. Anticipated personal rejection turns into a new delight in freedom from shots and in unexpected respect from others who realize you are using advanced technology to improve your health. Better blood sugar control can be a great relief to users and families as well.

Some people fear that others will consider them different or as having a "disease" if they see their pump. The teen years and early twenties are particularly difficult ages to be different, so this concern may not be easy to overcome at these ages. Hesitation can also arise in those who are actively involved in contact sports. However, sports problems can often be worked out through easy detachment of infusion sets while playing the sport or by wearing a protective case for the pump during active times.

If you are interested in trying a pump but have concerns, see whether you can obtain a loaner pump to wear. The pump's reservoir can be filled with water or remain empty with the Teflon infusion line taped to the outside of the skin. (Barb Chafe of Insulin Pumpers of Canada says a yoyo with its string extended also works nicely as a pump substitute.) A trial run can help you decide about the comfort and acceptability of a pump. Even if you decide against wearing a pump at this time, you will be more familiar with it for future consideration.

Ketoacidosis

Although a long-acting insulin creates some problems because of its variable activity from day to day, its longer action time does protect against ketoacidosis. A pump uses no long-acting insulin but instead delivers small amounts of rapid insulin under the skin through the day. If this delivery is interrupted for any reason, the blood sugar can start to rise 90 minutes later, and in three hours, the blood insulin level will have fallen to about half its original level.

As the insulin level falls and glucose is no longer accessible as fuel, cells start to use more fat for fuel. As more and more fat is consumed, a variety of acidic by-products called ketones begin to rise in the blood. Four to five hours following the interruption of insulin delivery from a pump, a dangerous acidic state called ketoacidosis begins.[27]

In studies done in the early 1980s, an emergency room or hospital visit for ketoacidosis occurred once in every six and a half years of pump use.[28] Since then, advances in pump therapy have decreased the risk for ketoacidosis.[29] In seven research studies that looked at this risk between 1985 and 1990, ketoacidosis had dropped to once for every 10 to 25 years of pump use.[30] Even so, ketoacidosis remains a higher risk on a pump.

On a pump, infusion site and set problems are the most common cause for ketoacidosis, followed on rare occasions by bad insulin or incorrect programming of the pump. Frequent blood sugar tests (four or more a day) are critical to catch these problem before they reach a critical stage.

Site Issues

The skin provides our most important defense against infection. When an infusion set or needle breaks through the skin, a door opens through which bacteria can enter. Skin infections are almost never seen with injections, but infection risk is greater on a pump because an infusion set remains in place for two or three days.

A mild infection may require an antibiotic, but if an infection progresses to an abscess, it must be lanced and drained. A severe infection may require hospitalization. Fortunately, such problems are rare and site infection can be prevented with good technique and appropriate hygiene, covered on pages 105 and 106. For prevention of infection, it is also important to change the infusion site every two to three days.

A particular infusion set may also cause irritation to the skin near the insertion site. Though designed to minimize skin problems, a particular set and individual may not mix well. Fortunately, there are a wide variety of infusion sets to choose from to replace a set if there is a problem. Various ways to minimize skin irritation are discussed in Chapter 9.

When a site needs to be changed can also be an issue. Most pumps provide a wide window of time during which the current infusion set can be replaced. This enables a user to wait a day or two if they are unable to replace a set right away because they forgot to order, they became stranded in an airport, etc. Being prepared is a useful talent in diabetes, but things do happen, such as an infusion set getting ripped out by a door-knob. Wearable pumps get around the infusion line problem, but they also have a much narrower time, currently 0 to 8 hours, during which the site must be changed before delivery stops. Your choice of a particular pump may depend on how organized your life is, but all pumps will generate some site choice and site change issues.

Expense

The initial cost of a pump and the ongoing cost of pump reservoirs and infusion sets make insulin pumps more expensive than multiple injections. It is important to have the financial support of good health insurance or to find some other way to meet these expenses.

1.8a An Optimal Control Checklist

This checklist provides a good guide toward optimal pump use. Find the source of problem areas in your current control by answering these questions. If you answer "Yes" to a question, go on the next question. If you answer "No" to a question, correct your control at that step by reviewing the indicated chapters before proceeding. For example, if your basal doses have not been set correctly, correct this before attempting to set your carb boluses.

Review & Check

**Check here
if OK:**

Review

Overnight Basal Dose

☐ Can you go to bed with a blood sugar of 90 to 120 mg/dl (5.0 to 6.7 mmol), eat little or no snack and wake up in the morning with a target reading?　No ➡ Chapters 10 & 11

Yes ↓

Daytime Basal Dose

☐ With a target blood sugar before a meal, can you skip that meal, take no carb bolus and have your blood sugar rise no more than 15 mg/dl (0.85 mmol) and fall no more than 30 mg/dl (1.7 mmol)?　No ➡ Chapters 10 & 11

Yes ↓

Carb Counting

☐ Can you accurately determine how many grams of carbohydrate are in the foods you eat by counting carbs?　No ➡ Chapter 7

Yes ↓

Carb Boluses

☐ With a target blood sugar before a meal, can you cover carbs with a carb bolus so that your blood sugar is at target 4 to 5 hours later?　No ➡ Chapters 10 & 12

Yes ↓

Correction Boluses

☐ When you have a high blood sugar, can you take a correction bolus so that your blood sugar returns to target 4 to 5 hours later?　No ➡ Chapters 10 & 13

Yes ↓

Bolus On Board

☐ When you give 2 or more carb or correction boluses within 5 hours of each other, can you avoid insulin stacking and return to your target?　No ➡ Chapter 5

Yes ➡ **Continued on next page**

1.8b An Optimal Control Checklist - continued

Review & Check

Check here if OK:

Review

Troubleshooting Low Blood Sugars

□ Can you identify patterns of and causes for lows, and make appropriate dose or lifestyle changes to have fewer of them and prevent rebound highs? — No → Chapter 15, 16, 18

Yes ↓

Troubleshooting High Blood Sugars

□ Can you identify patterns of and causes for highs, and make appropriate dose or lifestyle changes to reduce your glucose exposure and stabilize your readings? — No → Chapters 15, 19, 20

Yes ↓

Exercise

Can you adjust your insulin doses and carbs so you can exercise without causing a high or low blood sugar? — No → Chapters 23

Yes ↓

Terrific! No problems! Check again later!

Summary

Pumps provide distinct advantages for blood sugar control. When set up and used well, they allow a more consistent, flexible and precise delivery of insulin which keeps your blood sugar close to your target. As your control improves, your risk of developing health problems related to diabetes lessens.

A well-trained person on a pump with correct settings can skip meals, eat late, and cover variations in carb intake without losing control. When elevated blood sugars, exercise, or unexpected illnesses occur, a pumper can push the buttons on their pump to quickly adjust their insulin. The simplicity of giving and adjusting insulin makes a pump simpler than taking injections. Because a pump closely copies the functioning of a healthy pancreas, it creates freedom for the person wearing it.

Pumps have drawbacks. For example, the risk of ketoacidosis and infection can increase for some. Attachment to an external device can be a perceived drawback or a real one to be dealt with by those who swim or play contact sports. A pump can only be as successful as the ability and effort of the person responsible for its use.

When a pump is used well, the wearer feels better, lives more freely, and is far less likely to have diabetes-related health problems. Confidence about good diabetes management enables the wearer to feel more in control of daily living. "My friends (family, co-workers) say that I look healthier and more alert" is a frequently heard comment. The improved sense of well-being and the better quality of life that come from improved control motivates many people to do even better as time goes on. When the pros and cons are carefully weighed, a pump clearly offers significant advantages for people who want a healthy and enjoyable life.

Will improved health and happiness be enough to make you take on the challenge of using a pump for better blood sugar control? We hope so. Not only will tomorrow's health look rosier, but right away you feel better physically and emotionally because your blood sugars are close to where they need to be.

A normal blood sugar is important to both physical and mental health, so understanding how to make this happen pays tremendous benefits. This book assists you in becoming a pro with your insulin pump. It helps you set and achieve reasonable blood sugar goals, and guides you in using all the tools available. With awareness and experience, you can reduce blood sugar swings, feel better, and prevent or reverse complications. You cannot prevent diabetes once it has occurred, but you can prevent the miseries caused by poor control.

Facts do not cease to exist
because they are ignored.
Aldous Huxley

1.9 Complication Risk In Type 1 Diabetes

These percentages indicate average risk for developing each complication in someone with Type 1 diabetes whose A1c is about 9.7%. These values reflect data obtained prior to the DCCT Trial completed in 1993.

Organ	Lifetime Risk (unless noted)
Eyes	
Cataract	25-35%
Cataract removal	3-5%
Retinopathy	
any degree	90%
proliferative retinopathy	50% (15 yrs)
laser treatment	40-50%
blindness	3-5% (30 yrs)
Frozen Shoulder	10%
Trigger finger (DuPuytren's)	10%
Kidneys	
End stage renal disease	35%
Nerves	
Gastroparesis symptoms	1-5%
Peripheral neuropathy	54%
Autonomic neuropathy	
Bladder dysfunction	1-5%
Impotence	25%
Diarrhea	1%

For each 10% reduction in A1c, the risk of eye and kidney problems drops about 35% and may be similar for other complications.

Adapted from D.M. Nathan, Chap 5 in Atlas of Clinical Endocrinology Vol. 2: Management and Prevention of Complications in Type 1 Diabetes. Ed: C.R. Kahn, Current Medicine, Inc., Philadelphia, 2000

High Glucose Complications

Damage to the eyes, kidneys, nerves, and heart results from high or unstable blood sugars over a long period of time. Although other factors play a role in who gets complications and how quickly they develop, the most toxic factor is the presence of excess glucose. Maintaining relatively normal blood sugar levels is the best way to prevent unwanted diabetes complications.

This chapter explains

- How damage occurs
- Glucose exposure and variability
- A good A1c may not be enough

Benefits Of A Normal Glucose Level

A major goal of any diabetes treatment program is to keep the blood sugar as close to normal as possible. Large, well-designed research studies like the DCCT, EDIC, UKPDS and Kumamoto have proven beyond a doubt that a lower blood glucose level leads to fewer medical problems.[31-34] They have shown that keeping glucose levels close to normal is the best way to avoid complications and stay healthy with diabetes.

High blood sugars cause cell damage that leads to retinopathy, kidney damage, nerve damage, or heart problems over time. Beginning at a submicroscopic level, excess glucose creates toxic interactions with proteins and enzymes that increase oxidation, raise harmful protein kinase C levels, and reduce energy flow.

Blood sugars that go up and down in wide swings are also harmful. They do not make people feel great, but this loss of well-being is often least apparent to the person in poor control who has forgotten what normal blood sugars feel like. In Type 2 diabetes, the loss of control is less apparent as blood sugars gradually rise above normal over the typical 10 year period before a diagnosis is finally made. In the United Kingdom Prospective Diabetes Study Group (UKPDS) in which over 5,000 people with newly diagnosed Type 2 diabetes were screened, one or more early complications were already present in half of these individuals by the time they were diagnosed.[35]

Damage from high readings remains hidden for years and lulls many into thinking their control is adequate. The immediate task of preventing lows may take precedence, while highs do not appear as threatening. During this time many people become blasé about the risk they face down the road or they may start to believe they cannot change their readings or their fate. By the time symptoms occur that can no longer be ignored, the person may have developed advanced organ damage that cannot be reversed. High blood sugar readings will warn of future damage long before these complications become obvious. Yet many people ignore their readings or do a poor job of controlling them.

Though complications create no symptoms for years, specialized tests can indicate that a specific complication is underway. These include a urine test for microalbumin to detect early kidney disease, a dilated eye exam to identify retinopathy, and an exam of the feet for loss of nerve conduction. Everyone with diabetes should have these tests done regularly to catch problems early and keep them at bay. Prevention is less expensive and less traumatic than treating a problem that has already become serious.

The DCCT Study And Its Aftermath

Determining whether complications could be reduced or prevented through better blood sugar control was the goal of the ten-year Diabetes Control and Complications Trial. Starting in the mid–1980s, the study involved 1,441 people with Type 1 diabetes. Half of the group received conventional treatment using urine testing and one or two injections a day, while the other half received intensive treatment using multiple injections or an insulin pump and blood sugar tests several times a day. Frequent feedback via telephone and clinic visits helped the intensive control group adjust their insulin doses.

When the study ended in 1993, the intensive control participants had brought their A1c values down from an average of 9.3% to 7.2%. This improved control resulted in a 25 to 32% reduction in various complications for each 1% reduction in their A1c values compared to the conventional control group.

An even more surprising result came from a 12-year followup study of the DCCT participants called Epidemiology of Diabetes Interventions and Complications or EDIC. This study followed most of the original participants and found that heart attacks, strokes, and cardiovascular deaths were 57% less likely in the original intensive control group even though their A1c levels following the DCCT were identical to those of the original control group for 11 years after the study ended.[36] The reduction in A1c level during the six and a half years that participants averaged in the study accounted for 97% of the cardiovascular protection, far more than provided by reductions in blood pressure or cholesterol in this younger population.

Despite overwhelming proof from the DCCT and EDIC studies that control matters, blood sugar control has not improved significantly since the DCCT study was completed. Diabetes remains the leading cause of blindness and kidney disease in this country. In total, 5,000 new cases of blindness are caused by proliferative retinopathy (new vessel growth in the retina) per year, and 56,000 cases of blurred or impaired vision are caused by macular edema each year in the U.S. in people with diabetes.

If you have moderate background retinopathy or more advanced retinopathy, eye damage can temporarily worsen if you rapidly improve your control. Worsening of existing eye damage is caused by a rise in vascular endothelial growth factor (VEGF), which results from a rise in levels of protein kinase C (PKC).

When control is improved rapidly after a long period of poor control, a rise in PKC and VEGF causes new blood vessels to grow. Several angiogenesis inhibitors, which reduce the formation of new blood vessels are in trials for the treatment of cancer and diabetic retinopathy. These drugs appear promising for the prevention and treatment of diabetic retinopathy if side effects are shown to be acceptable.

If your previous control has not been great, your physician may advise you to improve gradually during the first few weeks of pump use to lessen the release of VEGF. Another approach is to use high doses of vitamin E for a few months. Unrelated to its antioxidant properties, vitamin E becomes a VEGF inhibitor at high doses. Usually 1,200 or 1,500 units a day are needed to prevent the rise in PKC levels and eliminate the abnormal blood flow that causes new vessels to grow. [37-40]

However, vitamin E is not benign. It has been associated with an increase in one type of stroke caused by bleeding. It also may block some of the action of the statin class of drugs that lower cholesterol levels. Discuss these issues with your physician or ophthalmologist before improving your control rapidly.

If you have existing retinopathy, you want to be followed by an experienced ophthalmologist to avoid a worsening of eye damage during early pump use. [41, 42] After 6 to 12 months of good control, retinopathy will usually stabilize and may slowly improve. Work with your ophthalmologist to make this happen.

Improved control can prevent at least 76% of the vision loss caused by diabetes[31] and is important for successful treatment of existing retinopathy.[43] If blood sugar control were improved so that the average A1c level among people with diabetes was brought down to 7.2%, similar to the level found in the DCCT, estimates suggest this would save $624 million a year in eye damage and extend vision by 112,000 person-years in the U.S.[44,45] Other complications show similar benefits from improved control.

Factors other than improved blood sugar levels also lessen complication risks. Lower blood pressure, regular exercise, an improved diet with reduced fat and protein intake, not smoking, and better cholesterol levels have all shown major benefits. Work with your physician on all these areas to improve your health, and keep in mind that the improved control possible with a pump helps stabilize or even reverse complications.

Why High Glucose Damages Cells

Some cells and organs receive little damage from high blood sugar levels while others bear the brunt of destruction. When the blood sugar is high, a cell that depends on insulin to move glucose into its interior does not have a high glucose level inside because the insulin is low. Muscle, liver, fat and other cells that depend on insulin stay relatively protected. On the other hand, cells that are more prone to damage, like those in nerves, blood vessels, eyes, and kidneys, do not rely on insulin for glucose transfer because they require a steady supply of glucose. As the glucose level rises in the blood, it also rises inside these cells to cause damage.

As a simple example of glucose toxicity, consider a turkey cooking in the oven at Thanksgiving. Before being placed in the oven, a turkey's skin is tough and flexible. Once the turkey has spent about 4 hours in an oven at 325° F, proteins and glucose in the skin react to turn the skin brown, fragile, and easy to eat. This browning of a turkey skin is identical to the "browning reaction" that happens in everyone as a part of aging when glucose forms irreversible crosslinks between proteins in the body. The A1c test that your doctor has you get periodically measures only one of the proteins called hemoglobin that has undergone a browning reaction. Compared to the four hours that a turkey spends in the oven, the human body has a much lower "oven temperature" that allows it a longer "cooking time". The chemical reaction, however, is the same.

Our understanding of how damage occurs to cells and organs in diabetes has gradually advanced as a result of thousands of research studies conducted over the years. Four major mechanisms have been identified that damage the body when it is exposed to excess glucose. These include excess glycosylation of proteins and enzymes, increased hexosamine pathway activity, increased sorbitol pathway activity, and activation of protein kinase C. These abnormalities damage cell structures and enzymes, redirect energy away from normal repair and healing, and cause abnormal blood flow.

Over the years, different drugs have been designed to block one of the four mechanisms in an attempt to stop organ and blood vessel damage. This approach has produced mixed results. When a drug affects only a single mechanism, such as blocking

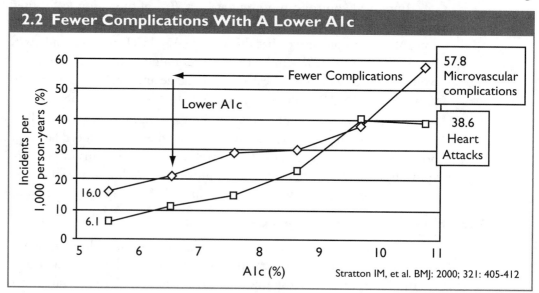

2.2 Fewer Complications With A Lower A1c

Stratton IM, et al. BMJ: 2000; 321: 405-412

the activation of protein kinase C, it may reduce eye damage, but it may also increase activity in the remaining three pathways and cause additional damage through them.

Some research suggests that a single process may activate all four mechanisms that harm body cells from high glucose levels. This silver-bullet theory suggests that high glucose levels cause oxidative damage to DNA in mitochondria, a component in cell nuclei that was borrowed from bacteria by mammals millions of years ago and is now the cell's major supplier of energy. Oxidation of mitochondrial DNA causes cellular energy production to fall, activating, in turn, the four damage mechanisms listed above.

To prove this theory, researchers have genetically modified mitochondria so they produce more of an enzyme called superoxide dismutase that protects mitochondrial DNA from oxidative damage. Cells and lab animals that have been genetically modified in this way appear to be protected from all four damage mechanisms when they are exposed to high glucose levels.[46]

These results appear promising and are supported by related research focused on the prevention of aging.[47] The hope is that more effective drugs or genetic modifications may eventually stop much or all of the damage caused by high blood sugars. However, it will take years to develop and test the first of these drugs, and this silver bullet theory may fail over time like many others before it. Currently, the easiest way to stop the damage caused by diabetes is to avoid high and erratic blood sugars.

Glucose Exposure And Glucose Variability

Emphasis is rightly placed on high blood sugar levels as a cause for damage, but evidence also points to up and down or unstable readings as an additional culprit. Glucose exposure, measured by an A1c test or by the glucose average from a meter, is clearly responsible for most of the damage caused by diabetes. But glucose variability, measured by the standard deviation in some new meters or pumps or when data from a meter is downloaded to software in a PC, is drawing attention as an independent risk factor.

Figure 2.3 shows the difference between glucose exposure and variability. Exposure is measured

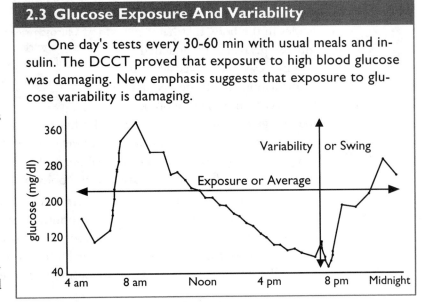

2.3 Glucose Exposure And Variability

One day's tests every 30-60 min with usual meals and insulin. The DCCT proved that exposure to high blood glucose was damaging. New emphasis suggests that exposure to glucose variability is damaging.

by the average glucose indicated by the horizontal line in the figure, while variability is measured by the up and down changes in glucose over time. Interestingly, glucose exposure and glucose variability don't necessarily occur together. In downloads of 256 consecutive meters brought in by patients to one physician's office, there was little relationship between A1c and glucose variability.[48] In other words, the variability in a person's blood sugar cannot be predicted by their A1c.

Ways To Measure Glucose Exposure

An A1c test measures the average exposure to glucose over the last six to ten weeks and is a good starting point to evaluate recent control. A normal A1c range is 4% to 6% at most labs. The American Diabetes Association recommends that people with diabetes keep their A1c below 7.0%,[49] while the American Association of Clinical Endocrinologists and the International Diabetes Federation recommend that they strive to keep the A1c below 6.5%[50] to prevent complications and heart problems. Living alone or having a history of hypoglycemia unawareness requires that A1c targets be set higher for safety, while pregnancy necessitates a lower target of 5.5% or less for the best opportunity to have a healthy child. Set realistic goals with your physician's help.

An A1c test measures the percentage of hemoglobin molecules in the body that have glucose permanently attached in a process called glycosylation or browning, mentioned earlier. Glycosylation of hemoglobin,

2.4 Estimated A1c From The Average Glucose On Your Meter		
Average Glucose On Meter*		**Est. A1c**
135 mg/dl	7.5 mmol	6%
170 mg/dl	9.5 mmol	7%
205 mg/dl	11.5 mmol	8%
240 mg/dl	13.5 mmol	9%
275 mg/dl	15.5 mmol	10%
310 mg/dl	17.5 mmol	11%
345 mg/dl	19.5 mmol	12%

* Glucose reading must be done before and 1-2 hours after meals to reflect a true average reading. The correlation used in this table was obtained from the DCCT study.

C.L. Rohlfing et al: Diabetes Care 25: 275-278, 2002

like the glycosylation of enzymes and other proteins, deforms their natural structure so they do not work well or at all. For instance, glycosylated hemoglobin does not release oxygen to cells in the way that normal hemoglobin does. The A1c test provides a good marker for harmful changes caused in the body by the browning reaction.

Ask your doctor for an A1c test every 3 to 4 months unless a sustained record of excellent control allows you to wait six months. Between A1c tests, your glucose meter can conveniently track your glucose exposure. A 14-day or 30-day average of your readings on your meter assesses your current control and guides you when you need to lower elevated blood sugars without waiting until the next A1c test is done.

Table 2.4 shows how to estimate your current A1c from a 30-day glucose average on your meter. A realistic goal for most people on a pump is to bring the average glucose below 150 mg/dl (8.3 mmol) when six or more tests are done each day before and after meals. Another realistic goal to have is to keep your blood sugar within your target range 75% of the time. Keep track of your glucose by recording the average from your meter once a week on your *Smart Charts*, logbook, or calendar.

A Good A1c May Not Be Enough

An A1c below 6.5% or 7% indicates "good" control, but the A1c test and the average blood sugar on your meter do not measure glucose stability. If your A1c is achieved through numerous ups and downs in your readings, this is not good blood sugar management, makes daily life unpleasant, and may increase the likelihood of complications.

Dr. Irl Hirsch, an endocrinologist at the University of Washington, has pointed out studies that suggest that glucose stability may improve health. Figure 2.5 shows the likelihood of eye damage progressing over time during the DCCT study. Both the upper and lower graphics in the figure show that a higher A1c level increases the risk of having eye disease worsen. However, people who were in the intensive control group on the bottom are shown separately from those in the standard control group on the top. What is striking is how much lower the risk of eye damage is for those in the inten-

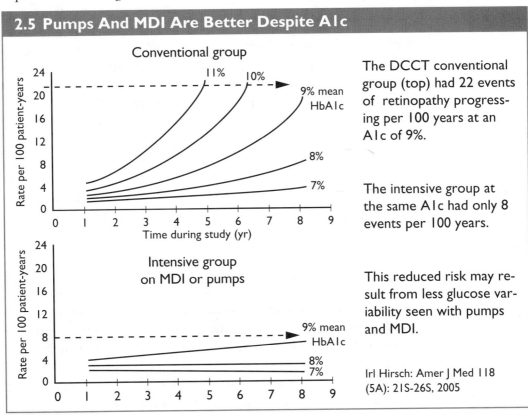

2.5 Pumps And MDI Are Better Despite A1c

Conventional group

The DCCT conventional group (top) had 22 events of retinopathy progressing per 100 years at an A1c of 9%.

The intensive group at the same A1c had only 8 events per 100 years.

This reduced risk may result from less glucose variability seen with pumps and MDI.

Irl Hirsch: Amer J Med 118 (5A): 21S-26S, 2005

21

sive control group **at the same A1c of 9%!** In the conventional control group, people with an average A1c of 9% had 22 events per 100 patient-years where existing retinopathy worsened, compared to the intensive group where only 8 events per 100 years occurred at the same A1c.

One explanation for this large reduction in risk at the same A1c is that there is less glucose variability with pumps or MDI compared to using 1 or 2 injections a day. Research with cell cultures demonstrates a possible link between glucose variability and eye damage. When human endothelial cells that line blood vessels

2.6 Causes For A High A1c
• Infrequent monitoring
• Infrequent bolusing
• Inaccurate carb counting
• Missed, incorrect, or misunderstood boluses
• Not logging enough data to improve control
• Fear of or over treatment of hypoglycemia
• Not adjusting doses for spontaneous eating
• Incorrect TDD, basal rates, carb factor or correction factor.
• Complexity of the challenge
• Unclear accountability

were exposed to glucose levels that vary between 90 and 360 mg/dl (5 to 20 mmol), they are two and a half times more likely to die than when the cells are left at 360 mg/dl (20 mmol) all the time.[51] More interestingly, activation of protein kinase C beta or PKC-beta, which is believed to cause retinopathy and vascular disease, is about 80% higher after 14 days when glucose levels vary between 90 and 360 mg/dl (5 to 20 mmol) compared to cells kept constantly at 360 mg/dl (20 mmol).[52] MDI and pumps have been shown to reduce glucose variability and this may lower levels of PKC-beta. This may explain the lower risk of having retinopathy progress as shown in Fig. 2.5. The safest environment for cells and humans appears to be a consistent glucose in the normal range.

Glucose variability can be measured by the standard deviation (SD) in a software program when meter readings are downloaded to a PC. They can also be read in some newer meters and pumps. At this early stage of tracking glucose variability, we suggest you keep your SD below 65 mg/dl (3.6 mmol) or try to keep it less than half of your average blood sugar at each time of day.

Summary

Complications in diabetes are preventable. The less variable your readings, the easier and safer it becomes to lower your A1c, so work to reduce both your glucose exposure and glucose variability. Some things that affect readings cannot be controlled. But keep in mind that the major cause for unwanted glucose exposure and variability originates in basals and boluses that are not yet adjusted to match need. Blood sugar control becomes easier, more systematic, and more understandable when a pump is used well. Having a better handle on control improves personal motivation. Strive to use your pump effectively so you can live a healthy life.

The Pancreas As Your Model

Normal glucose values for a person without diabetes range between 70 and 140 mg/dl (3.6 to 7.8 mmol), depending on when in relation to a meal a reading is taken. Someone with diabetes, even with excellent control, will have readings that go outside this ideal range.

No health professional expects perfect control, but years of clinical research and patient care have led those who specialize in diabetes to a single conclusion: the closer to normal and the more stable the blood sugar is, the better. For optimum control, a pump offers the best imitation of the action of the normal pancreas and is currently the best approach to replacing the pancreas.

This chapter describes

- How normal pancreatic insulin delivery works
- How to mimic normal insulin delivery with a pump
- Basal insulin and basal rates
- Bolus insulin and its uses

How The Pancreas Delivers Insulin

When questions arise about how to manage basals or boluses, consider how a normal pancreas would deliver insulin in the same situation.

Insulin release from the beta cells works as part of the body's system of checks and balances to keep the blood sugar in a narrow range. The brain and nervous system need the right amount of glucose in the blood at all times to fuel their vital functions. The beauty of normal beta cells is that they release exactly the right amount of insulin to move glucose into cells, and yet leave enough glucose in the blood to avoid hypoglycemia. If the blood sugar begins to fall, counter-regulatory hormones, like glucagon, epinephrine, growth hormone, and cortisol, move glucose from liver and muscle stores into the blood to provide the fuel the body needs.

Healthy beta cells release insulin into the blood throughout the day. This background or basal insulin as it is called in pump terminology enables stored fat and glucose to be released in the right amounts to support metabolism during times when we are not eating. A steady insulin level through the day regulates glucose production by the liver, the production and release of fat as fuel, and the entry of certain amino acids into cells for creation of enzymes and structural proteins. People without diabetes release about half of their total daily insulin dose through the day as background insulin to fulfill these needs.[53]

The top graphic in Figure 3.1 shows normal glucose levels, while the bottom graphic shows insulin levels. Note the relatively constant 24-hour release of basal insulin in the bottom graphic. Basal insulin levels may rise or fall during the day to balance changes in stress, activity, and levels of other regulatory hormones. Although basal insulin requirements will vary from person to person during the day, they remain relatively consistent from day to day in the same individual, unless external circumstances change.

The spikes in the bottom graphic show the remainder of the day's insulin being released at mealtimes to cover carbs. A large first-phase insulin spike occurs during the first 15 minutes as stored insulin is released from the beta cells, followed by a gradual second-phase release over the next hour and a half to three hours as insulin is produced to balance any rise in the glucose from digested carbs.

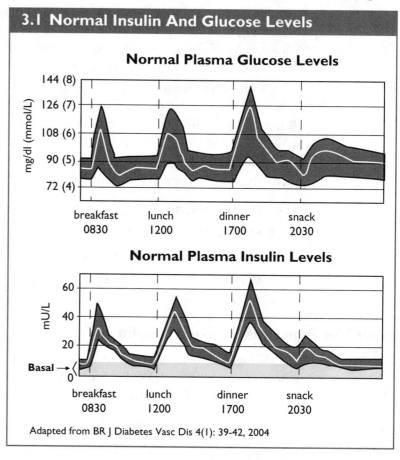

3.1 Normal Insulin And Glucose Levels

Normal Plasma Glucose Levels

mg/dl (mmol/L)

144 (8)
126 (7)
108 (6)
90 (5)
72 (4)

breakfast 0830 lunch 1200 dinner 1700 snack 2030

Normal Plasma Insulin Levels

mU/L

60
40
20
Basal →
0

breakfast 0830 lunch 1200 dinner 1700 snack 2030

Adapted from BR J Diabetes Vasc Dis 4(1): 39-42, 2004

On a pump the amount of bolus insulin required for a meal depends on how many carbs are eaten. A big stack of pancakes requires a large bolus, while a leafy salad may need none at all. Understanding the basal and bolus patterns of insulin release and how the pancreas uses each is critical for understanding how to use an insulin pump to control your blood sugar. You want your pump to duplicate both the basal and bolus functions of a normal pancreas well.

A Pump Mimics The Pancreas Better Than Injections

Injecting insulin doses once or twice a day does not provide adequate control in someone with Type 1 diabetes. An advisory panel from the Joslin Diabetes Center in Boston looked at data from the DCCT trial and stated that "three or more injections a day or use of an insulin pump should be recommended, unless clearly contraindicated."[54]

An insulin pump mimics normal insulin delivery better than injections because it provides more precise insulin delivery. A pump uses a single type of insulin like the body and can be programmed to deliver it when it is needed. Basal rates replace the background release of insulin from a normal pancreas. Unlike the long-acting insulins used in injections, basal rates can be adjusted every 30 minutes in increments as small as 0.05 unit/hr to balance the increased insulin need that many people experience before dawn or the decreased insulin need during long periods of exercise or activity. Basal rates can also be temporarily increased or decreased in 5% increments for a desired length of time (30 minutes to 72 hours) for illness, exercise or other situations.

> ## 3.2 Insulin Delivery On A Pump
>
> **Basal –** a continuous 24-hour delivery that matches background insulin need. The basal is given as units per hour, ranges between 0.4 to 1.6 u/hr for most adult pumpers, and usually makes up about half of the total daily insulin dose or TDD.
>
> **Carb Bolus –** a spurt of insulin delivered quickly to match the carbohydrates in a meal or snack. Most adult pumpers use between 1 unit for 5 to 25 grams of carb.
>
> **Correction Bolus –** a spurt of insulin designed to bring a high blood sugar back to normal. For most adult pumpers, one unit lowers the blood sugar between 20 and 120 mg/dl (1 to 6.7 mmol).

Boluses cover the carbs in meals or snacks and lower any high readings that may occur. The pump user enters into the pump how many carbs will be eaten, along with the current blood sugar, and the smart pump recommends a dose based on the personalized settings they and their health care provider have selected to match their needs.

Once a smart pump has been properly programmed, it provides the precise delivery that results in reasonable blood sugar control. Periodic testing and adjusting of basals and boluses is required to maintain long-term control, but this is much less difficult than using injections.

Even so, a pump is not a perfect system. An insulin pump cannot mimic first-phase insulin release and cannot deliver insulin into the portal vein that flows directly to the liver. Normally, as eating begins, a rapid rise in insulin in the portal vein activates enzymes in the liver that divert much of the meal's glucose into storage as glycogen. This keeps glucose levels much lower after meals.

When insulin is delivered under the skin by an infusion set and a pump, this greatly delays its arrival into the portal vein and its concentration never reaches the level seen when a healthy pancreas releases it directly. No first-phase insulin release is seen by the liver and mealtime blood sugars are more likely to spike because the liver does not divert as much incoming glucose into glycogen. On a pump, meal boluses must be given

well before eating to achieve optimum postmeal control. Other factors contribute to the abnormally high readings seen after meals. Chapter 15 discusses this, along with Symlin, a new medication used to improve postmeal readings.

Basal Insulin And Basal Rates

Basal delivery from a pump mimics nature with a steady delivery of small amounts of insulin around the clock. Basal rates are set to balance normal daily changes in counter-regulatory hormones and activity. Some teens to middle-age adults require a higher basal rate in the predawn hours to counteract a Dawn Phenomenon caused by a natural increase in growth hormone production at about 3 a.m. daily. If no extra insulin is provided at this time, the blood sugar rises and is high on waking. As a person ages, the Dawn Phenomenon and increased need for insulin often declines or disappears entirely, but a pump can be programmed to match anyone's need.

When the overnight and daytime basal rates are correctly set, the blood sugar stays level or drops only slightly overnight or when meals are skipped during the day. Basal rates are accurate when the blood sugar rises or falls no more than 30 mg/dl (1.7 mmol) during eight hours of sleep or during any five-hour period while awake.

Though basal insulin delivery usually makes up about half of the total daily insulin dose (TDD), people vary and effective basal rates may vary between 40% and 60% of the TDD. Carb boluses make up most of the remainder. A small percentage of the TDD, usually less than 8%, may be required for correction boluses.

Overnight Basals

Setting the overnight basal rates is the first thing done to establish optimum control by a new pumper or a pumper adjusting settings to solve control problems. If the blood sugar is under control on waking, the day will not be spent fighting high blood sugar levels.[55,56] On average, an increase in the basal rate of about 20% in the early morning hours is needed to offset a Dawn Phenomenon, but this will vary from person to person.[57] This 20% increase equates to an additional 0.1 or 0.2 u/hr over four to ten hours for most adults. For example, a middle of the night basal may be changed from 0.7 u/hr starting at 1 to 3 a.m. to 0.8, 0.85, or 0.9 u/hr until 9 to 11 a.m. A small increase in the basal rate started early will eliminate the need for a large increase later.

Once the overnight basal rate is correctly set, you can:

• Go to bed with a blood sugar in your target range, eat little or no bedtime snack, and wake up in the morning with a reading in your range. (This assumes there is no BOB active at bedtime and the day was not unusually active.)

• Correct a high glucose reading at bedtime and wake up with a reading in your target range the next morning. (To be sure this works, test at 2 a.m. or wear a continuous pump.)

• Rest peacefully during the night.

You, your spouse, parents, children, friends, roommates, and physician/healthcare team will all sleep better knowing you are unlikely to have a low blood sugar at night. Your day will start better when your fasting blood sugar is normal.

3.4 Advantage Of Flexible And Precise Basal Delivery From A Pump

Injections of a long-acting insulin cannot match everyone's physiology or lifestyle. In contrast, a pump can vary basal insulin delivery to match a persons need through any day.

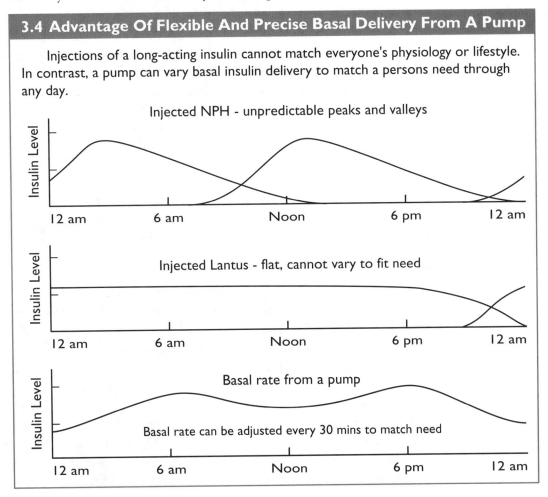

Life is not a matter of holding good cards. It's playing a poor hand well.

Robert Louis Stevenson

Daytime Basals

Setting basal rates during the day is the next step. Like night basals, daytime basal rates may have to be matched to different needs at different times of the day. Fortunately, the basal need is usually consistent from day to day. Specific steps for testing of night and day basals is covered in Chapter 11.

In contrast to the faster effect of a bolus, even a moderate or large increase or decrease in basal delivery has little impact on the blood sugar until 90 to 120 minutes have passed.[58] For example, a change in the basal rate at 2 a.m. will not begin to impact the blood sugar until a couple of hours later. If a basal rate is lowered or stopped entirely, the blood sugar does not begin to rise until 90 to 120 minutes later. For this reason, suspending basal delivery for a low blood sugar takes too long to have any effect. Eat fast-acting carbs instead.

Pumps also offer temporary basal rates and alternate basal profiles. Temporary rates can be increased to handle occasional illnesses or decreased during and after longer periods of exercise or activity. A user can also switch between alternate basal profiles if insulin requirements differ on weekends versus weekdays, or during menses for women. Some pumps now offer weekly scheduling to allow unique basal and bolus profiles to be set up and started automatically on different days of the week. This can be especially helpful for those whose activity varies from day to day, and can even include missed meal alerts when meal timing varies from day to day.

Boluses

Boluses are short spurts of insulin given to cover carbs or correct high blood sugar levels. They are not programmed ahead of time like basals but are given at the time they are needed for carb intake or to correct a high reading.

Carb Boluses

The amount of carbohydrate in a snack or meal determines the size of the carb bolus required to cover it. The more carbs, the larger the carb bolus will be, so accurate carb counting, described in Chapter 7, is a critical step for getting the most from a pump.

A personal carb factor is used to determine the bolus size for each meal and snack. Your carb factor is an insulin-to-carb ratio worked out by you and your health care provider. Setting your carb factor and testing its ability to give you accurate carb boluses is described in detail in Chapter 12. Enter your carb factor into your pump. You can program different carb factors for different times of the day if needed. A smart pump divides your meal or snack's total carbs by your carb factor to determine an accurate carb bolus for each meal and snack. Once you master this concept, you are on your way to reliable control such as you have never had before.

Boluses from a pump are not delivered directly into the blood like the delivery from a pancreas. Instead, the pump infuses insulin into fat below the skin from where it is gradually absorbed into the bloodstream. This delay in uptake means that carb boluses have to be given well before a meal begins to have their best effect. Although a meal bolus given right before eating may occasionally provide reasonable control, whenever possible give boluses 20 minutes before eating to get the best postmeal blood sugars possible. Do not do this if your blood sugar is low at the beginning of the meal.

When carbs are accurately counted and matched with a premeal bolus using an accurate carb factor, the glucose will not rise more than 40 to 80 mg/dl (2.2 to 4.4 mmol) and return to the target range 4 to 5 hours later.

Correction Boluses

A pancreas and the counter-regulatory system work so well that a healthy person has no high or low blood sugars, but delivery of insulin via basals and boluses from a pump will not be as effective. A high blood sugar occurs when too little insulin is given for basal or bolus coverage, although other causes will occasionally contribute. When a high blood sugar happens, a correction bolus is used to bring it down safely. The higher the blood sugar, the more bolus insulin needed to bring it down.

Your correction factor tells you how far your blood sugar will fall per unit of insulin. It is used to determine how much bolus insulin to take to bring a high reading down to your target without going too low. How to determine and test a starting correction factor is outlined in Chapter 13. Once the correction factor is programmed into a smart pump, correction boluses will be automatically calculated, with reductions made as needed for any active bolus on board (BOB).

Keep in mind that your pump must be thoroughly checked if a high blood sugar is unusual or unexplained. When an infusion site or mechanical problem may have occurred, take the correction dose by syringe or insulin pen. Ensure that you have taken action to lower your blood sugar before getting involved in troubleshooting the pump.

Your correction factor is accurately set when correction boluses consistently bring high blood sugars back to your target 4 to 5 hours later, and during any one week period, the correction boluses you need should make up less than 8% of your TDD.

Summary

Blood sugar control in diabetes is a complex process that requires good lifestyle choices as well as periodic changes in insulin doses. Decisions that affect your control are made several times a day and depend on data collection, management, and analysis. Compared to injections, an insulin pump allows a more normal daily life. It becomes easier to skip meals, exercise when you want, work varied schedules, eat late, and vary how many carbs you eat with less chance of losing control.

Testing and setting basal rates, carb factor, and correction factor should be completed within four to six week after a pump start. Once blood sugars are well controlled, occasional adjustments will be needed as weight, activity, or seasons change, or when blood sugar control is no longer optimal.

The time you spend learning, testing, adjusting and analyzing will be more than offset by a greater sense of well-being and more flexibility in your lifestyle. Most people find this approach offers clear advantages in the quest for a healthy future.

It is not at all uncommon for the careless person who has diabetes and lacks the initiative to self-manage to come abruptly to the recognition that a major complication has occurred without any detectable early warning. Diabetes can be silent for decades.

William M. Bortz, II, M.D., author of **Dangerous Diabetes**

Is Pumping For You?

CHAPTER 4

An insulin pump offers optimum control to those willing to make it work for them, but a pump is not suitable for everyone. This chapter helps you gauge whether your attitude, attention to detail, and dedication to self-care will lead to success. The person considering a pump, as well as the health care professionals, spouse, parents, and other support people who will be involved in day-to-day management will want to carefully consider these issues. At times your health care provider may not discuss wearing a pump with you or provide encouragement. In this case you may have to be your own advocate.

This chapter covers

- Questions to ask yourself about your readiness for pumping
- Questions for parents of a child or teen regarding pumping
- Skills you need to get ready
- Pump skills to learn for success
- Examples of people who became successful pumpers

An insulin pump may seem complicated or overwhelming before it is actually used. To help overcome this, pump companies and their representatives provide excellent information and training materials. Reading this information is a good beginning, but remember that it helps to have a skilled person walk you through the early stages. The pump company personnel can also explain and handle the financial procedures required by your insurance company. Your physician and nurse educator can assist you, as well as supportive family and friends.

Discuss any question or concerns you have with your health provider, a friend, a family member, or someone already wearing a pump. An open discussion can reassure you about whether you and a pump are a good match.

Are You Ready?

The questions below will help you determine your readiness for pumping. As another way to measure your readiness, take the self-assessment in Table 4.1.

Motivation

1. How well have you accepted your diabetes? Do you wear a medical ID? Are you comfortable testing your blood sugar in front of other people? Are you embarrassed using a syringe in public? Do you discuss recent diabetes news or research with friends?

   _____

   _____

2. Will wearing a pump be an uncomfortable reminder that you have diabetes? Do you think others will accept you as readily if you wear one?

   _____

   _____

3. Do you have special situations that make wearing a pump inconvenient, such as athletics, work environment, social events, etc.?
   ❏ yes   ❏ no   ❏ unsure

4. Who initially brought up the idea of you using a pump? _____

5. Why are you now interested in starting on a pump?

   _____

   _____

6. Who have you talked with about using a pump? Do you know anyone who has one?

   _____

7. Do you seriously want better control?
   ❏ yes   ❏ no   ❏ unsure

8. Do you know someone who has had problems with diabetes complications or do you have concerns about this yourself? Is this your motivation for wanting to pump?

   _____

9. Who will help you if problems arise? Who can you count on for emotional support?

   _____

Expectations

1. What do you expect a pump to do for you?

   _____

   _____

2. Does controlling your blood sugars on a day-to-day basis seem achievable to you?
   ❏ yes   ❏ no   ❏ unsure

3. Will better control improve your health?
   ❑ yes ❑ no ❑ unsure

4. Do you have confidence that an insulin pump is safe?
   ❑ yes ❑ no ❑ unsure

5. How will an insulin pump fit into your daily life?

   _____

   _____

6. Are your current and long-term diabetes goals realistic?
   ❑ yes ❑ no ❑ unsure

Need

1. What is your most recent A1c and how close is this to your recommended goal?

2. Are frequent highs or lows a problem for you?
   ❑ yes ❑ no ❑ unsure

3. Are your lows severe?
   ❑ yes ❑ no ❑ unsure

4. Do you have night lows or frequent morning highs?
   ❑ yes ❑ no ❑ unsure

5. Do you have hypoglycemia unawareness?
   ❑ yes ❑ no ❑ unsure

6. Do you use less than 30 units of insulin a day?
   ❑ yes ❑ no ❑ unsure

7. Do you travel frequently, have a varied schedule, or work split shifts?
   ❑ yes ❑ no ❑ unsure

8. Do you live alone and need safety features like Auto-Off and precise delivery?

   _____

9. If you have a vision problem or arthritis in your hands, are you able to push the pump buttons, fill the reservoir, and insert the infusion set yourself? Ask your health provider if you can try these techniques before you make a final decision.

   _____

   _____

Preparation

1. What other approaches to control have you tried? An insulin pen? Multiple daily injections? How well have these approaches worked for you?

   _____

Gauge Your Control

1. How motivated are you to control your blood sugars?

   not very   0   1   2   3   4   5   very   _____

2. Number of blood sugar tests you do each day:

            0   1   2   3   4   5   (or more)   _____

3. Number of injections per day:

            0   1   2   3   4   5   (or more)   _____

4. Do you record your test results?

            yes   (5pts)   no   (0 pts)   _____

5. Do you use your test results to adjust your insulin?

            yes   (5 pts)   no   (0 pts)   _____

6. Do you match your short-acting insulin to the carbs in each snack or meal by carb counting or other means?

            yes   (5 pts)   no   (0 pts)   _____

7. Do you use extra insulin to correct high blood sugars?

            yes   (5 pts)   no   (0 pts)   _____

8. Do you adjust your long-acting insulin doses?

            yes   (5 pts)   no   (0 pts)   _____

9. Do you get an A1c test to evaluate your control at least every 6 months?

            yes   (5 pts)   no   (0 pts)   _____

10. Do you call your doctor when control problems occur?

            yes   (5 pts)   no   (0 pts)   _____

Total = _____

© 2006 Diabetes Services, Inc.

Self Assessment

Points	0-9	10-19	20-29	30-39	40-49
Meaning	A bit casual	Honesty pays	You've got the idea	Minor changes will help	When do you start?

2. Are you knowledgeable about carb counting, exchanges, or some other method of matching food with your carb doses?
   ❏ yes   ❏ no   ❏ unsure

3. How often do you test your blood sugar? _____ times a day

4. Do you record or download your test results?
   ❏ yes   ❏ no   ❏ unsure

5. Do you regularly review your data?
   ❏ yes   ❏ no   ❏ unsure

6. Are you willing to test more often and keep records when this is needed?
   ❏ yes   ❏ no   ❏ unsure

7. Do you adjust your own insulin doses or the food you eat based on your test results? Can you work with figuring ratios and using measurements like ounces and grams? If not, are you willing to learn?
   ❏ yes   ❏ no   ❏ unsure

8. Are you willing to tackle any pump problems that arise and work toward solutions? Are your problem solving skills adequate to deal with the control or hardware issues that will arise?
   ❏ yes   ❏ no   ❏ unsure

9. Will your health insurance company, HMO, or Medicare cover the cost of pump therapy? Will out-of-pocket expenses fit in your budget?

   _____

Questions for Parents to Consider

These questions are specific for parents with children considering a pump:

1. Is your child or teen willing to wear a pump? Are you pushing the issue, and if so, why?

   _____

   _____

2. Does your child or teen's school cooperate with blood sugar testing and snacks?
   ❏ yes   ❏ no   ❏ unsure

3. Does your child learn new skills easily?
   ❏ yes   ❏ no   ❏ unsure

4. Does your child or teen participate in giving injections, counting carbs, determining carb boluses, and testing blood sugars with minimal help?
   ❏ yes   ❏ no   ❏ unsure

5. How do you feel about your child or teen gradually assuming responsibility for taking care of their diabetes?

   _____

   _____

6. Are you willing to be involved in your child or teen's pump program?

_____

_____

7. Will you have a trained diabetes professional available when you need help?
   ❑ yes ❑ no ❑ unsure

Discuss Your Decision

Whether you are considering a pump for yourself or a child, carefully consider your answers to these questions. If you (or your child) are not a good pump candidate, all is not lost. Say "no" to pump therapy if it does not fit well with you or your child's current desires or lifestyle. Discuss this decision carefully with your doctor, family, and friends before making a final choice. Their perspective may benefit you or your child more than you realize.

Getting Ready

You can never learn too much about diabetes, so speed your path to success:

- Read this book, your pump manual, and the training materials that accompany your pump before you start.
- Ask questions about any terms and procedures you do not understand. Ensure that you understand basal/bolus therapy and use of MDI therapy before you start on a pump.
- Learn and use carb counting for several weeks before you start to pump. You want to be able to match the carbs in your meals with appropriate boluses from injections before you start pumping. Accurate carb counting pays high dividends in improved control.
- Make an appointment with a dietitian to ensure the accuracy of your carb counts. Write down in a 3-day food diary the foods you eat, quantities, and your best estimate of their carb content. Bring this with you to your appointment. Be frank about your food choices and amounts to get the help you need. Listen carefully to the dietitian's recommendations and write down the changes you need to make.
- Make it a habit to chart blood sugars, carbs, basals and boluses, exercise, stress, etc., so that you and your doctor can see what has affected your readings.
- Nothing helps your control as much as an easy-to-review record of what is happening. The _Smart Chart_ shown in Figures 8.1 and 8.3 allows you to record all pertinent information on one page in a graphic format.
- Consider wearing a pump filled with saline for practice, if possible.
- Get comfortable with button pushing and pump operation. Learn how to troubleshoot problems that may arise and ask for help when needed.

4.2 Accountabilities For Success On A Pump

Health care provider will:

• train the pumper in good technical skills for pump use.

• assist in setting duration of insulin action, targets, alarms, and reminders

• set starting basals, carb factor, and correction factor and also show the user how to test and adjust them.

• teach problem-solving techniques to allow the pump user to make needed adjustments in case of highs or lows.

• make 24-hour contact available at first and daily contact possible later so that the pumper feels secure.

• gradually train a capable pump user in complete blood sugar management.

Pumper will:

• learn and use good technique in setting up the pump and connecting it to a well-placed infusion set.

• count carbs to improve control or use an equivalent diet method, and also record any carbs eaten.

• test at least 6 times a day at first and record blood sugar readings, particularly noting all hypoglycemic events and their relation to insulin dosages, exercise, and carbs counted.

• test basal rates and boluses as instructed.

• match basals and boluses to daily insulin need better by studying records, reviewing blood sugar goals, or contacting health professionals to become aware of blood sugar patterns and troubleshoot the ones that are causing problems.

Skills For Success

A number of skills are helpful during the first few months of pump use. Learn as many as you can before you start, but only the experience of wearing a pump long enough to respond to various situations can hone these skills. You want to learn:

• What your basal rates and boluses are designed to do, and what percentage of the TDD each typically represents

• How to set and test basal rates

• When to use temporary and alternate basal rates

• How to test your carb factor and boluses and your correction factor and boluses

• How to use Bolus On Board (BOB), also called insulin on board, unused bolus, active insulin, or residual insulin

• The DIA or duration of action time for your insulin

• How to analyze blood sugar patterns and correct unwanted ones

4.3 Myths And Truths Of Pumping

Myths	Truths
Pumpers have perfect blood sugar control.	Blood sugar control will improve as insulin is better matched to need, but no one's control is perfect with any method. For most people on pumps, a modest number of highs and lows routinely occur.
Pump therapy will prevent all complications.	Better control through skillful use of a pump can decrease the risk of complications greatly. However, some complications may still occur, depending on lifelong glucose exposure and variability.
A pump will be easier and take less time.	A pump becomes easier over time and ultimately is more convenient, but learning the techniques takes time. Aspects that are time-consuming at first become easier to do with repeated use. Like learning any task, the beginning is intense before rewards are seen.
Pumpers know what to do and understand what they are doing.	Pump therapy depends on analysis of patterns and use of formulas to improve control. Smart pumps track data, enable more accurate doses, and help prevent lows, but a pump cannot make every decision and assist in every situation. Mysteries and unexplained blood sugars will always occur, requiring "feel" or intuition in some circumstances.
Using a pump means diabetes is worse.	A pump is more physiologic and contributes to better blood sugar control. Use of a pump has nothing to do with "better" or "worse". Used well, a pump means you are taking better care of your diabetes.
A pump seems complicated. Isn't it better to use one unit for 15 grams of carb and a general correction scale.	Today's pumps have individualized carb and correction factors that are entered into the pump for easy bolus calculations. This leads to better control. The pump can precisely determine the dose you need based on your current blood sugar and the carbs you want to eat.
Using a pump to adjust your insulin doses based on what you eat is playing Russian roulette with your life.	Russian roulette is picking a random number and sticking to it. Pump therapy uses science, experience, formulas, and an increasingly sophisticated data management system to customize the pump program to match an individual's needs.

To learn basic pump skills, pay special attention to Chapters 10 through 13, the core material in this book that teaches how to set up a pump and test your pump settings. What you learn before you start will help tremendously as you program your new pump and begin to use it to improve your control. Talk to other pump wearers and your medical team about any issues that arise. All new users face some confusion and uncertainty that will resolve as successes and mistakes are processed and built on. Just don't give up before you reach the best control you have ever had.

People Who Became Pumpers

These four individuals, motivated by different circumstances, have all benefited from pumping. Their examples may help you identify and understand your own motivations and look ahead to potential benefits.

Amy

Amy is a software engineer and racquet ball fanatic in her late 20's. For most of the 12 years she has had diabetes, she has been plagued by repeated highs and lows. Her glucose variability is triggered by a high sensitivity to insulin and by irregular changes in her daily activities.

Her average total daily insulin dose is only 18 units and her blood sugar drops 140 mg/dl (7.8 mmol) for each unit of insulin. Her sensitivity to insulin makes it difficult to give safe doses with a syringe. She wanted to be able to deliver insulin in fractions of a unit, rather than estimating half units on a syringe. She also needed a way to adjust her background or basal insulin at various points during the night after she played racquetball vigorously that day.

Amy finally switched to an insulin pump after she was found unconscious behind the wheel of her car parked in a shopping mall parking lot. She was diagnosed with hypoglycemia unawareness and was warned that her unawareness and sensitivity to insulin made even small errors in dosing extremely serious.

Since starting on the pump, she marvels at the stability of her blood sugar. Being able to fine-tune her doses has given her a new sense of control. She has regained awareness that she is going low and is less fearful of going low. Her husband and coworkers are thrilled with her mellowed personality. "I now feel like a regular person," she says.

George

George is 66 and retired after selling his plumbing business. He has had Type 2 diabetes for 15 years. George added injections after 10 years of therapy when three oral agents could no longer control his morning blood sugar. After gradually increasing his doses to nearly 100 units a day, his fasting readings remained at 150 mg/dl (8.3 mmol) and over, well above the level he desired to maintain good health.

He considered a pump for more than a year before he finally agreed with his wife to try it. Three months later, with his A1c at 6.2% on only 60 units a day, George says, "Now I don't have to work so hard to have a good day. I wake up in the morning with normal readings. I use half as much insulin, and my triglyceride levels are normal for the first time in years. I can give insulin whenever I need it. I really love my pump."

Josh

Josh is a tile layer who has had Type 1 diabetes for 37 years. In the past, he blamed work and family obligations for not visiting his physician regularly. After he developed nerve damage with tingling in his feet and numbness up both calves, he finally admitted to his doctor that he had been making up most of the blood sugar records he had turned in over the years. He started to take his testing and control seriously when he could no longer get to sleep because of shooting pains in his legs that medication could not completely stop. When he finally got an A1c test, his value came back at 10.7%.

Once Josh started dealing with his diabetes, his doctor recommended that he try an insulin pump. He was told that this might help his neuropathy. With a pump, he could also quickly adjust his doses when his work changed from carrying, cutting, and cementing tile to less strenuous periods of grouting and polishing.

After ten months on his pump and many adjustments, his basals and boluses are finally matched to his true blood sugar readings. Now Josh is able to sleep through the night without a neuropathy medication. "The feeling in my feet and legs is definitely better. This has made all the effort worth it," he says.

Lisa

Lisa, who is five years old, developed diabetes when she was three. On injections, she went low at night due to the erratic peaking activity of her long-acting insulin. She is also a picky eater, which caused frequent highs after meals because her parents could not give an injection until they knew how many grams of carb she had consumed. She complained about having to take so many injections, and her parents were frustrated with trying to give her doses in fractions of units. When they tried to give larger premeal injections to avoid having to give corrective ones later, Lisa often went low.

Three months after starting, Lisa's parents noted that she sleeps more soundly at night due to the precise dosing allowed by her nighttime basal rates. Her parents have less fear of night lows. They can now give boluses quickly and easily when needed before or after meals. By having the pump give an alert two hours after each bolus, they can retest at that time. If needed, they can provide a small correction bolus or carb snack to stabilize her blood sugar. This has improved her control greatly and Lisa no longer worries about having to take injections. Lisa's parents and Lisa now smile a lot.

Summary

After considering this material, you may see you could benefit from a pump and are willing to put in the effort required to make it work for you. If so, check with your doctor about pump choices and how to begin, but keep in mind you will want to start at a time when your life is not undergoing turmoil. You'll need a clear head and more time than usual to devote to managing your diabetes.

In times of profound change, the learners inherit the earth, while the learned find themselves beautifully equipped to deal with a world that no longer exists.

Al Rogers

Smart Pump Features And Their Use

Today's smart pumps are full of new features that can help you improve your control more than classic pumps. First available in late 2002, these smart features include built-in complex math calculations to improve dose accuracy and better regulate blood sugar control, helpful alarms and reminders, easy and more accurate bolus calculations, and comprehensive memory recall. Continuous monitors are coming into wider use and have significant impact on diabetes control.

Smart pump features and how to use them:

- Carb factor and carb bolus types
- Correction factor and blood glucose targets
- Duration of insulin action (DIA) and Bolus on Board (BOB)
- Reminders, alerts, and weekly schedules for alternate basal profiles
- Basal/bolus balance
- Correction bolus percentage of TDD
- Pump-meter combos
- Wearable pumps

As well as other new and projected developments:

- Automatic basal and bolus testing, Super Bolus, Eating Alerts, pattern recognition
- Micro pumps, inhaled and oral insulin, and peritoneal delivery
- Continuous monitors and pumps

Two metastudies have been done to analyze several controlled trials in which people were randomly assigned to MDI or a classic pump. One study compared 600 people from a dozen smaller studies who were randomly assigned to either a pump or MDI. The average A1c for those on pumps was 0.51% lower compared to those on MDI. They also experienced less glucose variability and required 7.6 fewer units of insulin per day.[59] A second meta-analysis of 20 studies found that the A1c fell by 0.61% on pumps compared to MDI while daily insulin requirements fell by 11.9 units per day.[60]

Unfortunately, neither those using MDI or classic pumps were able to lower the average A1c below 8.2% to 9% in these studies. This is well above the goal of 7% or less recommended by the American Diabetes Association and considerably higher than the 6.5% goal jointly recommended by the American Association of Clinical Endocrinologists and the International Diabetes Federation.[49,50]

New Pump Features

Compared to classic pumps, today's smart pumps simplify the management of complex interactions between insulin levels, blood glucose, and carbs. This allows users to achieve desirable glucose levels with less effort, but the pump user still has to learn and apply rules and judge situations well to improve their control. This book assists the reader in doing this.

As pumps and devices become more intelligent, smart pumps combined with continuous monitors, software that assists in trend analysis and pattern recognition, plus other helpful aids will gradually make it easier to achieve better control. Though pumps contain many new features and reminders, many wearers do not use them. Only by learning and using these features to simplify dose decisions and increase accuracy will pump wearers improve A1c test results, glucose stability, and overall health.

1. Carb Factor

A personal **carb factor** programmed into the pump makes carb coverage easier and more accurate. The carb factor is how many grams of carb one unit of insulin will cover for you. One carb factor may be programmed for the entire day or different ones for specific meals of the day. When the number of carbs to be eaten is entered, the pump calculates the bolus needed to cover them, while compensating for any BOB (see #6). Some pumps offer a built-in **carb database** that simplifies carb counting. Users can create their own list of favorite foods and the exact carb count of these foods. Simply choose a food from your personal list in the database, select the serving size, and the pump determines an appropriate bolus. How to determine your carb factor is covered in Chapter 12.

2. Carb Bolus Types

Besides standard carb boluses, there are two additional **carb bolus types**. One is called an extended or square wave bolus, and the other a combination or dual wave bolus. These are used to match carbs with a low glycemic index or combination foods that digest slowly, or cover a time of prolonged snacking and grazing. They are also helpful when digestion that has been slowed by gastroparesis. For instance, a bolus may best match the digestion of a specific food as a combo bolus with part of the bolus given immediately and the rest given over the next 90 or 120 minutes.

Extended or square wave boluses are also useful with medications like Symlin or GLP-1 inhibitors like Byetta. These drugs slow food digestion and are extremely helpful for lowering postmeal glucose values to stabilize control. Pages 181 to 183 have more information on use of these medications.

3. Correction Factor

A personal **correction factor** (called insulin sensitivity factor or ISF in some pumps) makes it easier to correct high readings. Enter a correction factor for how far your blood sugar drops on one unit of insulin, along with a glucose target for different times of the day. The pump will then determine the precise bolus required for a high reading or a reduction for a below-target reading as it compensates for any BOB (See #5 and 6 below.). Bringing a high reading down becomes easier with less risk of going low. How to determine your correction factor is covered in Chapter 13.

4. Blood Glucose Target

A personal **blood sugar target or target range** can be entered into your pump for each meal and at bedtime so your pump knows the glucose level to aim for. This range is NOT the same as similar personal ranges that signify acceptable clinical goals. In contrast, the target range on a pump is the glucose the pump is attempting to achieve on a future blood sugar test, usually 3 to 5 hours later. The pump adjusts the current insulin dose to aim for this target at a later time. For example, if a reading of 140 mg/dl (7.8 mmol) is desired for bedtime at 10 p.m., this target should be set into the pump by 6 p.m. to allow time for the pump to achieve this goal.

Setting a single target, such as 100 or 140 mg/dl (5.507.8 mmol) is preferred. With a single value rather than a target range, more insulin will be given for any reading above this value and LESS for any reading below this value. On a pump, the wider a target range, the less able the pump is to zero the blood sugar toward a target. A wide target range means less insulin is added for readings above the target, but also that LESS IS SUBTRACTED for readings below the bottom of the target range. For low readings, the pump subtracts the current reading from the lower target value and reduces the carb bolus appropriately. If a target range is used rather than a single target, for safety the bottom of this range should be no lower than a single target that would otherwise be chosen. A higher target or a larger correction factor can be chosen at bedtime or at other times of the day to reduce the chance of having a low.

5. Duration of Insulin Action

One unanticipated challenge that faces those on smart pumps is how to select a duration of insulin action (DIA or how long a bolus lowers the blood sugar) that works for them and does not cause problems. Many pump users and health care professionals do not realize the importance of this setting. An accurate DIA helps prevent insulin stacking when boluses are given close together and overlap because insulin from previous carb and correction boluses is still active in the body. The time for your DIA must be accurate to allow BOB or bolus on board to properly calculate subsequent carb and correction boluses once the first bolus of the day has been given.

It takes a minimum of 4 to 6 hours for all of the insulin action from a recent bolus to stop lowering the blood sugar. Many people choose to set the duration of insulin action to short values such as 2 or 3 hours because they falsely believe insulin works very quickly for them, not realizing that this short time can make lows more likely because it hides bolus insulin action. Today's rapid insulins are not that fast. They have

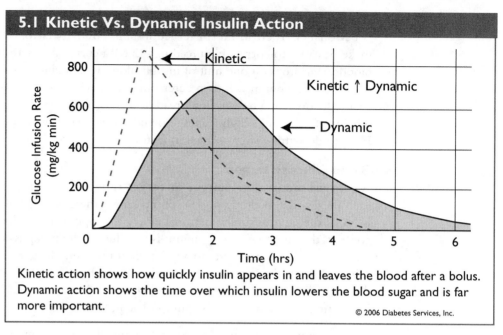

5.1 Kinetic Vs. Dynamic Insulin Action

Kinetic action shows how quickly insulin appears in and leaves the blood after a bolus. Dynamic action shows the time over which insulin lowers the blood sugar and is far more important.

© 2006 Diabetes Services, Inc.

little effect on the glucose for the first 15 to 20 minutes, reach a halfway point in activity at just over two hours, and have the other half of activity tail off over about 5 to 6 hours or more after the bolus is given.

Insulin sales are competitive, so insulin companies all claim a DIA of "3 to 5" or "4 to 5" hours. This time more closely matches the time it takes insulin to disappear from the blood (called its kinetic action) than it does the longer and more important time over which insulin lowers the blood sugar (called its dynamic action as shown in Fig. 5.1.) Today's pumps allow a wide range of times to be selected for the DIA, from 1.5 to 8 hours. This range is designed to handle faster genetically-engineered insulins that may appear in the future, as well as older Regular insulin. Unfortunately, people on pumps may not realize that this range is far wider than the action time for the insulin they use. Every pump comes with a default setting for DIA. This default setting can often be changed to a more effective and sometimes safer setting.

Insulin action varies between individuals. In a well-controlled study using Novolog® insulin, researchers found about a 25% variation in how long a rapid insulin works between different users.[61] A 25% variation means that insulin duration will normally fall within 45 minutes on either side of an average DIA. Assuming a total average duration of 5.5 hours, which includes the tailing off of all insulin activity, a generous variation between different pumpers would be 4 hours and 45 minutes to 6 hours and 15 minutes, not the outlying values in the 2 to 8 hour range available in pumps. (Do NOT select a DIA for YOUR pump until you have read this entire section!)

Bolus size also affects the DIA. Large boluses delay insulin action. Figure 5.2 shows how a larger bolus relative to one's weight will lower the blood sugar for a longer period of time. If a bolus twice the size of a normal bolus is given, the DIA of this bolus will be longer. Current pumps do not take this variation into account, so it is best to select a duration that matches your average bolus size relative to your weight.

It is easy for users to think their insulin is fast. If they feel normal before a meal and take a carb bolus, then a few minutes later begin to shake, sweat and have trouble thinking, they may believe their insulin works very fast. However, their symptoms will almost always be caused not by the bolus just taken, but by an earlier bolus or by excess basal delivery or by recent exercise. The timing of the low causes the recent bolus to get the blame, but it is almost never the cause. If a carb bolus is taken and someone goes low a couple of hours later, rather than having fast insulin, the person is more likely to not have accounted for all their active insulin when they took the bolus, or they overestimated the carbs in the meal or consumed carbs with a low glycemic index. On excess insulin, frequent lows make the insulin appear fast but it is simply excessive basals or boluses. Much of insulin's apparent "speed" is caused by dosing errors, not by any speed of action.

Given all this, any increase in physical activity does speed up insulin absorption and reduce its duration of action. When more active, children and adults may experience a faster onset of action in their insulin. Temperature also affects DIA, so exercise on a hot day would speed up insulin action even more.

Setting the duration to 2 hours is far shorter than the action time of today's insulins (Novolog®, Humalog®, and Apidra®). This setting makes the pump report in a BOB screen that none of a previous bolus activity remains 2 hours after it is given. A pump set up with a DIA of 2 hours makes a breakfast bolus given at 7 a.m. appear to have no activity after 9 a.m., even though it continues to lower the blood sugar for another two to four hours. If a blood sugar taken at 9 a.m. is high, the correction bolus recommended by the pump at that time will be larger than needed. This leads to insulin stacking and hypoglycemia.

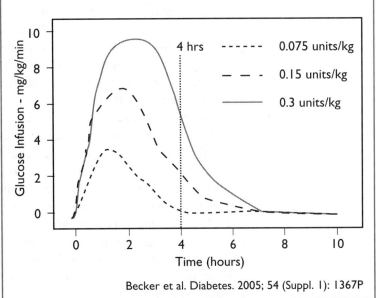

5.2 Bolus Size Affects Duration

Larger boluses increase the duration of insulin action.

For 110 lb (50 kg) person:

0.075 = 3.75 u   0.15 = 7.5 u   0.3 = 15 u

4 hrs - - - - - 0.075 units/kg

- - - - 0.15 units/kg

——— 0.3 units/kg

Becker et al. Diabetes. 2005; 54 (Suppl. 1): 1367P

5.3 Duration Of Insulin Action For Children

Parents of children with diabetes are vulnerable to a belief that their child's insulin has a short action time. Children can easily go low because they require small doses. Parents get convinced their child's insulin works fast, rather than that they may have received a half unit too much.

The limited research available at this time shows no difference in insulin action between children and adults. Dr. Bruce Buckingham, a pediatric endocrinologist at Stanford University, looked at how quickly rapid insulin worked in a small group of young children. In his study of 4 children between three and a half and six plus years, he found that rather than working quickly, their insulin action was slightly slower than found in published reports for adults.[62] Although the number of children was small, Dr. Buckingham found that these children still had active insulin working when the study ended at five hours.

From a study of Novolog insulin in 18 children and adolescents between 6 and 18 years of age, Novo-Nordisk concluded that: "The relative differences in pharmacokinetics and pharmacodynamics in children and adolescents with Type 1 diabetes between NovoLog and regular human insulin were similar to those in healthy adult subjects and adults with Type 1 diabetes."[63] Although children use smaller boluses, the size of their boluses relative to their weight is not terribly different from adults. For example, a 2-unit bolus for a 50 lb. child and an 8-unit bolus for a 200 lb. adult are the same size relative to weight, so the duration of insulin action for each bolus will be the same.

When insulin duration is too short, excess amounts of unrecognized bolus insulin accumulate whenever boluses overlap, usually between noon and midnight, to cause lows. The hidden bolus stacking may make the pump wearer assume that low readings are caused by a high basal rate, since their BOB appears to be small or nonexistent. If they lower the basal rate, high readings will occur more often and again be treated with excess correction bolus doses, especially when the blood sugar is checked more often. Unless the source of the problem is recognized as a duration of insulin action that is too short, control problems continue.

The question, of course, is what time should you select as your duration of insulin action? This is made difficult for clinicians and users alike not only because of the wide range of times allowed in pumps, but also because different pumps calculate DIA differently, and each pump has a different default setting for the DIA!

Medtronic's Paradigm 5xx/7xx pumps have a default DIA of 6 hours that can be changed in 1 hour increments over 2 to 8 hours. This DIA is calculated in a curvilinear fashion that follows the lines shown in Fig. 5.4. with the last 5% of insulin action ignored to keep the DIA time reasonable. This 6 hour setting is a realistic default setting. The Animas 1250 pump offers a default of 4 hours that can be changed in 30 minute increments between 1.5 and 6.5 hours. This DIA uses a curvilinear decay that extends to 100% of insulin action. The Deltec Cozmo has a 3 hour default for the DIA that can be changed in 15 minute increments between 2 and 8 hours. Omnipod also has a 3 hour default that can be changed in 30 minute increments over a range between 2 and 6 hours. Rather than a curvilinear method, both Deltec and Omnipod use a straight line method to calculate the DIA. For instance, a 4 hour DIA in these pumps assumes that 25% of the bolus will be used each hour. Like the Paradigm pump, this

linear method tends to ignore some of the late tailing off action of the insulin, and requires use of shorter times for the DIA.

The grey boxes at the bottom of Fig. 5.4 show suggested DIA's for each pump based on how each pump measures insulin action. Visit www.diabetesnet.com/diabetes_technology/dia.php to view any updates on minimum and maximum recommended times for new pumps that may use different methods to calculate residual insulin action or a new and faster insulin.

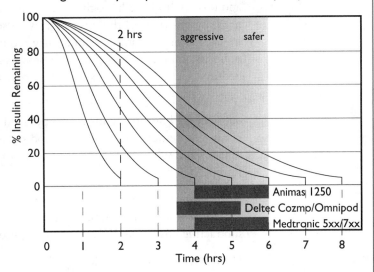

5.4 Insulin Activity For Various Pump DIAs

Current pumps allow DIAs of 2 to 8 hours. An accurate choice can significantly affect overall control. The grey bars show optimal timing for today's rapid insulins in different pumps.

Visit www.diabetesnet.com/diabetes_technology/duration_of_insulin_action.php for the latest updates on suggested DIAs for new pumps or insulins.

Test Your Duration Of Insulin Action

After testing your basals in Chapter 11 to ensure they keep your glucose level when you are not eating, find the real speed of your insulin action. Give an appropriate correction bolus the next time your blood sugar is above 250 mg/dl (13.9 mmol) and it has been at least 5 hours since the last bolus. Test your blood sugar every 30 to 60 minutes over the next 5 to 6 hours to see how long it takes for the high reading to **return to target and remain flat**. This shows the speed of your insulin and its true duration of action. If you go low before five hours have passed, the correction bolus was either too large or your basal rate is too high, not that your insulin works fast. See pages 158 and 159 for more information.

6. Bolus On Board (BOB)*

Frequent boluses are easy to give on a pump. This can benefit the user by lowering the A1c and reducing glucose variability, but frequent boluses can also lead to insulin stacking. When a carb bolus is given for dinner, another for an unplanned dessert, and then a correction bolus is needed for the high reading that follows, the resulting insulin pileup can be confusing when you need to determine how much bolus insulin remains in the body to act.

When a blood sugar test has been done and entered into the pump and a correction bolus is to be given, today's smart pumps automatically take into account bolus on board or BOB, also known as insulin on board and active insulin. This prevents hypoglycemia caused by insulin stacking. It is especially helpful for those who live alone and those who have hypoglycemia unawareness or a history of frequent lows. Knowing how much BOB there is can prevent someone from giving too much insulin. For instance, a high bedtime reading may require no correction bolus if enough residual bolus insulin remains to bring the blood sugar down, while a target blood sugar at bedtime may be dangerous if excess bolus insulin is still active.

If your meter does not automatically communicate readings to your pump, be sure and enter all readings into your pump by hand so your pump can accurately calculate your bolus requirements. Any time a blood sugar test is done, check to see how much BOB remains and whether a correction bolus or additional carbs may be needed. (see Clever Pump Trick 5.5)

All current smart pumps subtract the current BOB from correction boluses when the current blood sugar is high. The pump recommends a smaller correction bolus after subtracting any active BOB, which is appropriate.

However, current pumps do not all subtract BOB from carb boluses. Although they offer alternatives, the Paradigm 512 through 722 pumps and the Omnipod do not subtract BOB from any carb bolus displayed in a recommended dose, unless the blood sugar is already below target. Whether this is helpful depends on the situation. Consider a person whose carb factor is 1 unit for each 10 grams who recently took 10 units for 100 grams of carbs in a meal. If they decide later to also cover an unplanned dessert of 30 grams at they end of the meal, it would be appropriate to give 3 units for this dessert.

But if it is now two hours later and the blood sugar is 100 mg/dl (5.6 mmol) due to having overestimated carbs, not eating all of them, or being more active than usual, the BOB or active insulin at this time will be 4 to 6 units. If the person plans to eat a snack of 30 grams, a Paradigm pump or an Omnipod pump will recommend giving another 3 units and disregard the active BOB which may be sufficient to cover 40 to 60 grams of free carbs. The current Paradigm and Omnipod pumps subtract BOB from correction boluses but not carb boluses. The Omnipod has a feature called reverse corrections that can be turned "On" to subtract BOB from carb boluses but only when the current blood sugar is below the user's Target Blood Glucose. Other pumps in the

---

* BOB was introduced in the first edition of **Pumping Insulin** in 1989 as the Insulin-Used Rule.[64]

5.5 Clever Pump Tricks

Bolus Tipping To Prevent Lows

Each time you test your blood sugar, check whether your pump recommends that you give a bolus. If no bolus is needed, you still have insulin working from a previous bolus.

Your pump can tell you how many grams of carb you will need to offset the remaining insulin to prevent a low or how many carbs are needed to treat one if you are having one. Enter a small number of grams of carb as a meal bolus and check whether your pump recommends a bolus. Gradually increase the number of carbs until your bolus tips, i.e. the pump switches from recommending no bolus to recommending one.

When the bolus tips, the number of carbs you just put in will closely approximate how many carbs you need to eat to prevent a low reading later or to treat a current low. Remember that the DIA in your pump must be accurately set for this estimate to work. Some pumps now provide an automatic readout of your current carb deficit or insulin deficit every time a glucose test is taken that makes it clearer which action needs to be taken.

example above would recommend that no bolus be given to avoid hypoglycemia that could occur as a result of insulin stacking.

As long as the user knows how their pump works, they can select appropriate boluses for each situation. For an unplanned after dinner dessert, the Animas and Cozmo recommendations can be easily bypassed so the pump covers these carbs. When BOB is present on a Paradigm pump, rather than immediately giving the recommended bolus, hit the down arrow three times on that screen to reveal the food, correction, and active insulin amounts. Add the food and correction boluses together and subtract the active insulin or BOB to see how this matches the dose recommended by the pump. If the BOB is larger than the correction dose, a smaller bolus or additional free carbs may be needed to prevent a low. One pump already calculates the current carb or insulin deficit each time a blood sugar is taken and suggests how many carbs may be needed to avoid a low or how many units may be needed based on the Blood glucose and BOB. Again, an accurate DIA is needed for this to work.

A good rule of thumb when trying to decide whether or not to cover carbs is to cover extra unplanned carbs that are eaten within an hour or so of a meal bolus. Beyond this time, it is safer to check your blood sugar and allow your pump to compare your current blood sugar against any active BOB and let your pump calculate whether you need a correction bolus or carbs, or calculate this need yourself.

To check whether your pump subtracts BOB from carb coverage, the next time you give a meal bolus for 20 or more grams, wait a minute and then enter a carb amount of 15 grams along with a blood sugar equal to your target. If your pump recommends that no carb bolus be given, your pump is subtracting the carb bolus from your BOB (the safer method in some situations). If your pump recommends that you cover the 15 grams with a normal bolus (which you do not want to give, of course), it does not subtract the carb bolus from your active insulin or BOB. Remember, in some situations this will be appropriate and in others it will not.

Children and teens (and some adults) eat frequently and often have meals and snacks less than 2 hours apart. If a child seems to run frequent high blood sugars and their pump does discount BOB from carb boluses, the discounting will not be the source for the high readings. Instead, their insulin doses are too small. Either basal rates need to be raised, carb counting needs to improve, or the carb factor number needs to be lowered to make carb boluses larger.

See www.diabetesnet.com/diabetes_technology/dia.php for a more detailed discussion of how the latest pumps handle BOB and DIA.

7. Reminders And Alerts

Reminders and alerts on smart pumps can be customized for safety and to improve control. For instance, a postmeal reminder can be set to recheck your blood sugar an hour and a half or two hours after a bolus has been given. Testing at this time allows the meal bolus to be evaluated as to whether extra carbs are needed to prevent a low or a correction bolus is needed because the meal bolus was too small. This helps prevent lows and speeds correction of highs.

Reminders can also be set to ensure that boluses are given at specific times of the day. If a meal bolus is forgotten at lunch, some pumps can be set to alarm if no bolus is given at the usual time, such as between 11:45 a.m. and 12:30 p.m. This time can also be scheduled at different times on different days of the week, similar to a personal calendar. If a bolus is started but not completed because a user gets distracted, a smart pump can sound an alert that the bolus was not finalized. Another reminder can be set to alarm when the next infusion site change is due. Others will automatically remind the user to retest the glucose 15 or 20 minutes after a low blood sugar to ensure the treatment used has corrected the low, or 90 to 120 minutes after a high reading to ensure a correction bolus is working. Helpful reminders like these minimize human error and improve control.

An auto-off feature can be a lifesaver for those who travel or live alone. When auto-off is activated, the pump turns itself off if you do not press one of your pump buttons within a certain amount of time, such as 8 or 9 hours overnight. This protects you from continuing to receive insulin if you become incapacitated due to hypoglycemia.

Table 5.6 contains information on various reminders and alerts.

8. Weekly Schedule or Alternate Basal Insulin Profiles

Current pumps allow about four different basal profiles to be entered into a pump, such as a weekend profile to accommodate an increase or decrease in activity at this time or a profile for women during menses. However, these alternate profiles currently adjust only basal rates, not the carb and correction factors that accompany them. Fu-

5.6 Reminders and Alerts (varies from pump to pump)

Reminder or Alert	Function	Range	Default
Low Battery Alert	Warns when battery needs changing.	24 hrs	none
Low Cartridge Alert	Alerts when a selected # of units of insulin are left in the reservoir so a site change may be planned.	5-50 u	20 u
Alerts for Special Features	Alerts when alternative bolus delivery is still active, temporary basal is on, block feature is on.	24 hrs	none
Delivery Limit Alarm**	Warns when more than a selected number of units of insulin are gone in 1 hour.	1-150 u	40 u
Glucose Reminder Alert* (can set 4 custom alerts)	Reminds you to test your blood sugar at the time you select following a bolus.	1-4 hr (15 min increments)	2 hr
Low Blood Glucose Alert* **	Reminds you to test your blood sugar at the time you select following a low blood sugar reading.	Time: 5 min-1 hr BG Limit: 50 -100 mg/dl	15 min 70 mg/dl
High Blood Glucose Alert* **	Reminds you to test your blood sugar at the time you select following a high blood sugar reading.	Time: 30 min 2 hrs BG Limit: 150 - 300 mg/dl	200 mg/dl
Automatic Off Alarm*	A safety feature that turns the pump off if no button has been pushed during this time.	1 - 24 hrs	8 hrs
Site Reminder Alert* **	Reminder to change infusion set.	Usually at a certain time of day in 2-4 days.	none
Missed Meal Bolus Alert* ** (can set 4 custom alerts)	Alerts you that a meal bolus was not given at a certain time of day.	Set a time window, such as 11:45 a.m. to 12:15 p.m.	none

*These reminders and alerts often have a default of "OFF". Often better to set to "ON".

** Not available on all pumps

ture pumps will allow these factors to be adjusted along with the alternate basal profile. For routine basal profile changes, such as weekday to weekend, these would automatically be done at the same time each week so they are not forgotten.

Some pumps now offer weekly schedules to allow unique basal profiles and reminders and alerts to be set up and started automatically on different days of the week. This can be especially helpful for those whose activity varies from day to day. These schedule changes can even include missed meal alerts when meal timing varies from day to day.

9. **Basal/Bolus Balance and Correction Bolus Tracking**

Basal and bolus doses have to be balanced for optimum control. Your **basal/bolus balance** can be calculated from your average insulin doses per day or provided directly by the pump as a way to check your insulin usage and help spot where problems may be coming from. For adults with Type 1 diabetes, glucose control is usually best when basal insulin delivery makes up 40% to 65% of the TDD. If control problems occur, check your pump's memory to determine what percentage of your TDD you are currently using for basal rates, carb boluses, and correction boluses. Discuss your basal/bolus balance with your physician if you need help adjusting the ratio. Pages 123 and 124 provide more information about basal/bolus balance.

Many smart pumps separately track the insulin used for carb and correction boluses to let you know **how much correction bolus insulin** was used over the last 2 to 30 days to bring down high blood sugar readings. Tracking of correction boluses allows you and your health care professional to quickly determine if too much of your daily insulin dose is being diverted to lowering high glucose readings. Normally, correction boluses should make up less than 8% of the TDD. When more than 8% of your TDD is being used to bring down high readings, some of this insulin needs to be shifted into basal or carb bolus doses to reduce the number of high readings. When correction bolus amounts go above 8%, you can determine how much to shift back into basals or carb boluses by reviewing page 156.

10. **Pump-Meter Combos**

Some pumps have an associated meter that sends blood sugar readings directly into the pump for calculations. This means that your pump can calculate an accurate correction bolus to prevent insulin stacking. Direct entry of glucose values ensures accurate data entry, reduces human error, speeds bolus calculations, and ensures that every blood sugar reading is used to suggest appropriate boluses accounting for BOB. If your meter does not automatically enter readings into your pump, be sure to do this yourself each time a test is taken. Only by entering your blood sugar into your pump can you benefit from your pump using BOB for bolus calculations.

11. **Wearable Pumps**

One wearable pump, the Omnipod, is now on the market. It is a small disposable pump in the shape of a pod that is attached directly to the skin. This eliminates the need for an infusion line. The automated insertion of the cannula creates an easy and consistent application. Each pod is entirely discarded after 48 to 72 hours of use.

A personal data manager, completely separate from the pump pod, communicates with it via radio waves. The data manager provides a sophisticated and intuitive interface that guides users through setup, adjusting basals and boluses, calculating and delivering boluses, and other adjustments. It also contains the history of all management decisions, including a carb database,

5.7 BOB Will Not Work After An Injection

Even when wearing a pump, injections may still be needed. When a blood sugar is unexpectedly high due to an infusion site problem or when only enough insulin remains in your reservoir to cover the basal rates, an injection can be used for a correction or carb bolus.

However, when an injection is used in these situations, your pump will not know it and cannot determine the true BOB. After an injection, this insulin remains active for about 5 hours. The BOB from an injection can be tracked the old-fashioned way by estimating that 20% to 25% of this injected dose will be used each hour.

carb and correction boluses, and blood sugar readings. Similar to the meter built into the Deltec Cozmo pump, the Omnipod data manager has a built-in Freestyle meter that provides blood sugar readings directly into dose calculations. Review pages 46 to 49 for how the Omnipod deals with DIA and tracks BOB to adjust its carb and correction boluses.

The user can customize an expiration alert setting to alarm between 1 and 18 hours before pump use expires at 72 hours. Once 72 hours is reached, the pump alerts hourly for another eight hours to remind the user to change the pump. Once 79 hours is reached, the expiration alert repeats every 15 minutes until the pump expiration occurs at 80 hours and the pump goes into a continuous audible alert.

One drawback is that the data manager is separate from the pump and must be available to give boluses or change basal rates. If the controller is forgotten, an insulin pen or syringe is required to give boluses, though basal delivery will continue as normal. Users can purchase a second manager to have available in the car or at work.

Although wearable, this pump has a raised profile compared to an infusion set. The current pod measures 2.5 x 1.75 x 0.75 inches, so its raised profile may limit use for some. This increases the chances for getting bumped and becoming detached. However, many people report that they exercise while wearing their pump and it does not come off.

Future Developments

Future pumps will look and act different. They may be smaller, start simple and allow features to be turned on when desired, or provide a dual delivery system in which other drugs, such as Symlin or glucagon, can be given along with insulin. Ease of use, accuracy, better calculations, integration of data, data management, and reminders will eventually be integrated into a fully automated control system on the path toward an artificial pancreas. Table 5.8 lists some anticipated features in future pumps and how these features may impact control.

Automatic Basal And Bolus Testing

Besides delivering precise insulin doses, pumps provide data storage with several thousand events typically stored in memory. If sufficient blood sugar testing is done, such as six or more tests a day, this data could be analyzed by computer software or by the pump itself to automatically test basal rates and boluses and point out changes that might improve control. One pump is already providing basal testing feedback and another allows blood sugar readings to be marked as a basal test for later review.

As an example, when a bedtime test is done, a pump knows how much BOB is still active and how far the blood sugar is likely to fall from any residual bolus insulin. If conditions are appropriate, a pump could request that no bedtime snack be eaten and that a blood sugar test be done in the middle of the night (The pump would alarm to awaken the user at this time). From the results of the bedtime, middle of the night, and breakfast readings, an intelligent pump could suggest an appropriate basal adjustment for any unwanted rise or fall.

The accuracy of a carb factor can be checked by reviewing how previous carb boluses have performed. Assuming that carb counting is accurate or even ignoring this, if the carb bolus is routinely not covering the carb count, a pump could suggest a more appropriate carb factor. Similarly, after a few correction boluses have been given, a more accurate correction factor can be estimated by the pump. The pump can also suggest how much insulin to move into basal rates or carb boluses when correction boluses make up an excessive amount of the TDD, such as over 8%.

Pattern Recognition

Today's pumps and meters contain all the data needed to identify blood sugar patterns. Future pumps will identify unwanted patterns, such as excess lows, excess highs, highs or lows, high-to-low, and low-to-high, or excess variability at a particular time of day, and suggest ways to correct them. A pump might say "you are having too many lows before breakfast" or "your basal rate could be reduced by 0.05 u/hr between 10 p.m. and 6 a.m. to stop these breakfast lows" or "your blood sugar may go low in about 37 minutes." A gradual automation of blood glucose control will take place as insulin pumps, meters, PDAs and cell phones become partners in data management.

Time-To-Eat And Delayed-Eating Alerts

When a well-controlled user has a premeal blood sugar near their target, a meal bolus could be given about 20 minutes before eating begins. This delay provides time for the bolus to begin to work so it better matches the rapid rise in glucose following a meal. Future pumps could offer a **Time-To-Eat Alert** that would sound when 20 or so minutes has passed to allow time for a bolus to begin working with less risk of delaying eating too long. Because a pump tracks BOB, it could also determine whether a delay in eating might be too long when excess BOB is present.

If a blood sugar is high before a meal, a pump user can take a combined carb and correction bolus to bring the reading down quickly if eating can be delayed until the

5.8 Upcoming Pump Features And Potential Impact On A1c		
Feature	**Benefit**	**Improve A1c?**
Automatic basal/bolus testing	Basal rates and boluses can be automatically tested.	Yes
Current carbs or insulin deficit	Every time a blood sugar test is taken, the pump recognizes whether there is a carb deficit or insulin deficit based on the current reading. Recommends corrective action.	Yes
Correction bolus %	When correction boluses become excessive as % of TDD (over 8%), a pump can recommmend shifting some of the excess into basals or carb boluses.	Yes
Integration with a continuous glucose monitor	Speeds awareness of high or low BGs and their causes. Prevents lows and lessens time spent with high readings.	Yes
Super Bolus	Speeds fall in high glucoses, safely provides more insulin average for large carb meals and high GI foods.	Yes
Delayed Eating Alert	Allows food intake to be delayed until a high glucose has been lowered. Pump uses artificial intelligence to measure insulin activity and estimate when glucose will be close to target, then alerts user to retest and eat.	Yes
Insulin lookback	Lets user clearly see basal and bolus activity over last 5 hours. Faster identification of which insulin is deficient or in excess.	Yes
Indentification of blood sugar patterns	Faster recognition of insulin mismatches and more accurate basal and bolus adjustments.	Yes
Rank intensity and duration of planned exercise, along with your current blood sugar.	Pump suggests an increase in carb intake or a basal or bolus reduction to balance planned exercise based on BG and BOB.	Yes
Rank the day's activity on a 1-5 scale at day's end	Pump can suggest a lower night basal if increased activity is indicated.	Maybe
Messaging	Speeds communication between parent and child or pump user and physician for convenience and safety.	Maybe

In the book of life, the answers aren't in the back.

Charlie Brown

blood sugar falls to an acceptable range. Here, an intelligent pump could use the bolus information to predict when the blood sugar will reach an acceptable range where eating would not cause excess glucose exposure. This **Delayed-Eating Alert** could alert the user when their blood sugar is likely to have reached a target blood sugar, such as 150 mg/dl (8.3 mmol) or 120 mg/dl (6.7 mmol), for a recheck of the blood sugar in preparation for eating. Combined with a Super Bolus, this could lower a high blood sugar faster while avoiding much of the risk of a low. An intelligent device could even use the second blood sugar result to gradually improve the accuracy of its predictions.

Insulin Lookback

When a high or low reading occurs, one very helpful tool is to look at how much basal and how much bolus insulin has been active in the previous five hours. For instance, when a low blood sugar occurs before breakfast, the amount of basal insulin will almost always be larger than bolus insulin over the previous five hours unless a bolus was used to correct a high reading during the night. When a high or low occurs during the daytime and both basal and bolus insulin have been delivered, a lookback at insulin activity over the last five hours would be helpful. By quantifying basal versus bolus doses, the wearer can more accurately determine which insulin was responsible for a particular high or low and decide appropriate dose changes that may be needed.

A Super Bolus

A Super Bolus could provide more insulin at present when you need it by shifting future basal insulin into an immediate bolus to bring a high blood sugar down faster or to reduce glucose exposure when a meal has more carbs or contains foods with a high glycemic index. To balance the larger bolus, a temporary basal reduction equal to the extra insulin given in the Super Bolus would be automatically programmed. The temporary basal reduction would prevent a low from occurring later.

For example, the basal rate could be lowered to a half or a third of its normal rate for two to four hours using a temporary basal rate, and the insulin taken from basal delivery would immediately be given as a Super Bolus on top of the normal carb and correction bolus that would be given. This Super Bolus given right away provides faster coverage for a high reading or a high GI meal, while the basal reduction prevents a low.

Future pumps could automatically shift insulin between basal and bolus delivery to best serve the user's needs. One option would be to lower the basal rate when excess BOB is present to lessen the need to eat carbs in order to avoid a later low. In certain circumstances, such as where a bedtime blood sugar is already at 90 mg/dl (5 mmol) but there is excess BOB, a basal reduction would be too slow to prevent hypoglycemia. Here, an intelligent pump might suggest how many carbs are needed to counteract any immediate BOB as well as a basal reduction when appropriate.

Micro Pumps

Several companies are working to miniaturize pumps for size reduction and to make attachment to the skin easier. One approach involves Micro-Electro-Mechanical Systems or MEMS devices. A MEMs pump would be significantly smaller in size than today's pumps. MEMs pumps are created from silicon chips that undergo micromachining. This results in an ultra-miniturized size and precise delivery.

Silicon is a transition metal that is quite different from its cousin silicone, used as a lubricant and as filler in breast implants. Silicon in micro-pumps appears to be biologically safe but after being micromachined in a chemical process, it is chemically changed to a more active form that interacts with insulin. Research is underway to find a secondary treatment that would keep the silicon inert and unreactive with insulin. The gates through which insulin passes are extremely small and constantly moving, so the piezoelectric gates used now require large amounts of electrical energy to move enough insulin through. New types of gates are being designed to increase battery life. More research will be needed to document both the safety and feasibility of MEMS pumps.

The small size of MEMS pumps allows dual delivery devices to be built that have two pumps in one. The second pump could deliver a medication like Symlin to improve postmeal control, or to help create a "closed loop" that would deliver small amounts of glucagon as needed to raise the blood sugar quickly to avoid lows altogether.

Major advantages of MEMS micropumps include mass production at low cost and very accurate insulin delivery. The insulin cartridge used in today's pumps would be replaced with a small bladder of insulin in an ergodynamic pump body. Although compact, these pumps would still require the user to have a separate controller available at all times.

Another approach that may evolve sooner than MEMS is to apply pressure to an insulin bladder and use this pressure gradient to precisely measure insulin delivery. This approach eliminates the need for a motor and syringe-type reservoir, enables precise delivery of insulin and other medications, and could also be used as a dual delivery device. With a precise pressure delivery system, it might be possible to detect leakage of insulin between the hub and the infusion site, something that is not currently possible.

5.9 Clever Pump Tricks

Reduce Basal To Offset BOB

With today's pumps, many pumpers will sometimes use a temporary basal rate reduction to offset excess BOB. For example, if someone has 3 units of BOB still active at bedtime and their blood sugar drops 50 mg/dl (2.8 mmol) per unit, a bedtime reading of 150 mg/dl (8.3 mmol) would likely be followed by a low during the night if nothing is done. One alternative to eating a bedtime snack is to use a temporary basal rate reduction equal to 2 units over the next two or three hours.

Peritoneal Insulin Delivery

When insulin is delivered into the peritoneal cavity, it is more directly absorbed into the portal vein than injected or infused insulin. This provides better postmeal readings with much less hypoglycemia. Currently, there are two investigational approaches geared toward achieving this more physiologic delivery of insulin.

The first approach is to implant an insulin pump beneath the skin with a tube to deliver insulin through the abdominal wall into the peritoneal cavity. The peritoneal cavity is a sack-like structure that holds the intestines, stomach, liver, and other organs. About half the insulin delivered into the peritoneal cavity is absorbed into the portal vein and goes directly to the liver. Enough insulin is absorbed in this way to greatly dampen glucose excursions after meals and reduce hypoglycemia that can result from the long action time of bolus insulin from a pump.

Implantation of a pump involves surgery and requires the wearer to visit a physician's office every two to three months to refill the pump with a special insulin. Even more problematic, current implanted pumps are large, clearly visible beneath the skin, and require periodic surgical replacement.

A second, simpler approach is to place on the skin in the abdomen an external port attached to a tube that delivers insulin into the peritoneal cavity. A standard insulin pump can then be used to deliver insulin through this port. This approach creates the improved control of peritoneal delivery using a less intrusive procedure than implantation with a more pleasing cosmetic effect.

Fast and safe peritoneal insulin delivery makes a port a more realistic way to close the loop for an artificial pancreas than implantation. Research is underway to lessen infection risks and determine ideal placement for the tube within the peritoneal cavity.

You campaign in poetry, you govern in prose.

Mario Cuomo

Continuous Monitors And Pumps

One exciting development in diabetes is the availability of continuous monitoring devices or con mons. Using a sensor placed through the skin, the blood sugar is read out every 1 to 5 minutes on a screen on a device that must be within about 5 feet (2 meters) of the sensor. Trends in the blood sugar readings can be acted upon to significantly reduce the number of highs and lows. The wearer's awareness of glucose trends quickly improves basal and bolus doses, and enables lifestyle modifications that free a user from worrisome and dangerous episodes.

The typical response by users is how much they learn about the effects that different foods have on their blood sugar. They can clearly see how often the blood sugar spikes within an hour or two of eating. Also surprising to many is how variable their blood sugar is during the night while they sleep.

A con mon lets the wearer see the current blood sugar and the direction it is moving in. A trend line is shown over various combinations of the last 1 to 24 hours, depending on the device. A trend arrow in some con mons shows whether the blood sugar is stable, going higher, or dropping lower. If an unwanted reading is seen on the monitor and verified by a fingerstick reading, action can be immediately taken to prevent an upcoming problem. High and low thresholds can be set to alert the user when the blood sugar reaches one of these limits to prevent a high or low reading. Some monitors will even warn that the blood sugar is trending low before it happens.

The first con mons require calibration with a standard fingerstick and meter. Because they read glucose in interstitial fluid rather than blood, the readings lag behind a fingerstick test, especially when a blood sugar is changing quickly to a low or high reading. Early con mons can be inexact or erroneous, so readings must be verified with a standard fingerstick before action is taken. The number of fingersticks per day may not fall dramatically at first after starting on a con mon, but there is tremendous value in trends and alerts.

A con mon will not be as accurate as a glucose meter because it is calibrated from readings obtained from a standard meter. All standard meters have some inaccuracy and a con mon multiplies this inaccuracy. A con mon may be late in detecting low blood sugars if the low threshold is set to a reasonable level, such as 70 mg/dl (3.9 mmol) because the blood sugar as shown by a fingerstick may already be lower than this. Expect at least a variance of 10 to 40 mg/dl between the con mon reading and a fingerstick reading. To catch all lows, the low threshold may need to be raised into a normal blood sugar range, for example 80 mg/dl or 100 mg/dl (4.4 or 5.6 mmol), which unfortunately increases the number of false alarms.

One blogger who wears a con mon found that he needed to retrain himself to make the best sense out of his data. At first he compared readings from his con mon with those from his glucose meter and was disappointed at how much they differed. This raised doubts and made him wary of trusting the monitor. But when he changed his attention to using the trends it provided, he realized that this gave him much more information to improve his control. He says he would prefer accurate readings but he values highly the predictive help that trends provide.

Early con mons can be tempermental. Skips in data may occur if the receiver is not close enough to read the blood sugar from the sensor or if it is unsure of a value because the glucose is rapidly going up or down. A continuous monitor cannot be totally relied on to detect hypoglycemia, especially at night if the wearer does not notice an alarm and sleeps through it. The receiver should be worn in the pocket of sleepwear, on a belt around the waist, or near the head while sleeping so that a vibrating alarm will be felt or an audible one heard. When control is erratic, the device will sound warnings more often, so patience is required as the wearer works toward readings that have fewer highs and lows.

Use of a con mon requires that a sensor be worn on the skin and the readout has to be viewed by the wearer on either a pump screen or a screen on a separate device. One pump already shows the reading and trend from a con mon on the pump screen to reduce the number of devices required, although this screen is smaller than screens on a separate device. Despite some shortcomings, most users of con mons are thrilled because they know their approximate blood sugar at any time, where it went during the night, and in what direction it is now headed.

Prevent And Quickly Correct Lows And Highs

The blood sugar trend on a con mon warns of upcoming lows and enables preventive action. Keep in mind that the reading on a continuous monitor tends to be about 20 minutes behind your actual blood sugar. This means that you should take action at the first sign of an upcoming low. A blood sugar reading on a con mon cannot yet be completely relied upon in situations such as driving or other activities. The reading should be confirmed with a fingerstick. If this cannot be done, sufficient glucose or candy should be consumed before turning a car on or participating in certain activities. Patience is also required after treating a low to allow the monitor reading to catch up with your actual blood sugar. Devices differ as to whether one or two low blood sugar alerts can be selected to sound or vibrate when the blood sugar has fallen or may fall below these levels.

When a low happens or is upcoming, it is helpful to look at the BOB on the pump to see if insulin is still active to determine how many carbs may be needed to prevent or treat a low. Following treatment, patiently watch the trend line to ensure treatment worked and the blood sugar is rising. If your treatment is generous and a sharp rise is seen in the blood sugar trend, a correction bolus can be taken early to minimize the blood sugar rise.

Used properly, a con mon can greatly reduce the number of high readings. A warning can be set to alert the wearer when the blood sugar rises above a selected upper limit. If a carb bolus was inadequate and a rapid rise in the blood sugar follows, an

5.10 Tips For Using Rapid Insulin In A Pump

- Always keep fast carbs, such as glucose tablets, available to use for treating low blood sugars. This is a basic requirement for anyone who uses rapid insulin.

- Do not suspend or detach from your pump as a way to treat a low blood sugar. Even a complete suspension of the pump will not allow the blood sugar to rise until an hour or more later. Instead, eat quick carbs for all lows.

- Do not delay a meal more than 20 minutes after bolusing if your blood sugar is within your target range.

- When you eat some complex carbs or low glycemic index foods, you may want to use a combination bolus, such as taking half the bolus now and half over the next hour or two, or an extended bolus that extends insulin release over time.

- Be safe, not sorry. Switch to an injection when you have two consecutive blood sugars above 250 mg/dl (13.8 mmol) or at the FIRST high blood sugar reading over 300 mg/dl (17 mmol). Inject the insulin you need, then research the problem with your set or pump.

- Call your pump manufacturer right away if you suspect faulty delivery. Their trouble shooters will calm your anxiety and lead to a faster resolution of the problem.

experienced user can select an appropriate correction bolus shortly after the sharp rise is detected on the trend screen or indicated by the alarm. An inexperienced user, on the other hand, may at first overreact to these rises or be impatient that their readings are not brought down as quickly as they would like. Acting too early will cause unnecessary lows.

Always check your current BOB on your pump when deciding whether a correction bolus is needed. A con mon can be helpful to ensure that a low does not occur once a correction bolus is given. Remember, though, that today's con mons cannot be totally relied upon to be working at the time they may be needed. A sensor may have timed out or a reading may not be displayed for other reasons.

Trends And Patterns

A con mon reveals short-term trends in the blood sugar as they happen. You can see the direction your blood sugar is taking in the last 1, 3, 6, 9, 12, or 24 hours, depending on what times the monitor offers. Short-term trends help identify and predict immediate control problems. Trends enable early treatment to minimize or eliminate symptoms.

Trends make basal and bolus testing very easy because the effects of insulin action become clear. Basal testing is as simple as looking at whether the blood sugar stays level when nothing is eaten. Bolus testing is easier because you can watch the trend until the action of the bolus insulin has ended. Complete steps for basal and bolus testing with a continuous monitor are included in Chapters 11-13.

Short-term trends picked up by a con mon are certainly helpful, but long-term patterns are perhaps more important to control. Long-term blood sugar patterns can best be analyzed after downloading several days or weeks of data to a PC. Patterns can only be seen when several days' readings are reviewed by the user and their health provider. This data is analyzed in order of its importance: patterns in the overnight blood sugar, then premeal readings, and finally postmeal readings. The wearer and their care provider need to use good judgment to find more effective doses, more appropriate foods, or other approaches to reduce the number and severity of highs and lows. A con mon, just like frequent fingerstick meter testing, is designed to break the cycle of highs and lows by alerting the wearer to the need to make appropriate long-term insulin and lifestyle changes.

A con mon helps avoid highs and lows to improve control, but only when wearers are willing to spend time analyzing their trends for an appropriate response. Early con mon research suggests that occasional use of a con mon does not seem to lower the A1c, as it does when used continuously.

Helpful tips:

- Insulin is slower than carbs, so do not overreact when a reading is high.
- A con mon will have a 15 to 20 minute delay, so the blood sugar appears slow to respond when a low has been treated.
- Always back up any questionable readings with a fingerstick before taking action.
- Never totally rely on a con mon to catch lows or highs.
- Use your con mon to test basal rates and carb and correction boluses.

Progress is underway to combine pumps and con mons into a closed loop system, although this is still several years off. It may never be totally feasible until faster insulins or faster delivery of insulin becomes possible.

Several improvements could help users in the mean time. An alert could tell the user when their trend is changing rapidly and help them know when to pay more attention. This would reduce the need for looking at the trend screen repeatedly. Continuous blood sugar readings could be sent to the pump for more accurate BOB calculations by the pump, as well as accurate bolus and basal testing. Insulin use data from a pump could be combined with the blood sugar results from a continuous monitor to quickly identify problem patterns and needed adjustments. For example, the user could be told that "carb boluses taken for dinner are leading to a high blood sugar at bedtime. Consider adjusting the dinner carb factor." Also foods could be recorded in detail instead of only carb counts so that troublesome ones could be identified and eliminated.

Angels fly because they take themselves lightly.

Robert Louis Stevenson

Select A Pump, Infusion Set, And Insulin

If you are just beginning to pump or are switching to a new pump, take the time you need to make a good choice. You will depend on this pump for four to five years, so discuss different pumps and pump options with your doctor and health care team to select the features that will be most helpful. Research the features listed in the marketing information you receive, as well as those at each pump company's web site and at other web sites like www.diabetesnet.com/diabetes_technology/insulin_pump_models.php.

What this chapter covers

- Questions to ask when choosing a pump
- Considerations for infusion sets
- Insulin for your pump

Ask lots of questions when choosing a pump. Get a list of local pump representatives and call them to get a demonstration of their pump. Discuss the advantages of each pump and assess the support provided. Look for a pump support group or go to a diabetes conference where pumpers are present and pump vendors are showing their products. This may take some time, but you will be better informed and able to make a better decision.

The pump company will prepare the paperwork to submit to your insurance carrier or Medicare to cover their share of the pump and supplies. They can also help you deal with any insurance problems that may arise.

Considerations In Choosing An Insulin Pump

Insulin pumps differ in their features and ease of use. Your needs may make one pump a better choice than another. When selecting a pump, consider the following:

1. What appeals to you about the pump? Look, feel, and color, features, accessories?
2. How easy is the pump to program and use?
3. How many infusion set choices do you have?

4. How easy are the buttons to push? A bolus should be easy to deliver, but giving a bolus accidentally while gesturing, reaching into a pocket, or displaying the pump to inquisitive friends should not.

5. What type of reminders and alarms does the pump have?

6. How finely can basal rates be programmed for children and insulin-sensitive adults who require low basal rates? How often does basal delivery occur?

7. How easy is it to stop a bolus? If the pump is for a child, can a caregiver easily learn to stop the pump in an emergency?

8. Can you hear or feel the alarms? Will you know if your insulin delivery has stopped?

9. How much information is stored in the pump's memory? How easy is it to access? This is important if you get distracted and forget to bolus, or if you want to check on your current BOB or active insulin, or if a parent wants to verify bolus delivery by a child.

10. If required, can the pump survive rough use? Is the pump waterproof? Is it easy to disconnect before showering or swimming?

11. What level of customer service is provided by the manufacturer? 24-hour telephone support? Assistance with insurance coverage? Warranty? Trial period? Shipment of temporary supplies to different addresses? How soon will a replacement arrive if needed?

Questions To Ask

Your Doctor And Diabetes Educator

1. How many pumps have they prescribed in the last year?

2. Which of the current pumps and infusion sets do they prefer and why?

3. How familiar are they with the pump you want?

4. Have they or users had problems with any pump that they are aware of?

5. What pumps have people who recently started using one recommended?

6. Is a loaner pump available for a trial?

Your Insurance Company Or Medicare

1. Do you fit their qualifications for pump use?

2. Which insulin pump or pumps will they cover? Many HMOs have a contract with only one or two pump companies.

3. If you prefer a particular pump that is not currently approved under your plan, how can you obtain coverage for this pump?

4. Do you have DME coverage? How much of the pump and supply expenses will this cover?

5. How often do they cover a new pump?

6. If you are not happy with the pump coverage provided by your current insurer, are you able to switch to another company in the near future that would provide better coverage.? You may want to wait until you have better coverage before buying a pump.

7. If you are turned down by your insurance company, ask your pump representative to help you with your paperwork.

Other Pumpers

1. Is there a local pump club or someone you know on a pump that you can talk with? You can also join a forum or chat room on the internet to seek information and advice.

2. Some pumpers have worn several pumps. Which pump would they recommend?

3. What features do experienced pumpers feel are most important?

4. What advice would they give you from their experience?

5. Have they had particular issues that caused problems in their control?

6. Have they needed to contact the pump company's 24-hour support line? What necessitated the call and did they get the support they needed?

After You Decide On A Pump

Once you choose a pump and infusion set and have your doctor's approval, your doctor will write a prescription and a letter of medical necessity. The letter helps you get insurance approval and may make it easier to choose a pump that may not be on your insurance provider's preferred list.

Once approved, your pump and pump supplies will be delivered to your door or to your doctor's office. A certified pump trainer from the pump company or from your doctor's office will train you on using the pump. Your doctor will review and assess your skills and guide you in setting initial basal rates and bolus factors, as well as the programmable pump features you choose to start with.

Your pump trainer and health care professional will be available by phone or appointment to help with any problems that may arise. They know this can be confusing and will help you succeed. Ask for an emergency phone number and use it if you need help.

Considerations For Infusion Sets

Using an infusion set that works well for you is one of the most important steps in making your pump experience successful. The infusion set and site are the weakest link in pumping. If a particular set causes skin irritation, falls off when you swim or sweat, or is easily dislodged, problems with your control will occur. For a satisfying pump experience, the infusion set you wear must be reliable and comfortable.

When Selecting An Infusion Set, Consider:

- How much body fat do you have?
- Which sites on your body are best to use?
- Do your belt or clothing choices limit wearing a set near the waist?
- Does your activity level limit you to certain sites?
- Which type and size infusion set will work best for the body locations you prefer?

- Can you detach the pump easily for showering? Is the disconnection technique hard for you to handle? Some sets disconnect right at the infusion site, while others have a separate connector located a few inches away.
- Will you need a device to aid with insertion of the infusion set?
- Straight-in metal sets are reliable and easiest to insert, even using only one hand. Slanted Teflon sets may be more reliable for some users than staight-in Teflon sets. Inserters tend to work best with straight-in sets.
- Suggested set sizes: for children under 12 and very lean adults with a body mass index or BMI less than 24 or 25, try 6 mm straight or 13 mm slanted sets. For a BMI less than 27 or so, use 8 mm straight or 17 mm slanted sets. For a BMI over 27, try 10 mm straight or 17 mm slanted sets. Visit www.diabetesnet.com/diabetes_tools/ tools_bmi.php to find your BMI.

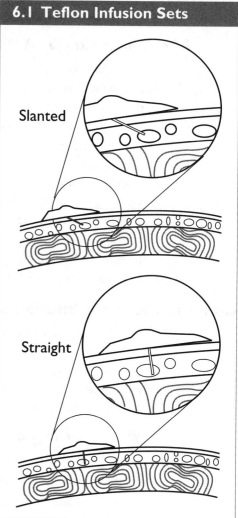

6.1 Teflon Infusion Sets

Slanted

Straight

The set you receive with your pump may or may not turn out to be the best choice for you. When your pump arrives, it will come with sets recommended by your physician or nurse educator, or Teflon infusion sets manufactured by the pump company, along with samples of a few other sets in the pump box itself. If possible, wear different infusion sets before deciding which one is comfortable, easy to use, and stays in place. Insertion devices are available for inserting Teflon catheters through the skin.

Many pumps have a standard Luer™ connection between the reservoir and infusion set. A standard connection allows you to choose from about 20 different types of infusion sets. Other pumps have a proprietary connection between the reservoir and the infusion set. This limits your choice to their infusion sets or a few others from small manufacturers. If you need to find an infusion set that works better for you, your health team can provide samples and offer suggestions, or you can call different infusion set manufacturers and request samples of their products.

Finding the right infusion set can have a major impact on the satisfaction you get out of pumping. Various infusion sets are shown in Table 6.2 and others can be seen at www. diabetesnet.com/diabetes_technology/infusion_sets.php.

6.2 A Wide Variety Of Infusion Sets To Choose From

Name(s)	Type*	Needle	Tubing	Base	Disconnect	Inserter
Accu-Chek® Ultra Flex	Straight Teflon, LL	8, 10 mm 25/27 gauge	24, 31, 43 inches	Cotton Adhesive	At Site	No
Medtronic Minimed Quick-Set®	Straight Teflon, LL, P	6, 9 mm 25/27 gauge	23, 43 inches	Cotton Adhesive	At Site	Yes
ICU Medical® Orbit 90	Straight Teflon, LL	6, 9, 12 mm 26 gauge	24, 31, 42 inches	Translucent Tape	At Site	No
Unomedical® Inset	Straight Teflon, LL	6, 9 mm 25/26 gauge	23, 43 inches	Cotton Adhesive	At Site	All in one
Simple Choice® Easy (Pro)	Slanted Teflon, LL, P	12, 17 mm 25/27 gauge	23, 43 inches	Waterproof Adhesive	At Site	Yes
Smiths Medical® Cleo 90	Straight Teflon, LL	6, 9 mm 27 gauge	24, 31, 42 inches	Transparent Adhesive	At Site	All in one
Medtronic Minimed® Silhouette	Slanted Teflon, LL, P	17 mm 25/27 gauge	23, 43 inches	Cotton Adhesive	At Site	Yes
Accu-Chek® Tender	Slanted Teflon, LL	13, 17 mm 25/27 gauge	24, 31, 43 inches	Cotton Adhesive	At Site	No
Unomedical® Comfort	Slanted Teflon, LL	13, 17 mm 25/27 gauge	23, 31, 43 inches	Cotton Adhesive	At Site	No
Accu-Chek® Rapid D	Straight Metal, LL	6, 8, 10 mm 28 gauge	24, 31, 43 inches	Cotton Adhesive	Short Tail	No
Unomedical® Contact Detach	Straight Metal, LL	6, 8, 10 mm 25/27 gauge	24, 31, 43 inches	Cotton Adhesive	At Site	No

* LL = Luer Lock Connection, P = Paradigm Connection   Visit www.diabetesnet.com/diabetes_technology/infusion_sets.php for links and information.

Many of today's metal needles are as comfortable as Teflon sets. Accu-Chek's® Rapid-D™ and Unomedical's® Contact sets have a fine-guage 0.36 mm wide metal needle that is easier to insert than 0.50 mm Teflon sets. Their reliability often reduces infusion site problems in children and lean adults. Longer needles work better in padded areas of the abdomen, while shorter ones may be more comfortable in less padded areas like the thigh or biceps.

Reliability is the most important feature of any infusion set. Most infusion sets work well, but problems like a tendency to detach, Teflon crimping during insertion, or a series of unexplained high blood sugars caused by set failure will not be apparent until a set is worn for some time. A particular infusion set may cause a skin rash or irritation while another one will not. A trial run with various sets is likely to pick up most of these problems. Do not continue to wear a set that causes problems. You have many good choices.

Steps to troubleshoot problems arising from an infusion set are covered in Chapter 21. Keep in mind that pump supplies, including infusion sets and reservoirs, are rarely available at a local pharmacy. Order ahead of time!

Insulin For Your Pump

Multiple injections rely on both rapid and long-acting insulins, but a pump uses only a rapid insulin. A slow release of rapid insulin through the day provides the background insulin that replaces the long-acting insulin. Boluses or a quick release of the rapid insulin covers carbs and lowers any high readings. On a pump, one rapid insulin covers all your insulin needs.

6.3 Insulin Storage Tips

- If you have an unexpected high, do not automatically assume it is your fault. It could be bad insulin.

- Keep insulin out of direct sunlight.

- The bottle of insulin you are using in your pump may be stored at room temperature for 30 days.

- Keep a backup supply of insulin refrigerated or cooled at all times, but no cooler than 36 degrees Fahrenheit. Freezing destroys insulin's potency.

- If your insulin is shipped through the mail, or by a delivery service, demand that it be insulated and cooled against temperature extremes during shipment.

- Do not leave insulin in a car for an extended length of time in freezing or hot weather.

The different rapid insulins that can be used in a pump are similar in action. Currently, the rapid insulins that are available for pumps include:

- Novolog® (aspart) by Novo Nordisk was released with pump approval in 2001

- Apidra® (glulisine) by Aventis was released and approved for pump use in 2004

- Humalog® (lispro) by Eli Lilly and Company was released for injections in 1996 and approved for pump use in 2004

Before everything else, getting ready is the secret to success.

Henry Ford

Carb Counting

One benefit of wearing a pump is the ability to eat the carbs you want and cover them with an accurate bolus at any time of day. Carbs can be matched by the flexible, precise and convenient insulin delivery of a pump once you've learned to count carbs accurately.

If you are not already using this great tool, this chapter shows how to count carbs to maximize your success on a pump. If you currently count your carbs, review this chapter to sharpen your skills. Periodically check your accuracy to stay on top of this valuable tool. Make sure you bolus for the right amount of carbs in a meal to ensure good control you can count on.

This chapter describes

- What carbs and grams are
- How to figure your daily carbohydrate needs
- Three methods for carb counting
- The bigger nutrition picture
- The glycemic index and glycemic load

An accurate carb count tells you how much a meal will raise your glucose. This enables your pump to determine the size of the carb bolus you need. Some pumps include their own carb database to simplify carb counting or have one in an accompanying PDA or smart phone. Matching your carbs well with insulin accounts for half the day's blood sugar control. To splurge occasionally on foods like ice cream, cake, pie, or candy, you just need to match all the carbs with a carb bolus using the carb factor in your pump.

Food contains three main nutrients: carbohydrate, fat, and protein. Although the whole story is more complex, carbs and fats are used largely as fuel, while protein provides structure to cells and enzymes.

Carbohydrate is the primary nutrient in food that affects the blood sugar. Over 90 percent of the carbs derived from starches and sugars end up as glucose that moves through the blood to your cells. Small amounts of protein turn into glucose that seldom affects the blood sugar. Certain fats indirectly affect the blood sugar by making cells resistant to insulin. See Textbox 7.1 for a discussion of these effects.

Carbohydrate has the greatest effect on blood glucose but the other main food components – fat and protein – can have a small effect, as well. For instance, the fat in certain foods will delay the absorption of carbohydrate from the intestine. This causes a smaller or slower than expected rise in the glucose.[65] For example, old-fashioned ice cream gives the ice cream a low glycemic index. This slows the rise its carb content indicates, which may lead to confusing readings afterward.

On the other hand, certain high fat meals create a higher state of insulin resistance for 8 to 16 hours, making the blood glucose rise more than expected.[66, 67] For example, the fats found in many chips and pizzas can cause a rise that is later and longer lasting than expected.

Normal portions of dietary protein have little impact on blood glucose.[68] Making up only 10 to 20 percent of calories in most diets, protein affects less than a tenth of the total blood sugar control. Large portions of protein, however, can create a gradual rise in glucose because half of the calories in protein are slowly converted to glucose over several hours. A high-protein dinner, such as an eight-ounce steak or a bean burrito, may cause glucose levels to rise 4 to 12 hours later, creating an unexpected high reading the next morning.

Talk with your doctor or dietitian if you think your intake of fat or protein may be causing your control to be less stable than you want it to be. A pump with its extended bolus ability may be a help here.

To maintain control, carbs in a meal must be balanced by insulin or occasionally by exercise that helps clear them from the blood. To determine the size of a carb insulin bolus, you want to first determine how many units of insulin will cover one gram of carb in your body. This is your carb factor. Enter this into your pump so that you can count the grams of carbohydrate in any food you eat and balance them with a correctly-sized bolus.

Carb counting is well worth the effort to learn when you consider the impact it has on your control. How else can you match carbs and insulin well? Carb counting might seem difficult, but hang in there. It is the best control tool to use with a pump.

Where's The Carb?

To start covering carbs with insulin or exercise, you want to know which foods contain enough carbs that they require counting and which can be ignored.

Carbohydrate is found in:

- Grains (breads, cereals, crackers, and pasta)
- Fruits and vegetables
- Beans, lentils, and peas

- Root crops (carrots, beets, potatoes, sweet potatoes, and yams)
- Beer, wine, brandy and liquors
- Desserts, candy, cookies, cake, and pie
- Milk and milk products, except cheese
- Regular soft drinks, fruit juices and drinks
- Sugar, honey, syrup, sucrose, and fructose

Carbohydrate is not found in significant amounts in animal proteins such as meat or eggs, or in tofu or nuts. It is not present in fats such as oils, margarine, or butter. Most vegetables contain so few carbs that they can be ignored unless the carbs add up to more than 15 grams or you find your blood sugar rises when you eat them.

Healthy Carbs

In a healthy diet, most carbohydrate comes from nutrient-dense foods like whole grains, fruits, legumes, vegetables, nonfat or low fat milk, and yogurt. These foods contain a high volume of micronutrients, such as vitamins, minerals, fiber, and protein in proportion to their caloric content. These allow glucose to be processed correctly and prevent the development of deficiencies that generate "carb craving." Some nutrient rich foods are high on the glycemic index, but they tend to be lower on the glycemic index causing less spiking of the blood sugar.

Nutrient-poor foods like candy and regular sodas contain carbs from simple sugars but lack the other nutrients your cells require for health. These carbs tend to rank high on the glycemic index and are likely to spike the blood sugar. They are best eaten in small amounts. Nutrient-dense foods like brown rice and broccoli are more filling and are better for your health and your blood sugars. All vegetables are nutrient dense and when counting carbs most contain such a low proportion of carbohydrate that they can be ignored unless large quantities are eaten. Some vegetables such as beets, carrots, peas and corn contain enough carbohydrate that they should be counted.

7.2 Metric Conversions	
1/2 oz	= 14 grams
1 oz	= 28.4 grams
2 oz	= 57 grams
3 1/2 oz	= 100 grams
1 fl. oz	= 30 mls
1 cup (8 fl oz)	= 240 mls
33 fl. oz	= 1 liter (volume)

What Are Grams?

Carbs are counted in grams. Like ounces, a gram is a unit of weight, but its small size makes it more useful to accurately measure food components. There are 28 grams in one ounce. Memorize this simple fact so that gram measurements in books and on labels will not be confusing when you need to calculate carb boluses.

How Many Carbs Do You Need A Day?

Your daily carb requirement is based on your daily calorie need. A person who needs 2000 calories a day ideally would get 50% to 60%, or 1000 to 1200, of those calories from the carbohydrate in breads, grains, vegetables, fruits, low-fat milk, and so on. Each gram of carbohydrate contains four calories of energy. This means a person eating 2000 calories a day needs 250 to 300 grams (1000 to 1200 calories divided by 4 calories per gram) of carb with the rest of their calories coming from protein and fat.

To get an idea of how many grams are in your current diet, eat your usual meals for a few days and keep a record of how many carbs you actually take in. Use this chapter and carb references, books, labels, and perhaps a computer software program to help you analyze your diet. Sit down with a nutritionist and reviewing your diet diary to confirm that it provides a healthy balance of nutrients. Use Workspace 7.3 to calculate a recommended daily carb intake. If you are eating significantly less carbohydrate than this recommended amount, try increasing your carb intake by 10%. Reduce fat and protein calories by the same amount. Remember that carbs and proteins have four calories per gram, while fat has nine. The same number of fat grams will have more than twice as many calories.

Carb amounts play a major role in setting your carb boluses. It is best to make gradual changes in how many carbs you eat and adjust your insulin gradually as you go. An abrupt change in the number of carbs you eat a day can make blood sugar control more difficult. Also, fast changes in food choices seldom become permanent ones.

A food's weight does not tell how much carbohydrate it contains because most foods are not pure carbohydrate. For example, even though 224 grams (one cup) of milk, a 160-gram slice of watermelon, a 14-gram rectangular graham cracker (two squares), and 12 grams (one tablespoon) of sugar have different weights, they all contain exactly 12 grams of carbohydrate. Only the sugar is all carbohydrate. The other foods contain water and other ingredients.

Despite their different weights, these foods all require the same carb bolus to cover them. Knowing the total number of grams of carb in a food tells you what you need to enter into your pump to calculate an appropriate bolus. Knowing your carb factor or how many carb grams are covered by one unit of insulin completes your calculation needed for precise insulin dosing.

Three Ways To Count Carbs

Carbs can be counted directly from food labels, by looking up the carb content in a book that lists carbs, or by weighing a food on a gram scale and multiplying its weight by its carb percentage.

Like any new skill, counting grams of carbohydrate will take a couple of weeks to understand and apply easily. To learn this, you will need to weigh and measure foods consistently. As you look up foods in resources, make a list that you commonly eat for

7.3 Determine Your Carb Requirement Per Day

Follow steps 1 through 4 to find your daily carb requirement.

1. Current Weight or Desired Weight?

Enter your current weight or desired weight in pounds below. If overweight, a 10% reduction in weight is an ideal goal.

My current weight   =   _____   lbs

or

My desired weight.   =   _____   lbs

2. Choose a Calorie Factor

From the table below, choose a calorie factor that best describes your activity level.

My calorie factor = _____

Daily Calorie and Carb Need

3. Find your daily calorie need by multiplying your weight by your calorie factor.

4. To determine how many grams of carb you need a day, divide your daily calorie need by 10 if you want 40% of your calories to come from carbs.

_____ lbs. X _____ = _____ / 10 = _____ **grams of carb/day**
$\quad$ weight $\qquad\quad$ calorie factor $\quad$ calories per day

* Divide by 8 for 50% or by 6.67 for a 60% carb diet.

Calorie Factors For Levels of Activity

Activity Level	Calorie Factor male	female
Very Sedentary: Limited activity, slow walking, mostly sitting.	13	11.5
Sedentary: Recreational activities include walking, bowling, fishing, or similar activities.	14	12.5
Moderately Active: Recreational activities include 18 hole golf, dancing, pleasure swimming, etc.	15	13.5
Active: 20 minutes or more of jogging, swimming, tennis or similar activities over three times per week.	16	14.5
Super Active: An hour or more of vigorous activity (football, weight training, full court basketball) four or more days per week.	17	15.5

easy reference. Keep your list next to your *Smart Charts* or logbook, and use it to figure the carbs in every meal before you decide how much insulin to take. Do this by first selecting the meals you like and eat them most of the time. After you have learned

7.4 Carb And Nutrition Resources Online

A great resource for carb and nutrition information is the USDA National Nutrient Database at http://www.nal.usda.gov/fnic/foodcomp/Data/. The database can be searched, or you can download an alphabetical list of every food you can think of along with its carb content.

these basics in your food plan, it will be easier to count carbs in your entire diet.

As you keep at it, your eye becomes trained to estimate serving sizes and weights more accurately, whether eating out or at home, and you will remember how much insulin it takes to cover that food. Eventually, you'll be able to look at a piece of fruit, a bowl of pasta, or a plate of stir-fried veggies and rice, estimate its carb count and take an accurate bolus for it. This, of course, is easier if you often eat the same things, as many people do. Be patient and persistent. When you can adjust your boluses precisely to the carbs you eat, you'll know it was worth all the effort.

1. Weighing And Measuring To Determine Carbs

Accurate carb counting requires equipment for weighing and measuring, such as a gram scale (which often measures ounces as well), and measuring cups and spoons. Scales measure weight, while cups and spoons measure volume. For some foods there is a big difference between volume and weight. For example, 1 1/4 cups of Cheerios® is 10 ounces in volume but only one ounce in weight (28 grams). Many nutrition labels and food composition tables give both measures. Since all your carb counting will be done in grams, the metric conversions in Table 7.2 can be helpful for calculating foods specified in ounces.

Measuring cups and spoons are available at most grocery and kitchen supply stores. A glass measuring cup with marked lines that you can sight across is helpful for measuring liquids.

Using A Gram Scale Or A Computer Scale

Many foods, like fruit, cooked pasta, or a casserole have no food label. You can estimate the carb content of these foods from a list in a nutrition book if you can accurately measure serving sizes. However, a more accurate way to calculate the carb content in these foods is to weigh them on a gram scale and multiply the weight by the percentage of the weight that is carbohydrate. Appendix A at the end of the book provides a list of the carb percentages in different foods. You can also use a computerized gram scale which has built-in nutritive breakdowns for a variety of foods. Based on a food's weight and its specific food code, a computer scale will provide the carbs, calories, fat, and protein it contains.

With a standard gram scale and carb factors list:

1. Zero out your plate on the scale, then place the amount of cooked spaghetti you want to eat on it.

2. Let's say your portion weighs 200 grams on the scale. From Appendix A, you find that cooked plain spaghetti has 26 percent of its weight as carbohydrate.

3. Multiply the spaghetti's total weight by its percentage of carbs.

Example

$$\underset{\substack{\text{weight of} \\ \text{spaghetti}}}{\underline{200\,g}} \quad \times \quad \underset{\substack{\text{carb} \\ \text{percent}}}{\underline{.26}} \quad = \quad \underset{\substack{\text{total carbs} \\ \text{in this portion}}}{\underline{52\,g}}$$

4. When you eat 200 grams of cooked spaghetti, you eat 52 grams of carbohydrate.

With a computer gram scale:

Computerized gram scales already contain programmed information about the nutrition content of spaghetti and other foods.

1. Zero out your plate on the scale.

2. Enter the food code for spaghetti into the scale.

3. Place the amount of spaghetti you want to eat onto your plate.

4. Press the carb key on the scale to find out how many grams of carbohydrate are in the spaghetti.

Gram scales are available at kitchen supply stores and www.diabetesnet.com.

Advantage: Convenient for measuring carbs in odd-sized foods like fruits, unsliced bread, soups, or pasta.

What you need: A computer gram scale, or a standard gram scale, a calculator, and a list of carb percentages that can be found in Appendix A at the back of the book. See Table 7.5 for details on how to find a food's carb content with a gram scale.

Sometimes it is helpful to carry your gram scale and list of carb percentages with you to restaurants. Weigh your food to calculate the grams of carbohydrate the meal contains. Don't worry. People do strange things in restaurants. Pretend you are a food inspector or food critic. Your self-consciousness will be more than offset by your improved control and the extra service you receive from the waiter.

2. Nutrition Books, Cookbooks, and Software Give Carb Counts

Nutrition books, software in a PDA or Palm device, and cookbooks list the amount of carbohydrate in a typical serving of different foods. If what you eat varies from this serving size, you may need to weigh or measure your actual serving and do some minor calculations to convert your serving into grams of carbohydrate.

Advantage: Nutrition books, cookbooks, software, or a pump or PDA database can improve the accuracy of carb counts. This makes it easier to look up brand name foods and restaurant meals. Most cookbooks provide the carb count per serving, which makes counting carbs easy when using these recipes at home.

What you need: Books or software programs or a pump or PDA with a food database. You may also need measuring cups, spoons, and scales to determine serving size.

What To Do: Look for nutrition books and cookbooks in the "Nutrition and Diet" section of your local bookstore, library, at online sources like the American Diabetes Association (www.diabetes.org) or order from the Diabetes Mall (www.diabetesnet.com/ishop/), where you can get helpful suggestions about which books may fit your needs. Online sources and diabetes product guides from diabetes magazines, such as *Diabetes Health* and *Diabetes Forecast*, provide helpful lists of software or books. Recipes in the "Food" section of your local newspaper and in health magazines list the carb content per serving.

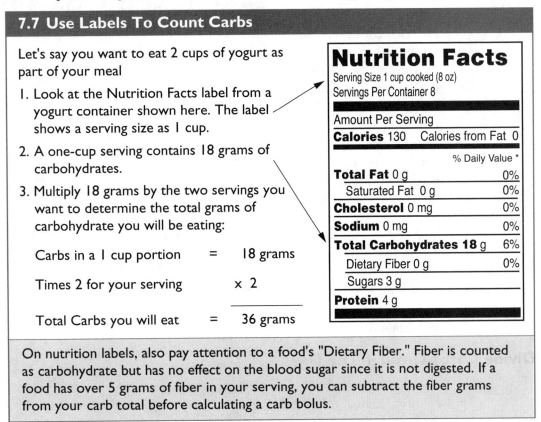

7.7 Use Labels To Count Carbs

Let's say you want to eat 2 cups of yogurt as part of your meal

1. Look at the Nutrition Facts label from a yogurt container shown here. The label shows a serving size as 1 cup.

2. A one-cup serving contains 18 grams of carbohydrates.

3. Multiply 18 grams by the two servings you want to determine the total grams of carbohydrate you will be eating:

Carbs in a 1 cup portion	=	18 grams
Times 2 for your serving	x	2
Total Carbs you will eat	=	36 grams

Nutrition Facts

Serving Size 1 cup cooked (8 oz)
Servings Per Container 8

Amount Per Serving

Calories 130   Calories from Fat 0

% Daily Value *

Total Fat 0 g	0%
Saturated Fat 0 g	0%
Cholesterol 0 mg	0%
Sodium 0 mg	0%
Total Carbohydrates 18 g	6%
Dietary Fiber 0 g	0%
Sugars 3 g	
Protein 4 g	

On nutrition labels, also pay attention to a food's "Dietary Fiber." Fiber is counted as carbohydrate but has no effect on the blood sugar since it is not digested. If a food has over 5 grams of fiber in your serving, you can subtract the fiber grams from your carb total before calculating a carb bolus.

3. Food Labels Give Carb Counts

Packaged foods have nutrition facts on their label that gives the size of a standard serving and how many grams of carb each serving contains. The food label also gives the number of calories in a serving to assist weight loss, the amount and types of fat, such as saturated fats and trans fats, and other nutritional information, such as the grams of protein. People with kidney disease need protein information, and those with heart disease or diabetes need to regulate their fat intake and avoid hydrogenated or trans fats.

Fig. 7.7 shows how to calculate the carbs in a serving of food from a label.

Advantage: Relatively easy, occasional calculations are required.

What you need: If you eat the serving size on the label, the label is all you need. If you eat a different amount, you will need to use the food label, a measuring cup or gram scale, and a calculator to calculate the carbs in the amount you actually eat.

What To Do: Food labels contain all the information you need to do carb counting. Just be sure your serving is the same size as the serving described on the label.

Cafeteria Style And Combination Foods

Combination foods can vary greatly in their carb content depending on the recipe. Table 7.8 provides an estimate of the carbs per portion size for a variety of combination foods. You can also conduct your own test. Eat the same amount of a particular food made from the same recipe several times and take a carb bolus based on its estimated carb count. Test your blood sugar at 2 hours and again at 4 hours. Keep a record and use your best estimate from then on.

Divide Carbs Through The Day

Although carb counting matches the flexibility of a pump very well, some people may want a regimented system that spreads the carbs through the day. You may prefer to eat set amounts of carbs for each meal or snack of the day and cover these with fixed carb boluses, or you may need to adjust your boluses to match changing carb counts. Either way will work if your carb count is accurate and your pump is programmed with the proper settings.

7.8 Sample Values In Cafeteria Style Foods

Homemade recipes vary greatly in their nutritive values, so do not rely on the carb values below until you have tested them yourself.

Food	Cals	Fat	Carbs
Beef Stroganoff, 5 oz	195	13	7
Beef Stroganoff w 4 oz noodles	350	14	36
Chicken Lasagna, 1 piece	300	11	32
Chicken Chop Suey w 4 oz rice	245	4	37
Deep Dish Burrito, 7 oz	265	13	20
Grnd Beef Casserole, 2 scp, 6 oz	245	13	17
Italian Meat Sce for Spagh, 5 oz	150	9	9
w 5 oz Spaghetti	350	10	49
Lasagna, 1 piece	275	11	25
Meatloaf, 3 oz	205	13	4
Ranch Beans, 2 scp, 6 oz	350	11	45
Red Beans & Rice, 7 oz	280	9	37
Scalloped Potato/Ham, 2 scp, 6 oz	160	6	20
Stuffed Shells in Sauce (1)	105	3	17
Swedish Meatballs (3)	205	12	9
Sweet & Sour Pork/Rice, 9 oz	240	3	40
Swiss Steak w/Mushr Gravy, 5 oz	280	11	4
Tator Tot Casserole, 2 scoops, 6 oz	260	15	20
Tenderloin Tips/Mushr Gravy, 5 oz	210	13	3
w 5 oz noodles	395	15	38
Tuna Noodle Casserole, 2 scp, 6 oz	180	6	17
Turkey Tetrazini, 2 scp, 6 oz	195	7	17
Vegetable Lasagna, 1 piece	250	13	21

7.9 Grams Of Carb Divided Through The Day

Meal	Example 1	Example 2	Example 3	My Carbs
Breakfast	75 grams	30 grams	75 grams	_____ grams
Morning Snack		15 grams		_____ grams
Lunch	75 grams	45 grams	70 grams	_____ grams
Afternoon Snack		30 grams		_____ grams
Dinner	75 grams	75 grams	40 grams	_____ grams
Bedtime Snack		30 grams	40 grams	_____ grams
Total Carbs	225	225	225	_____ grams

Example 1 divides 225 carbs evenly into 3 meals. Example 2 starts with a light breakfast and lunch, with snacks between meals, and ends with a big dinner. Example 3 starts with a large breakfast and lunch and finishes with a light dinner and bedtime snack.

Once you know how many carbs you need a day from Workspace 7.3, divide your own total carbs per day into different meals.

© 2006 Diabetes Services, Inc.

For a well-balanced carb routine, divide your total daily allotment of carbs among the meals and snacks you eat each day. Base this distribution on your personal preferences and needs. If it isn't personalized, you won't follow it very long. Consistent eating helps when you first go on a pump or anytime you need to bring blood sugars into better control. Table 7.9 shows ways to distribute total daily carbs through the day. Use this table to set your carbs at each meal and snack.

The Bigger Nutrition Picture

Once you master the art of carb counting and accurately determine your carb factor, you become an expert in balancing your insulin with your food intake for optimum control. As important as this is, however, it is not the only health goal you have. Your overall health depends on eating a wide variety of nutrient-rich foods.

Healthy eating guidelines:

* Eat a variety of healthy and nutritious foods
* Reduce fat, particularly trans and saturated, and protein to reasonable amounts
* Balance carbs with bolus insulin or exercise

The amount and type of fat in your diet is very important to health. A high intake of saturated, trans, or partially hydrogenated fats can increase risks for heart disease and cancer. Heart disease is especially common in people with diabetes, who have a two- to six-fold increase in risk over those without diabetes. A fat intake of no more than 20% to 30% of total calories is recommended by the American Heart Association and the American Dietetic Association, and the preferred fats are unsaturated or monounsaturated. Reducing the intake of saturated and hydrogenated or trans fats has helped to gradually reduce heart attacks in this country over the last two decades.

To lower your risk of heart disease, lower your intake of foods like chips and crackers made with hydrogenated fat, butter, margarine, sour cream, cheese, and shortening used for frying. Switch to monounsaturated oils (olive oil, avocado), polyunsaturated seed oils (safflower oil, sunflower oil, corn oil), and add nuts to your diet. Choose protein foods that are lower in fat or those that contain better types of fat and less fat, such as fish, skinless chicken, nonfat milk, and nonfat cheese products. Instead of butter or margarine on your waffle or pancake, have apple butter which contains some sugar but no fat, and add flavorful nuts.

About one of every three people with Type 1 diabetes develops kidney disease. Lowering the animal protein in the diet has been shown to lessen the risk of kidney disease as well as slow its progression once it has begun. Smaller red meat portions lowers the intake of harmful saturated fats and protects kidney function.

Sugar is no longer banned from coffee, nor jelly from toast, nor an occasional small piece of pie from the dinner table. This good news can help your quality of life. Research has shown it is possible to control blood sugars when eating reasonable quantities of splurge foods once

7.10 Don't Skip Meals

When someone eats only one or two meals a day, the body learns to store extra fat for quick release to enable survival when food intake is not consistent. The most accessible storage space is the abdomen.

During long hours of sleep, large abdominal fat stores can easily raise circulating free fatty acid and triglyceride levels in the blood. Higher free fatty acid levels raise insulin resistance and accelerate damage to blood vessels.

In contrast, by eating reasonable amounts of complex, low glycemic index carbohydrates through the day, you help minimize fat release into the blood and assist weight maintenance. A healthy "nibbling" diet helps lower triglycerides and LDL cholesterol levels, and keeps the glucose in better control.

7.11 Slow (Low GI) Carbs

Just like long-acting insulins, there are long-acting or slow carbs. Some carbs that digest slowly can be used at bedtime or during lengthy exercise to prevent your glucose from falling too far soon after you eat.

Examples of slow carbs include beans (lima, pinto, etc.), green apples, Power Bars, raw cornstarch, pasta al dente, barley, cracked wheat, parboiled long grain and whole grain rice, and whole-grain rye bread. Plus, these carbs work well because they have a low glycemic index.

you know how to match their carb content with insulin. This has become easier with today's rapid insulins which can more easily counteract the extra carbs found in desserts, ice cream, and candy.

No one really benefits from an excess of high-calorie, low-nutrient foods, yet small amounts of sweets can add flavor to a diet and, when chosen wisely, make avoiding fatty foods easier. Be careful though: sugar often travels with fat. Those sweet chocolate candy bars get about 60 percent of their calories from fat! Also, remember that when products have reduced sugar, they often have added fat and vice versa.

If you find that sweets are addictive and a little is never enough, you may decide to eliminate processed foods made with simple sugars entirely. A good cure for sweet craving is to eat only whole grain foods for six to eight weeks before gradually reintroducing small amounts of refined carbs into your diet. Another help is to eat fruit to satisfy sweet cravings.

Whether you include sweets in your meals or not, the key to blood sugar control is to determine the amount of carbohydrate in your food and cover it with an appropriate amount of insulin. Carb counting and eating a nutrient-rich, low-fat, low-protein diet is a vital part of any healthy lifestyle for those with diabetes.

7.13 Only Five Grams Of Glucose In The Blood

The human body holds five quarts (4.7 liters) of blood distributed through 60,000 miles of blood vessels, with a surface area equal to three tennis courts. When the glucose level is 100 mg/dl (5.5 mmol), the entire blood supply contains only five grams of glucose. Compare this to a 12-ounce can of soda which contains 40 grams of glucose, or eight times as much as the entire blood supply!

A healthy but carb-rich breakfast of pancakes or cereal that contains several times the amount of glucose found in the blood can challenge control. Whether you consume 15 or 150 grams of carb, matching basal and bolus doses to this carb intake is critical to maintaining a healthy glucose level.

Diabetes is like a box of chocolates. You never know what reading you're going to get.

June Biermann and Barbara Toohey

The Glycemic Index And Glycemic Load

The glycemic index lists various carbohydrate foods based on how quickly they digest and affect the blood sugar.[69-71] Glucose, the fastest-acting carbohydrate, is given a value of 100, and other carbs are ranked relative to that measurement.

A food's glycemic ranking is compiled from studies in which people eat a set amount of that food and researchers measure how it affects their blood sugar. Ripeness, cooking time, fiber, and fat content can all impact how a food affects the blood sugar, so a glycemic index ranking may vary somewhat in daily use, but its relative ranking is unlikely to change. If you have access to a continuous blood glucose monitor, you can create your own glycemic index through trial and error testing of the foods you eat. Personal testing takes time but pays off well in the years to come.

Fast carbs with higher numbers are good choices for raising low blood sugars, covering moderate or strenuous exercise, and speeding the restoration of glycogen stores following exercise. If your blood sugar is normal before a meal, you might choose to give your bolus earlier for a high GI food or to simply eat less of it. When your blood sugar is low or rapidly dropping due to exercise, you will need the highest glycemic index carbs to quickly raise the blood sugar.

Slow carbs with lower numbers are better choices for maintaining day-to-day control. They minimize unwanted spikes after meals and lessen the drop in blood sugar seen during long periods of activity. If your blood sugar often spikes after breakfast, try changing to a cereal or bread with a lower glycemic index, or reduce its quantity and add another carb with a lower GI. A low glycemic index snack at bedtime can ensure blood sugar stability during the night.

Eating a food with one glycemic index in a meal of foods with other rankings will produce an intermediate effect on your blood sugar. A wise use of carb counting along with the glycemic index has helped many people improve their control.

Glycemic Load

Glycemic load is a way to make the glycemic index practical. A food's glycemic load is its glycemic index times the grams of carbohydrate in a serving. The resulting number provides a way to see how different foods are likely to impact the blood sugar. A smaller portion of a high glycemic index food like hard candy can raise the blood sugar as much as a large portion of a low glycemic index food like popcorn. Portion size and the glycemic ranking of a food must both be considered.

The New Glucose Revolution provides information on glycemic index and glycemic load. The authors are respected dietary experts with 20 years of research regarding blood sugar responses to foods. They have also put together booklets, called the **Glucose Revolution Pocket Guides**, which cover heart disease, diabetes, weight loss, PCOS, and more, and can be found at bookstores or at www.diabetesnet.com/ishop/.

7.14a Glycemic Index

Foods are compared to glucose, which ranks 100. Higher numbers indicate faster absorption and a faster rise in the blood sugar, while lower numbers indicate a slower rise.

Cereals		Snacks		Fruit	
All Bran™	51	chocolate bar	49	apple	38
Bran Buds +psyll	45	corn chips	72	apricots	57
Bran Flakes™	74	croissant	67	banana	56
Cheerios™	74	doughnut	76	cantaloupe	65
Corn Chex™	83	graham crackers	74	cherries	22
Cornflakes™	83	jelly beans	80	dates	103
Cream of Wheat	66	Life Savers™	70	grapefruit	25
Frosted Flakes™	55	oatmeal cookie	57	grapes	46
Grapenuts™	67	pzza, cheese & tom.	60	kiwi	52
Life™	66	Pizza Hut™, supreme	33	mango	55
muesli, natural	54	popcorn, light micro	55	orange	43
Nutri-grain™	66	potato chips	56	papaya	58
oatmeal, old fash	48	pound cake	54	peach	42
Puffed Wheat™	67	Power Bars™	58	pear	58
Raisin Bran™	73	pretzels	83	pineapple	66
Rice Chex™	89	rice cakes	82	plums	39
Rice Krispies™	82	saltine crackers	74	prunes	15
Shredded Wheat™	67	shortbread cookies	64	raisins	64
Special K™	54	Snickers™ bar	41	watermelon	72
Total™	76	strawberry jam	51	**Pasta**	
Root Crops		vanilla wafers	77	cheese tortellini	50
French Fries	75	**Crackers**		fettucini	32
potato, new, boiled	59	graham	74	linguini	50
potato, red, baked	93	rice cakes	80	macaroni	46
potato, sweet	52	rye	68	spaghetti, 5m boil	33
potato, wht, boiled	63	soda	72	spaghetti, 15m boil	44
potato, wht, mash	70	water	78	spaghetti, prot enriched	28
yam	54	Wheat Thins™	67	vermicelli	35

7.14b Glycemic Index - continued

Breads		Beans		Soups/Vegetables	
bagel, plain	72	baked	44	beets, canned	64
banana bread	47	black beans, boil	30	black bean soup	64
baquette, French	95	butter, boiled	33	carrots, fresh, boiled	49
croissant	67	cannellini beans	31	corn, sweet	56
dark rye	76	garbanzo, boiled	34	green pea soup	66
hamburger bun	61	kidney, boiled	29	green pea, frozen	47
muffins		kidney, canned	52	lentil soup	44
apple, cinnamon	44	lentils, gr or br	30	parsnips, boiled	97
blueberry	59	lima, boiled or frozen	32	peas, fresh, boiled	48
oat & raisin	54	navy	38	split pea and ham	66
pita	57	pinto, boiled	39	tomato soup	38
pizza, cheese	60	red lentils, boiled	27	**Cereal Grains**	
pumpernickel	49	soy, boiled	16	barley	25
sourdough	54	**Milk Products**		basmati white rice	58
rye	64	chocolate milk	35	bulgar	48
white	70	custard	43	couscous	65
wheat	68	ice cream, vanilla	60	cornmeal	68
Drinks		ice milk, vanilla	50	millet	71
apple juice	40	skim milk	32	**Sugars**	
colas	65	soy milk	31	fructose	22
Gatorade™	78	tofu frozen dessert	115	honey	62
grapefruit juice	48	whole milk	30	maltose	105
orange juice	46	yogurt, fruit	36	sucrose	61
pineapple juice	46	yogurt, plain	14	table sugar	64

If it's true that we are what we eat, then I am fast, easy and cheap.

Barbara Johnson

Let Records Work For You

8

Changes in diet, activity or schedule can all require a change in insulin doses. These may need to be adjusted for the seasons, with a rise or fall in activity, when weekdays turn into weekends, with a change in level of stress, and as diet selections shift.

How well you match basal rates and boluses to your lifestyle over time determines your control. As life and choices change, you want to compensate to maintain smooth control with a minimum of highs and lows. To track your insulin and lifestyle match so you can adjust when necessary, keep good records.

This chapter reveals

- Benefits of graphing the rise or fall of your glucose
- What to record to maintain control
- Sample charts and analyses

Charting Benefits

Frequent testing leads to better control only if you personally learn from your results. To do this well, you want to keep accurate and detailed records when you go on a pump and at any time your blood sugars go out of control. Recording blood sugars and the other factors that affected them lets you spot patterns and optimize basal and bolus doses. To improve control, frequent testing combined with charting or logging your results is your most effective tool.

Your records provide the critical information you and your medical personnel need to solve problems when your control is not what you want. Charts and records show interactions between your basal rates, boluses, food choices, carb counts, exercise, and blood sugar readings. Good charts and records help reduce glucose variability, improve quality of life, and free yourself from worry about internal damage.

Compared to the longer view of an A1c test or the glucose average on your meter, accurate charting allows you to reduce glucose variability immediately by showing what changes your blood sugar from day to day. Unhealthy glucose patterns can be corrected quickly. When you encounter a high or low reading after a food or lifestyle change, its cause can be immediately identified.

Charting lets you to eat, work and exercise the way you want. Over time, a detailed chart or record reveals whether you are getting where you want to go and whether the changes you make are really helping. Visual learners find graphing blood sugars helpful, while those who are number oriented may find that an enhanced logbook works best. Both approaches are used in this book to guide you to better control.

To test whether your basal rates and boluses are appropriate, you want to record blood sugar results, carb boluses, correction boluses, foods with their total carbs and when they are eaten, times of known and suspected lows, what was eaten to treat lows, extra exercise or activity, and changes in your basal rates.

It helps to keep records before you start on a pump, for several weeks after you start, and whenever control problems reappear so you can quickly determine optimum basal rates and bolus factors. Record books, such as the *Smart Chart* in Figure 8.1, let you build confidence as a new pumper because they are immediately available to review what may have led to a high or low.

Software downloads from your pump and meter can also be helpful in displaying the data in a graphic format. There is no software currently that pulls it all together as well as the *Smart Chart*. However, software has some unique features, such as showing the standard deviation of your blood sugars so you may track and evaluate how much your glucose varies. You can also download your meter numbers to software in a computer or send them over the internet to a central location.

Now more widely available, continuous monitors display your current glucose and its trend over the past few hours. Seeing the trend allows you to take action to prevent many highs and lows. Unfortunately, many continuous monitors do not record other details like carb intake, bolus sizes, or activity. This makes it more difficult to identify what led to the glucose pattern that is seen. At present, nothing beats writing things down as they occur. For self-management to succeed, good written records are vital.

What To Record On A *Smart Chart*

One tried and true rule is that the more information you put on your charts, the easier it is to control your blood sugars. Charting lessens the daily mental strain of trying to remember later what led to a high or low. Keep records handy to enter and review data easily. Mark all high and low readings with symbols or colored markers to highlight unwanted patterns and the effect of various foods, activities, and events on your blood sugar. As soon as a high or low reading occurs, treat it, then look at your chart or record book to review what may have led to it. Write your comments down right away. Look at Sam's Sample chart in Fig. 8.1 for these key items you want to record:

Activity

With an ink pen or felt pen, block in the time and intensity of activity, exercise, or work that is greater than normal in the activity area at the top of the graph. Add a word or two to specify what it was that you did.

8.1 Sam's Sample Smart Chart

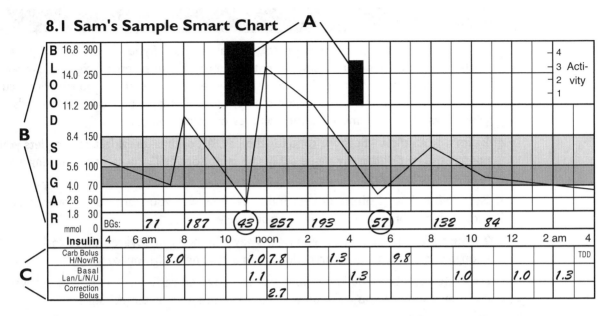

	A												
BGs:	71	187	(43)	257	193	(57)		132	84				
Insulin	4	6 am	8	10	noon	2	4	6	8	10	12	2 am	4
Carb Bolus H/Nov/R		8.0		1.0	7.8	1.3		9.8					TDD
Basal Lan/L/N/U				1.1		1.3			1.0		1.0	1.3	
Correction Bolus					2.7								

Blood Sugar axis: 16.8/300, 14.0/250, 11.2/200, 8.4/150, 5.6/100, 4.0/70, 2.8/50, 1.8/30, mmol 0

Activity: 4, 3, 2, 1

B - Blood Sugar

	Breakfast			**Lunch**			**Dinner**	
Time	Food	Carb Grams	Time	Food	Carb Grams	Time	Food	Carb Grams
7:00	Cheerios	40	1:00	1 c nonfat milk	13	6:00	pasta and clams	64
	1 c nonfat milk	13		tuna sandwich	34		green salad	11
	strawberries	10		apple—154 gms	23		Chardonnay	6
	2 rye toast	30			70		vanilla ice cream	17
	applebutter	8						98
	poached egg	0						
	Morning Snacks	101		Afternoon Snacks			Evening Snacks	
11:00	2 blueberry muffins	70		crackers	12			
	banana	25		cheese	4			
	diet soda	0		glucose tabs	10			
		95			26			

Day: **Saturday** Wt: ___ Comments: *Biked 21 miles in am, ate too much! Noon, blew my*
Date: **03/10/07** *fuse at nursery store clerk? 4 pm - helped Fred load dirt into his trailer.*

© 1994, 2003, 2005, 2006 Diabetes Services, Inc.

A - Activity and exercise   B - Blood glucose readings   C - Insulin doses
D - Foods and carbs   E - Comments

Fill in the grid to rank your activity on a personal 1 to 5 scale. A "1" is used for a mild increase in activity, while a "5" is given to activities that are far more strenuous than usual. For instance, if you usually sit behind a desk but you spend the day moving your files and records to a new office, you would block in an area probably between 2 and 5 during these hours, based on the extra activity this move required.

Testing guides you to good control, but cannot help if you want to please your doctor by getting good numbers. Do not skip a test if you suspect a high or low reading. This is the most valuable time to test. Only testing can turn a problem with a current reading into a better reading on the next test. Testing when low also records when lows occur and improves the accuracy of insulin adjustments.

Before breakfast - Sets the tone for the day. An optimal breakfast reading lets you control the rest of the day more easily. If it is not optimal, you can start making adjustments at breakfast.

Before lunch and dinner - Lets you know how well your carb bolus covered the carbs eaten at breakfast and lunch, respectively.

2 hours after meals - Tells you right away whether you covered those carbs well enough and enables a fast correction when a reading is high or low.

At Bedtime - Lets you know how well you covered carbs at dinner. Helps prevent night lows and lets you wake up with your glucose in your target range.

Occasionally at 2 am - Prevents middle of the night lows, tells you whether your night basal is too high or low, and lets you make adjustments that lead to great breakfast readings.

Before driving and hourly during longer trips - Keeps you safe.

Before, during, and after exercise or activity that last longer than I hour - Maximizes performance and safety. Be sure to check at 2 am that night!

Any time you think you are low or high - Speeds corrections.

Before and after drinking alcohol - More safety and less embarrassment. Again, be sure to check during the night.

After any change in basal rates or bolus doses - Tells you if you need further adjustment. Alerts you to a correction that may lead to lows.

Record insulin doses, blood sugars, food choices, carb counts, and activity in Smart Charts or a comprehensive logbook. Bring your written records and meter to each clinic visit.

If you start a running program and become quite winded as you run, you might mark a 5 on your chart. After you run the same route for a few days, the activity may no longer be as strenuous and would be listed progressively as a 4 and then a 3.

Area A in Figure 8.1 gives an example of how to chart physical activity.

Blood Glucose Readings

Write your blood sugars at the time they happened on the BG (blood glucose) line of the blood sugar section of the *Smart Chart* and graph the readings in the area above to reveal patterns that may require a readjustment of your basal rates and boluses.

8.3 Smart Chart

BLOOD SUGAR																				Activity
16.8 300																				4
14.0 250																				3 Acti-
																				2 vity
11.2 200																				1
8.4 150																				
5.6 100																				
4.0 70																				
2.8 50																				
1.8 30																				
mmol 0 BGs:																				
Insulin	4	6 am	8	10	noon	2	4	6	8	10	12	2 am	4							
Carb Bolus H/Nov/R																				TDD
Basal Lan/L/N/U																				
Correction Bolus																				

Breakfast			Lunch			Dinner		
Time	Food	Carb Grams	Time	Food	Carb Grams	Time	Food	Carb Grams
Morning Snacks			Afternoon Snacks			Evening Snacks		

Day: _____   Wt: ____   Comments: _____

Date: _____

Discuss how often to test your glucose with your physician. You can test and record anytime on a *Smart Chart*. The more testing you do the better you will understand your insulin needs. When you start on a pump or have control problems, four tests a day before meals and at bedtime are the minimum required to adjust basal rates and boluses. Seven or eight tests a day with aftermeal testing gives you more information for a faster return to control. To see how different foods affect your readings, test two hours after meals, with an occasional test at 2 a.m. to prevent night lows.

Always try to test when you believe your blood sugar is low, unless symptoms are so severe that waiting to test would be dangerous. Excitement, fatigue, stress, anxiety, and even a high blood sugar can all mimic the symptoms of a low blood sugar. Testing confirms that what you are experiencing is actually caused by a low glucose.

Record all suspected lows, even if monitoring is not done at that time. Put a mark, such as SL for suspected low, on your chart every time your think you are low but do not test. If you often suspect low blood sugars at work or during the night but do not routinely test when that happens, recording this in detail gives you and your physician a better basis for adjusting your doses. Highlight all verified and suspected lows on your charts with a circle, an arrow, or a specific color. Show the severity of each low blood sugar by the size of the mark. For instance, if symptoms are mild, use a small circle or arrow, while, if severe, use a large one.

> ### 8.4 Causes For Lows
>
> - Too much basal or bolus insulin
> - Delayed or skipped meal for which a bolus was taken
> - Eating fewer carbs than planned
> - Being more active than expected

Never hesitate to show all your highs and lows. If your physician has only an elevated A1c test to judge your control by, he or she may not realize that many of your highs are caused by an excess of insulin that results in frequent lows that are being overtreated but not recorded, or that you are simply forgetting to bolus before meals. Problem solving is hard enough when all the facts are known. Without the facts, it can be impossible.

Area B in Figure 8.1 shows a graphic record of blood sugars with the readings listed below on the BG line. Connect all the dots of blood sugars tests so that the direction of the blood sugar is easy to recognize.

Insulin Doses

The three rows of squares below the graph area near the middle of the *Smart Chart* are used for recording basal and bolus doses. On the top row, record how many carb bolus units you take for each meal and snack. Basal insulin doses can be recorded every few days on the middle row. The third row is for recording correction boluses used to lower high blood sugars. Log your correction boluses separately from carb boluses so you know how much extra insulin you are using each day to correct high readings. Note the exact time each bolus is given by placing a dash or cross-hatch on the time line when that bolus is given.

Area C in Figure 8.1 shows insulin doses and when they are taken.

Foods and Carb Counts

Carb counting measures how much a meal or snack may raise your blood sugar. How to count carbs is covered in Chapter 7. It is easier than you think and is a very important step to good control, especially when using a smart pump. Start by recording the foods you eat and the number of carbs in them, being as specific as you can.

A general word like "cereal" won't do, as all cereals are not equal. Cheerios®, Grape Nuts®, Cornflakes®, and oatmeal affect the blood sugar differently. A sandwich can have a very different effect if it is a whole wheat/tuna/tomato sandwich with 32 carb grams, a white bun/hamburger/tomato sandwich with 45 carb grams, or an ice cream sandwich with 68 grams.

Record all the carbs you eat. If you do not record the four full-sized graham crackers (44 grams) and 16 ounces of milk (24 grams) that you took for a nighttime low, you won't know later why your blood sugar rose to 306 mg/dl (17 mmol) before breakfast. You may also want to record foods that have no carbs because some may affect your blood sugar for reasons other than their carb content.

Area D in Figure 8.1 shows foods eaten, portions, and carb counts.

8.5 Causes For Highs

- Too little basal or bolus insulin
- Eating more carbs than usual
- Being less active than usual
- Emotional or physical stress
- Infection or other illness
- Chronic or severe pain
- Certain medications like prednisone
- Outdated or bad insulin
- Loose or detached infusion set

Comments – Emotion, Stress, Pain, Medication, Etc.

At the bottom of the chart in the Comments section, record other information you feel is relevant to your control. A change in weight, emotions, stress, or illness can impact your glucose and should be noted. Your note might say "Asthma worse – used steroid inhaler," "I woke up with a headache, may have gone low during the night," or "I haven't changed my infusion site for five days."

An unusually high blood sugar before dinner might be explained by a comment like "a lot of stress at work today." Comments allow you and your doctor to identify variables besides diet and insulin that might have caused high or low readings that day.

Area E in Figure 8.1 shows an example of comments.

Sample Charts

The *Smart Charts* on pages 92 and 93 show four days in the life of Sam, our sample pumper. Sam weighs 160 pounds, leads an active lifestyle, and eats 2600 calories a day, with about 880 calories a day (equal to 220 grams of carb) coming from carbs. He uses one unit for every 10 grams of carb. For high blood sugars, he uses 1 unit for every 35 mg/dl (2.5 mmol) above 100 mg/dl (5.5 mmol) to bring down high readings. His premeal target range is 100 mg/dl (5.5 mmol) and his postmeal target range is to stay between 120 and 180 mg/dl (6.6 and 10 mmol) as much as possible.

Find the patterns in Sam's charts by marking all readings below 70 mg/dl (3.9 mmol) with circles and all readings above 130 mg/dl (7.2 mmol) before meals or above 180 mg/dl (10 mmol) between meals with triangles. Can you find reasons for his highs or lows? How might you change his basals or boluses to improve his readings? Write down your suggestions, then look at the short analysis that follows to confirm your thinking.

8.6 Sam's Charts

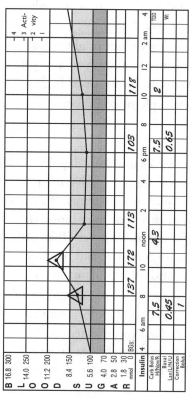

Tuesday

			B	16.8	300
			L	14.0	250
			O	11.2	200
			O		
			D	8.4	150
			S	5.6	100
			U		
			G	4.0	70
			A	2.8	50
			R	1.8	30
			mmol	0	

Insulin	6 am	8	noon	2	4	6 pm	8	10	12	2 am	4	TDD	Wt
BGs:	6.2	201	173			49		148					
Carb Bolus H/N/R			48			90		11					
Basal Lan/L/N/U	0.45					0.65							
Correction Bolus	2		2					1					

Breakfast

Time	Food	Carb Grams
8:00	2 waffles	30
	blueberry	12
	1 cup of milk	9
	Soy latte	11
	1/2 cup yogourt	
		62

Morning Snacks

Lunch

Time	Food	Carb Grams
12:30	lentil & veget. soup. 1 cup	24
	1/2 cup of beets	24
		48

Afternoon Snacks

4:00	apple	20
5:30	Sweet Tarts	16
		84

Dinner

Time	Food	Carb Grams
6:00	2 beef franks	4
	2 buns	48
	salad, greens	
	milk	12
	potato	26
		90

Evening Snacks

| 10:15 | 1/2 cup of ice cream | 26 |

Day: *Tuesday* Wt: \
Date: *05/20/03* \
Comments: *Packed supplies in heavy boxes and moved to another office at work. Made me low at 5:30. Ate Sweet Tarts to bring me up and then ate dinner. High at bedtime, added 1 unit to bring me down.*

© 1994, 2003 Diabetes Services, Inc.

Monday

			B	16.8	300
			L	14.0	250
			O	11.2	200
			O		
			D	8.4	150
			S	5.6	100
			U		
			G	4.0	70
			A	2.8	50
			R	1.8	30
			mmol	0	

Insulin	6 am	8	noon	2	4	6 pm	8	10	12	2 am	4	TDD	Wt
BGs:	137	172	113			103		118					
Carb Bolus H/N/R	7.5		4.3			7.5							
Basal Lan/L/N/U	0.45					0.65							
Correction Bolus	1		2			2							

Breakfast

Time	Food	Carb Grams
8:00	large muffin	36
	6 oz yogourt	30
	Soy latte	9
		75

Morning Snacks

Lunch

Time	Food	Carb Grams
1:00	4 crackers with peanut butter	20
	apple	23
	cheese	43
		75

Afternoon Snacks

| | 1 1/2 graham crackers | 16 |

Dinner

Time	Food	Carb Grams
6:00	roast beef	20
	2 bread	32
	potato	26
	carrots	8
	asparagus	5
	1 cup milk	12
		83

Evening Snacks

| 10:00 | 1/2 cup of ice cream | 26 |
| | | 102 |

Day: *Monday* Wt: \
Date: *05/19/03* \
Comments: *Good Day*

© 1994, 2003 Diabetes Services, Inc.

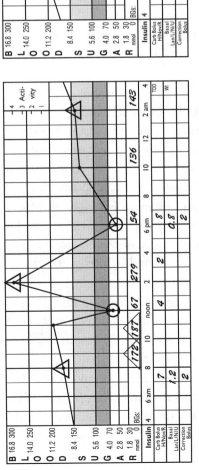

Thursday Chart

Insulin	4	6 am	8	10	noon	2	4	6 pm	8	10	12	2 am	4
B 16.8 300													
L 14.0 250													
O 11.2 200													
O													
D 8.4 150													
S													
U 5.6 100													
G 4.0 70													
A 2.8 50													
R 1.8 30													
mmol 0 BGS:		203		168	71	132		106		136	153		
Carb Bolus H/Nov/R		6			4		1	9		1	2		
Basal Lan/L/N/U		1.2						1.0		0.7			
Correction Bolus		3											

TDD ___ Wt ___
Acti-vity 4 3 2 1

Breakfast — Day: Thursday Wt: Date: 05/22/03

Time	Food	Carb Grams
7:30	Bagel	45
	1/2 cup yogurt	11
	Soy latte	9
		65

Morning Snacks

Lunch

Time	Food	Carb Grams
12:00	cottage cheese	5
	1 cup grapes,	
	blueberries, and	14
	raspberries, and	9
	Eng Muffin	26
		45

Afternoon Snacks

	1 1/2 graham crackers	16
		61

Dinner

Time	Food	Carb Grams
6:00	pizza	62
	6 oz pepperoni	
	1 cup of corn	34
		96

Evening Snacks

10:00	1/2 cup cherry	20
	garcia ice cream	
		20

Comments: High at 10:00 pm. took 2 units to bring it down overnight. got up at 1 am to check

© 1994, 2003 Diabetes Services, Inc.

Wednesday Chart

Insulin	4	6 am	8	10	noon	2	4	6 pm	8	10	12	2 am	4
B 16.8 300													
L 14.0 250													
O 11.2 200													
O													
D 8.4 150													
S													
U 5.6 100													
G 4.0 70													
A 2.8 50													
R 1.8 30													
mmol 0 BGS:		172	187	67	279			54		136		143	
Carb Bolus H/Nov/R		7			4		2	8					
Basal Lan/L/N/U		1.2						0.8					
Correction Bolus		2			2			2					

TDD ___ Wt ___
Acti-vity 4 3 2 1

Breakfast — Day: Wednesday Wt: Date: 05/21/03

Time	Food	Carb Grams
8:00	2 eggs	
	Eng Muffin	26
	Orange Juice	30
	Soy latte	9
	1/2 cup of yogurt	11
		76

Morning Snacks

Lunch

Time	Food	Carb Grams
12:00	salad, greens	2
	2 bread	32
	cheese	1
	milk, 1 cup	12
		47

Afternoon Snacks

	1 1/2 graham crackers	16
		63

Dinner

Time	Food	Carb Grams
6:15	1 cup rice stir fry	46
	veggies	11
	3/4 cup of carrot	1
	green beans, corn	12
	2 breads	32
		89

Evening Snacks

Comments: Tested at 2 am to check overnight blood sugar – about same as bedtime reading. Needed 2 units of Humalog before dinner to bring down a high ("Mary's BD party at work")

© 1994, 2003 Diabetes Services, Inc.

93

Analysis

On Monday, Sam's blood sugar control was fairly good after waking with a slightly high reading. The following day, he had a high reading when he awoke and remained high before lunch. Tuesday afternoon, Sam packed and moved his file boxes and office supplies at work to a new office. Because his blood sugar was high at lunch that day, he did not expect the extra activity to cause him to go low. That afternoon, he did go low after 4 hours of packing and moving boxes to his new office at work. By 5:30 p.m. when he finished, his blood sugar was at 49 mg/dl (2.7 mmol). He treated this low with 20 grams of glucose and waited 20 minutes before driving home.

During his drive, he realized he had not planned the move well by not lowering his lunch bolus nor stopping to eat extra carbs while he was carrying several heavy boxes up a flight of stairs to his new office.

On Wednesday, he awoke high again at 172 mg/dl (9.6 mmol). At 11 a.m., he took the correction bolus recommended by his pump for the blood sugar of 187 mg/dl (10.4 mmol), but his blood sugar rapidly fell to 67 mg/dl (3.7 mmol) just over an hour later. After eating too much for the low, he spiked to 279 mg/dl (15.5) and again took the correction dose his pump recommended, only to fall to 54 mg/dl (3 mmol) before dinner that evening.

From Wednesday night to Thursday morning, his reading rose 60 mg/dl (3.3 mmol) even though he had nothing to eat. Once his blood sugar came down at lunch on Thursday, the rest of the day went well.

Because of the rise in his overnight readings, Sam decided to check his overnight basal rates that night. He covered his dinner carbs so that he had a starting reading of 136 mg/dl (7.6 mmol) at bedtime five and a half hours later. He skipped a bedtime snack so that no rapid insulin would be active while he ran a basal test during sleep. When he awoke at 2 a.m., his blood sugar had remained relatively steady at 153 mg/dl (8.5 mmol), but by breakfast on Friday it had risen to 203 mg/dl (11.3 mmol).

When Sam reviewed his readings and counted his highs and lows at the end of the week, he found his major pattern was the rise in his overnight blood sugar results. Over seven nights, his breakfast reading averaged about 60 mg/dl (3.3 mmol) higher than his bedtime readings, and this was confirmed by the overnight basal test he had done on Thursday night.

For unplanned activity, such as moving boxes in his office on Tuesday, Sam decided it would be a good idea in the future to take time out and check his blood sugar an hour and a half or so into the activity even if high beforehand. He realized also that he needed to test as soon as any excess activity is finished.

Sam also reflected that he had probably made a mistake a couple of weeks earlier when he had again lowered his night basal rates to stop lows that were happening between 11 p.m. and 1 a.m. Looking back over his charts, he decided he would estimate how much insulin he had been getting from his basal rates versus his boluses in the six hours between 5 p.m. and 11 p.m. before the lows typically began. When he did this, he realized he had been getting about twice as much bolus insulin for dinner and evening snacks during this time than from his basal rates at the time.

He had lowered the wrong insulin to get rid of his lows! His carb factor number should have been raised to reduce his dinner boluses. After experiencing the two consecutive lows on Wednesday when he took the correction boluses recommended by his pump, Sam also suspected that his correction factor number was too low, making his correction boluses too large.

Over the weekend, he faxed his records to his doctor's office and got in touch with him on Monday afternoon. His doctor agreed with Sam's conclusion that he was getting too much bolus insulin and too little basal. Over several months, Sam had been tending to lower his basal insulin when he experienced lows and raising his boluses to rein in his highs. Because of his current basal/bolus imbalance, his doctor recommended a major realignment of his doses. His doctor suggested that Sam's carb and correction factors be raised to lower his carb and correction boluses and that his basal rates be raised to reestablish a better basal/bolus balance. Sam's current and new doses are shown in Table 8.7.

8.7 Sam's Old And New Pump Settings	
Old	**New**
Basals	
12 am 0.45	12 am 0.75
2 am 0.55	2 am 0.85
6 am 0.90	3:30 am 1.05
12 pm 0.65	11 am 0.85
9 pm 0.40	9 pm 0.80
Total 15.55	Total 21.55
Carb Factor	
1u /10g	1u/12g
Correction Factor	
1u /35 > 100	1u/45 > 100
TDD	
~41 units	~43 units

Sam's doctor suggested he test his new basal rates in the next couple of days, and then test the new carb and correction factors. He also recommended that Sam use glucose tablets for his lows to raise the blood sugar quickly, but check his BOB to see if more carbs may be needed to offset any remaining bolus on board.

Enhanced Logbook

Some people prefer to chart their readings on *Smart Charts* to visualize patterns, while others prefer an enhanced logbook where they can spot and add up numbers that fall outside their target range. Figure 8.8 shows Sam's *Enhanced Logbook*.

An enhanced logbook has space to record blood sugar results before each meal, one to two hours after each meal, and at bedtime, along with the times they occur, but has only limited space to record food choices and grams of carb eaten, length and type of exercise, and comments about things like stress or illness. Even though space is limited, record foods, especially carbs and the time they are eaten. Note the time and duration of exercise in the margin. Even short notes will help.

8.8 Sam's Sample Enhanced Logbook		Breakfast Before	Breakfast After	Lunch Before	Lunch After	Dinner Before	Dinner After	Night Bedtime	Night 2 a.m.
Sunday 5/18/03 (walk)/run/bike at _7_ am/(pm)	BG	167				181		93	
	Time	9:30				7:00		10:30	
	Carbs	88				66			
	Bolus	8+2				6			
Monday 5/19/03 walk/run/bike at ___ am/pm	BG	137	172	113		103		118	
	Time	8 am	10:30	1:00		6:00		10:00	
	Carbs	75		44		83		26	
	Bolus	7+1		4		7.5		2	
Tuesday 5/20/03 walk/run/bike at ___ am/pm	BG	201		173		49		148	
	Time	8:00		12:00		5:30		10:00	
	Carbs	62		48		90		26	
	Bolus	5.5		4+2				2+1	
Wednesday 5/21/03 walk/run/bike at ___ am/pm	BG	172	187	67	279	54		136	153
	Time	8:00	11:00	12:00		6:00		10:00	2:00 am
	Carbs	76		47	24	89		0	0
	Bolus	7+2		4	2	8+2		night basal test	
Thursday 5/22/03 walk/run/bike at ___ am/pm	BG	203	168	71	132	106		136	153
	Time	7:00	10:00	12:00	4:00	6:00		10:00	1:00 am
	Carbs	65		45	16	96		20	
	Bolus	6+3		4	1	9H+7UL		1+2H	
Friday 5/23/03 (walk)/run/bike at _4_ am/(pm)	BG	203	196	128		87	135	102	
	Time	7:30	10:00	12:30		6:15	8:30	10:30	
	Carbs	55		60		83		20	
	Bolus	5+1	1H	5.5		7+7UL		1H+3L	
Saturday 5/24/03 walk/run/(bike) at _7_ (am)/pm	BG	148		77		111		86	
	Time	8:00		12:30		6:00		10:30	
	Carbs	89		52		80		30	
	Bolus	8+1H		4H		7H+7UL	2H+3L		
# below target				1		2			
# above target		7	3	1	1	1		2	

Targets: before meals: _70_ to _130_ bedtime: _90_ to _140_
after meals: _120_ to _180_ 2 am: _90_ to _140_

Basals: ___ u/hr at 12 am ___ u/hr at ___ am/pm
___ u/hr at ___ am/pm ___ u/hr at ___ am/pm
___ u/hr at ___ am/pm ___ u/hr at ___ am/pm

© 2006 Diabetes Services Inc.

The *Enhanced Logbook* has a section at the bottom that helps you spot blood sugar patterns. At the very bottom, fill in your target blood sugars for different times of day. After you test and record for seven days, circle all the highs above your target range in one color and all the lows below the target range in another color. Total these highs and lows for each time of day and write them down in the pattern section at the bottom of the *Enhanced Logbook*.

Analyzing records for patterns is critical to make decisions that will improve your control. The more analysis you do, the easier and faster it becomes. When a reading falls outside your target range, be sure to write an explanation for it in the margin of your logbook or on the back of the page, using numbers to key each note to the log. Write down anything that might influence your blood sugar, such as extra stress, unusual exercise or activity, high carb meals, or delayed eating. Place notes close to the time it happens or draw a line to the margin where you have more room to write.

When high readings occur at the same time of day on three or more days or low readings occur on two or more days a week, seek reasons for these patterns. Unwanted patterns can often be corrected by adjusting basal rates and carb boluses, but keep in mind all the tools you can use to improve your control. If you are eating too many or too few carbs, engaging in more or less activity, feeling more or less stress, or in the midst of an illness, make the dose or other changes you need.

Summary

As you fill out *Smart Charts* or records, you may not record all the information you need. Recording get easier with practice and charting becomes a small distraction that has a big payoff by preventing lows and lessening the time spent with high blood sugars.

Common patterns will stand out as you flip *Smart Chart* pages back and forth or you review the readings that are above and below your target range in an *Enhanced Logbook* at the end of each week. Patterns that repeat but do not occur every day, such as low-to-high readings, will show up in weekly reviews rather than daily ones. Identify your unwanted patterns, so you can correct them. As your confidence increases you will better manage your diabetes.

Look over your records regularly for patterns. Share them with your physician and health care team. Bring a record of your readings along with your meter and pump to every visit with your physician or health care team to get the best advice possible. Share your records with others and listen to their suggestions. A professional is trained to see things that you may have missed and can be especially helpful. If you are unsure about how to correct an unwanted pattern, be sure to contact your physician or health care team. Use their knowledge and experience to simplify your path toward normal readings and to build on your current understanding and ability to control your own blood sugar.

Once you stabilize your readings through more appropriate basal rates and better-matched boluses, a fully detailed Smart Chart may be more data than you need. At this point, a simple logbook or a regular download of your meter or pump to your PC or to a site on the internet may do. But if your control begins to slip, go back to recording the full data you need in Smart Charts or another system. You want to get back the control you want quickly, and systematic recording enables you to do it.

The map appears more real to us than the land.

D. H. Lawrence

8.9 Enhanced Logbook		Breakfast		Lunch		Dinner		Night	
		Before	After	Before	After	Before	After	Bedtime	2 a.m.
Sunday ___/___/___ walk/run/bike at _____ am/pm	BG								
	Time								
	Carbs								
	Bolus								
Monday ___/___/___ walk/run/bike at _____ am/pm	BG								
	Time								
	Carbs								
	Bolus								
Tuesday ___/___/___ walk/run/bike at _____ am/pm	BG								
	Time								
	Carbs								
	Bolus								
Wednesday ___/___/___ walk/run/bike at _____ am/pm	BG								
	Time								
	Carbs								
	Bolus								
Thursday ___/___/___ walk/run/bike at _____ am/pm	BG								
	Time								
	Carbs								
	Bolus								
Friday ___/___/___ walk/run/bike at _____ am/pm	BG								
	Time								
	Carbs								
	Bolus								
Saturday ___/___/___ walk/run/bike at _____ am/pm	BG								
	Time								
	Carbs								
	Bolus								
# below target									
# above target									

PATTERNS

Targets:
before meals: _____ to _____ bedtime: _____ to _____

after meals: _____ to _____ 2 am: _____ to _____

Basals:
_____ u/hr at 12 am _____ u/hr at _____ am/pm

_____ u/hr at _____ am/pm _____ u/hr at _____ am/pm

_____ u/hr at _____ am/pm _____ u/hr at _____ am/pm

Get Ready And Start

An insulin pump is usually started in an outpatient setting, such as a doctor's office or medical clinic. This approach works well and allows basal rates and boluses to be set and adjusted to match an individual's normal daily routine. Alternatively, some physicians prefer to hospitalize new pumpers for a couple of days to establish pump use and evaluate their pump settings in an environment where professional help is available day and night. Carb counting can also be taught and verified during a hospital stay.

Work with an experienced health care team and pump trainer who can clearly explain how a pump operates and provide information on lifestyle issues, control factors, backup resources, and where to obtain the information or supplies you need.

What this chapter covers

- Pre-start day practice
- Tapering off injections
- Equipment you will need
- Programming the pump and reviewing its memory
- Preparing and filling the reservoir
- Choosing an infusion site, preparing the site and inserting an infusion set
- Monitoring the infusion site
- Follow-up
- Ideas on where to wear your pump
- How to take time off the pump

Get Ready

Your preparation is critical for a successful pump start. When you start, you will put into action all the things you have learned or practiced before that time. Training specific to your pump will be provided by a nurse educator associated with the pump company or by a health professional at your physician's office. Pump training includes ample time for questions, answers, and practice with your pump, usually two to six hours, depending on your familiarity with pumps and how prepared you are.

The things you need to know may seem intimidating at first, like how to insert a battery, the initial programming messages on your pump, filling and inserting the reservoir, attaching and priming the infusion line, inserting your infusion set, and programming your personal settings. Remember that hundreds of thousands of people have gone through these same steps before you over the last quarter century.

Make sure you are prepared for emergencies. Have a glucagon kit for injection and plenty of quick carbs on hand for lows, and have Ketodiastix or ketone testing materials available to monitor ketone levels should your blood sugar go high.

Practice First

A representative from the pump company or a health professional from your physician's office will spent time with you to review how to set up, program, and operate your pump. It helps to familiarize yourself with your pump prior to this training session.

To become comfortable with how to operate your pump, you want to set some basal rates, program pretend boluses, and review the pump's memory. If you do not have access to your pump before you start, most pump companies have online training that you can use. These early training steps lessen nervousness and fumbling when you start but should never be considered enough to start on a pump. Nothing can replace the hands-on training and advice of an experienced diabetes professional.

Table 9.1 lists common steps in pumping that you want to practice before you begin to pump. It helps to practice all these steps before starting. As soon as the pump arrives, take it out of the box, insert a battery, and start practicing. You cannot hurt the pump and becoming familiar with it makes it less likely you will encounter problems when you start.

Training Steps

1. Understand how to operate the buttons on your pump to give boluses, set basals, review history, and activate features like temporary basal rates, carb and correction factors, duration of insulin action, reminders and alerts.

2. Be comfortable with loading the reservoir with insulin and placing it into your pump, attaching and filling the infusion line, inserting and changing the infusion set.

3. Know the routine and non-routine times to test your blood sugar, as well as your personal blood sugar targets.

4. Know who to contact for technical problems and for control problems.

Review Chapters 9–13 in this book, read the user manual that accompanies your pump, and watch the manufacturer's training CD or DVD at least twice with the pump at your side to practice the steps as they are demonstrated. Push all the buttons to get a feel for how they work. Advanced features will take time to understand, so be sure to go back and review any steps that you need to. Ask a family member or friend to watch the video and work the buttons along with you. You want to feel at ease with your pump before you actually start delivering insulin.

9.1 Pump Proficiency Checklist

To sharpen your skills, practice with your pump several times before you start. Complete as many of these preparatory steps as you can. Place a check next to each item when you have mastered it.

Checklist

- [ ] insert a battery
- [ ] set the date and time
- [ ] fill a reservoir with old insulin or water
- [ ] attach an infusion set to the reservoir and prime the infusion line
- [ ] wash your hands and cleanse your skin at an infusion site with IV prep
- [ ] mentally practice inserting an infusion set while holding it comfortably and remove the metal needle (with Teflon sets) after "insertion"
- [ ] suspend and restart the pump a couple of times
- [ ] set a duration of insulin action for 4 to 7 hours

Practice basal and bolus programming by placing these values into your pump:

- [ ] program a target glucose of 120 mg/dl (6.7 mmol) or a target range of 100 mg/dl to 120 mg/dl (5.6 to 6.7 mmol)
- [ ] program start times and basal rates for at least 3 different basals, such as 0.6 u/hr at 12 am, 0.8 u/hr at 3:30 am, and 0.7 u/hr at 10 am. Then change these and program different ones. Check to see what your total daily basal is.
- [ ] program a carb factor or insulin-to-carb ratio of 1 unit for each 20 grams of carb. Give a carb bolus for 40 grams of carb which should equal 2 units. Finalize delivery and check how much BOB or active insulin you have (again should be 2 units).
- [ ] program a correction factor of 1 unit for 80 mg/dl (4.4 mmol) point drop. Give a correction bolus for a reading of 320 mg/dl (17 mmol). The pump subtracts your target of 120 from 320 to give 200 mg/dl (11 mmol) as your desired drop. The correction bolus should be about 0.5 units because you have 2 units on board (BOB).

- [ ] give a carb bolus for 40 grams of carb, plus a correction bolus for a blood sugar of 280 mg/dl (15 mmol). This should equal about 2 units after the pump subtracts the 2 units on board (BOB).
- [ ] set a temporary basal rate at 80% for 4 hours and then cancel it
- [ ] review the pump's history (basal rates, boluses, alarms, and daily insulin totals). These will be blank or show minimal data, but you want to know where the information resides.
- [ ] read through the list of alarms in your pump manual to become familiar with the messages you may encounter on your pump and what to do about them

2006 © Diabetes Services, Inc.

Unanticipated questions and problems often arise during the first week of pump use. If questions or problems arise about use, alerts, or errors arise, each pump manufacturer lists their 24 hour help line on the back of the pump. Call your health provider for control problems or dose questions.

Live as routine a life as possible during the first couple of weeks. Try to consume about the same number of carbs at breakfast, lunch, and dinner. As much as possible, exercise and sleep at your regular times.

When To Stop Your Long-Acting Insulin

Injections have to be stopped at some point before you start. A pump makes it easy to adjust the basal rates as the activity of your long-acting insulin tapers off. An easy scenario would be if Lantus is taken once a day in the morning. The last dose of Lantus would be taken the morning before the start day. Only short-acting insulin is used on the morning of the pump start to cover carbs and correct any high blood sugars that occur until insulin begins to be delivered by your pump.

If Lantus, Levemir, or NPH is taken at bedtime, skip it the night before the pump start. Wake up in the middle of the night to take short-acting insulin to cover the next four hours since no Lantus is working, plus what may be needed to correct a high reading. Alternatively, you can take Lantus that night and when you start on your pump the next day, use a temporary basal reduction to accommodate the action of the Lantus insulin that will not be gone until about bedtime that night.

Lantus will be gone about 24 to 30 hours after the last injection, while NPH will disappear 18 to 24 hours after the last injection. Often there is some long-acting insulin still active when you go on your pump. If so, a temporary basal reduction can be used to offset this residual insulin until it is gone. Table 9.2 shows options for stopping various injections prior to a pump start.

9.2 When To Stop Long-Acting Insulin For A Pump Start

Regular Day				Day Before				Start Day			
B	L	D	B	B	L	D	B	B	L	D	B
✓				✓			X[2]	X[1]			
✓		✓		✓		✓		X[1]		X	
✓			✓	✓			X[2]				X

✓ = take   X = skip

1. Temporary basal reduction may be needed until long-acting insulin is gone.
2. Supplemental correction boluses may be needed to offset loss of long-acting background insulin.

102

Start Day

Bring Everything You Need

Wear comfortable 2-piece clothing and confirm that you have these to bring:

• Meter, test strips, lancets and lancing device, or these plus a continuous monitor

• Recent blood sugars on charts or logbook, or a download of your meter readings

• A new bottle of rapid insulin – Novolog® (aspart), Humalog® (lispro), or Apidra® (glulisine).

• At least 3 reservoirs/cartridges

• At least 3 infusion sets (See Fig. 6.2.)

• A skin disinfectant, such as IV Prep® or Hibiclens® pads to kill bacteria on the skin at the infusion site

• Adhesive dressings, such as Opsite® IV 3000, Tegaderm™ HP, Polyskin™ II, or DuoDerm®

• A roll of 1" tape, such as 3M Micropore™ or Smith and Nephew Hypafix™

• Treatment for a low blood sugar, such as glucose tablets, candy, raisins, fruit juice

Program The Pump

Your physician will help you determine and program the pump doses you need to start: TDD, basal rates, carb factor, correction factor, duration of insulin action, and target blood sugar readings for different times of the day. These initial settings are tested and adjusted over the

9.3 Clever Pump Tricks
Avoid Champagne When cold insulin is used to fill a reservoir, small champagne bubbles often appear as the insulin gradually reaches room temperature. Avoid harmless champagne bubbles by filling your reservoir from an insulin bottle kept at room temperature. If you are passionate about New Year's eve celebrations, you can revert back to a bottle of cold insulin for the occasion.

first few days and weeks of use. Basal rates are always tested first. Carb and correction boluses can be tested once the basal rates have been set so they keep your blood sugar level when you fast.

Learn to program basal rates and boluses, clear alarms, and review your history of blood sugars and insulin use. After you start, your physician needs this information from your pump and meter during clinic visits or phone calls to evaluate your basal rates, carb factor, and correction factor. Keep written records with the information you need in one place so you and your physician will be on the same page regarding your treatment needs. As you learn more, this information will help you test the accuracy of your basal rates and bolus factors so you can adjust them appropriately.

Fill And Load The Reservoir And Prime The Infusion Line

1. Relubricate the O-rings in your reservoir as described in Textbox 9.3.

2. Insert an amount of air from the reservoir into the insulin bottle equal to the insulin you will withdraw.

3. Turn the insulin bottle upside down and fill the reservoir with insulin by pulling the plunger back slowly. Remove air bubbles by tapping them loose and working them out of the reservoir into the insulin bottle.

4. Insert the reservoir into the pump, following the procedure in your pump manual or CD. Firmly tighten the connection between the infusion line and the reservoir and then prime the infusion line by filling it with insulin.

9.4 Prepare The O-rings

Plastic pump reservoirs are precoated with a lubricant that provides a tight seal between the two O-rings and the barrel of the reservoir. When a reservoir sits in storage, however, the lubricant may pool at the bottom of the reservoir. This increases the chance of insulin leaking out the back of the reservoir past "dry" O-rings. Even a small leak between the O-rings can cause a rapid loss of control. Replace the reservoir with another one if liquid, mist or bubbles are noted between the O-rings. The picture to the right shows such a leak.

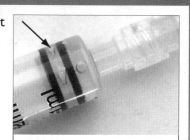

An insulin leak like this can cause unexpected highs.

To avoid O-ring leaks, recoat the reservoir wall with lubricant prior to use by freeing the plunger and pushing it completely into the barrel. Rotate the plunger a couple of times to recoat the O-rings; then carefully pull it back and forth two or three times in the reservoir to recoat the barrel. This redistributes the lubricant onto the O-rings and reservoir wall and helps prevent insulin from leaking out past the O-rings.

Select An Infusion Site

1. Anywhere you can "pinch an inch" can be used to insert the needle of an infusion set. Pinchable areas in the abdomen extend from just below the rib cage to just above the pubic area on both sides of the navel. The upper buttocks, thighs, and biceps also can be used, as shown in Fig. 9.4. The buttock area often works best for young children because it is a large skin area and out of sight.

2. Stay at least two finger widths away from the navel for good absorption, and above or below the belt line to avoid pressure on the set if you wear a belt.

3. For infusion sets that go straight in, different needle lengths may work better in different areas, depending on the depth of the fat pad, such as a 6 or 8 mm set for the thighs and a 10 mm set for the abdomen.

4. Change the location of infusion sites every 2 to 3 days to prevent infection, damage to the skin, scarring below the skin, and fat buildup from excessive use of one area.

5. Rotate areas, such as right upper quadrant of the abdomen to right lower quadrant to left lower quadrant to left upper quadrant. Sites may also be rotated in small steps, such as moving each new site about 2 inches from the last one. To remember to change your infusion site, put only enough insulin in the reservoir to last until the next site change. Today's smart pumps also have reminders that you can set to alert you when it is time to change a site.

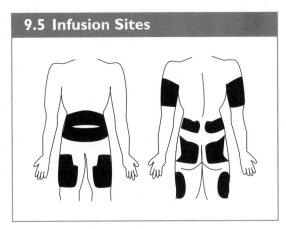

9.5 Infusion Sites

Prepare The Infusion Site

Bacteria are found on the hands, the breath, the skin, counter tops, clothing, and on everything you touch. If you have had even a small skin infection in the past or a history of inflammation and redness around cuts or wounds to the skin, you may be a carrier for one of the most dangerous bacteria, called staph aureus. Over 20% of people carry staph on their body at all times and another 25% intermittently carry it. People with diabetes are more likely to be a carrier. Those who carry staph have a higher risk for infection at infusion sites.

Staph may be carried in the nasal cavity or on the skin, especially in the armpits and between the legs or buttocks. Staph levels can be reduced using a combination of an antibiotic cream applied inside the nose and use of an antiseptic cleanser on the skin. All pumpers should routinely use sterile technique when setting up an infusion site. Staph carriers should attempt to minimize as much staph as possible on a regular basis. This prevents an infection or abscess and avoids unnecessary use of oral antibiotics, surgical drainage, or hospitalization.

9.6 Practice Sterile Technique

When you change an infusion site:

1. Wash your hands well.

2. Do not breathe or blow on your equipment or infusion site.

3. Do not touch your face or nose.

4. Eliminate bacteria from the skin with IV Prep®, Hibiclens®, or Betadine® prior to inserting the infusion set.

5. Place a bio-occlusive material like Opsite® IV 3000 onto the sterilized skin, then place the infusion set through it.

1. Reduce the bacteria count on your hands by washing them thoroughly with soap and water. Do not touch the reservoir needle, the open end of the reservoir, the end of the infusion set that goes through the skin, or the top of the insulin bottle.

2. For close viewing, hold your reservoir or infusion set at eye level above your nose. Many germs reside in the nose and breath, so do not breathe or blow directly on the pump, the reservoir, the infusion set or the infusion site.

105

3. An alcohol pad is not strong enough to cleanse the skin. Scrub the skin with an antiseptic product. IV Prep® wipes or Betadine™ pads are convenient, or you can use bottled products such as Betadine® Solution (iodine) or Hibiclens® (chlorhexidine). Start at the center and rotate the pad or swab in a circular fashion away from the center and do not go back. A cleansed area about three inches in diameter is needed.

4. Place a bio-occlusive adhesive like Opsite® IV 3000 over the site as soon as it dries. This prevents bacteria from gaining access to the skin around the infusion site. Most adhesive materials are not bio-occlusive.

5. Skin Prep™ often helps those who have tape allergies.

6. To keep insertion sets tightly attached with perspiration, use Mastisol®/Detachol®, Skin Tac H®, Applicare's Compound Benzoin Swabstick™, Drysol®, or an odorless antiperspirant (not a deodorant) spray. For excessive perspiration, put IV Prep down and while it is wet, stick the set over it. If this doesn't work, try using a fragrance-free antiperspirant spray. Use IV Prep on the skin first and while it is still wet, spray the antiperspirant on and put the set through. IV Prep may get "gummy" and lose its adhesion when it gets wet. Another remedy for sweating or swimming to keep your infusion set in place is Mastisol®. Try using it to adhere the set to the skin. For removal, Mastisol can be cleaned from the skin with a cleaner called Detachol®.

Insert The Infusion Set

1. Insert the infusion set through the Opsite® IV3000 adhesive and skin by hand or with an inserter. Have a qualified instructor demonstrate how to insert your set properly.

2. With Teflon sets, the metal needle used to insert the Teflon is pulled out gently and the empty space left behind by the needle removal is filled with a small bolus of insulin. Find out the size of the bolus you need to fill this space, usually 0.3 to 0.8 units, from your pump instructor or product insert.

3. After the infusion set is inserted and secured, place a piece of 1" Micropore or

9.7 Reduce Insertion Pain

Some people feel pain or discomfort when inserting needles or catheters. Luckily, there are ways to numb the skin to make needle insertion more comfortable. Numby Stuff® and LMX™ 4 cream can be used to reduce sensation, or Emla cream, a prescription numbing cream, can be applied to the skin about an hour before inserting the infusion set.

A handy solution for children and adults with a needle phobia is to place an ice cube or cold spoon on the site before insertion to trick the nerve endings into feeling cold instead of pain.

Many people find these aids unnecessary after the first few weeks or months of pump use. Keep in mind that if one infusion set seems to cause pain, there are many other types that can be tried. Automatic inserters also make it easier for many people to put an infusion set in place.

Showers and bathing

Detachable infusion sets allow the infusion line to be disconnected from the set so that the pump can be put aside temporarily. Be sure to reattach within 30-45 minutes after a bath or shower. Leave the pump in run mode to reduce the chance of having a clog and so that you do not forget to restart it.

Sleeping

Place the pump free on the bed, under a pillow, in a soft bag hanging from a neck ribbon, in a pajama pocket, or clamped to shorts or a soft belt. A wide variety of pump accessories are available that make wearing a pump at night a pleasurable experience.

Sex

If you and your partner are comfortable with the pump, put it in one of the above locations and let it take care of itself. Women may want to attach the pump to a garter belt by using the pump's belt clip. With detachable infusion sets, it is easy to detach from the pump for up to 45 minutes. Staying detached longer may cause the blood sugar to rise. Be sure to reattach your pump before falling asleep.

Hot Tubs and Saunas

High heat can make proteins like insulin lose potency. If a pump or infusion line becomes exposed to the heat in a sauna or hot tub, it can turn an enjoyable experience into high blood sugars or ketoacidosis. Disconnect your pump at the infusion set before entering a sauna, hot tub or hot shower. A hot tub or sauna may also mobilize insulin more quickly from the infusion site. Always test your blood sugar carefully after a hot tub or sauna to avoid having a severe low blood sugar or an unexpected high.

Durapore tape over the infusion line a couple of inches away from the site to keep the infusion set from being pulled out if the pump is dropped or the infusion line gets tugged. For added protection, make a loop of infusion line and tape this down.

Monitor The Site

1. Infusion site failure is a common cause of unexplained highs. Check your site regularly for irritation, redness, swelling or bleeding. Change the infusion set immediately if there is a problem at the site or any question about insulin delivery.

2. If your glucose is high twice in a row for no obvious reason, give a correction dose by injection and change your infusion set and rotate to a new site right away.

3. Test the blood sugar within two hours of changing your set. Monitor regularly over the next few hours to ensure that the new infusion set is working.

4. There is no perfect infusion set for everyone. If you experience unexplained highs that seem to disappear after the set is changed, consider trying a different insulin set.

Follow-up

After you go on a pump, close follow-up by health care professionals is essential for success. A followup visit in the first week and another one or two in the first month are the minimum needed to adjust basals and boluses appropriately. It is often not obvious to the pumper that a change is needed, so do not cancel appointments if things seen to be going well! To sort things out quickly, communicate clearly and tell your health provider about any problems you are having and why you think they may be occurring.

Bring your records or *Smart Charts* to every clinic visit. You can also use software at home to download information from your meter and pump to show trends and patterns. Your physician needs this to quickly evaluate blood sugar patterns and pump problems. Be sure to document all hypoglycemia and hyperglycemia, and tell your doctor what you did to treat them.

Give quick and concise information on carb and correction boluses, blood sugars, timing of the tests, carb intake, and activity. If you are in the office, be prepared to show your infusion site and review your pattern of site rotation. Point out any skin problems. Don't wait for the health professional to ask.

Bring a pen and note pad. Write down any recommendations you are given, new basal profiles, carb and correction factors, dates of follow-up appointments, what you

---

9.9 Follow-Up Contract After A Pump Start

After starting on a pump, know what your blood sugar targets are, who to contact if problems with the pump or blood sugar control occur, and when to call for help.

My target range is:

_____ to _____ mg/dl (mmol) before meals

_____ to _____ mg/dl (mmol) after meals.

_____ to _____ mg/dl (mmol) at bedtime.

I agree to call _____ at (____)_____ or (____)_____ if I have:

☐ more than _____ low blood sugars below _____ mg/dl (mmol) in any ____ day period.

☐ any low blood sugar below _____ mg/dl (mmol)

☐ more than _____ high blood sugar above _____ mg/dl in any ____ day period

_____   _____
Your signature   Your doctor's signature

On one of the first mornings after starting on her pump, Gwenn's breakfast reading was 87 mg/dl (4.8 mmol) and she was thrilled that her blood sugars were finally within her target range on waking. She thought her pump settings were perfect. Her doctor, however, disagreed. Although Gwenn's blood sugar was 87 mg/dl (4.8 mmol) at breakfast, her earlier reading at 2 a.m. had been 181 mg/dl (10 mmol). Even though she had not taken a correction bolus at the time, her blood sugar dropped more than 90 mg/dl (5 mmol) by dawn. Imagine if Gwenn's reading had been 90 mg/dl in the middle of the night!

Her physician pointed out this excessive drop during the night and emphasized the basal's role in keeping her blood sugar flat. Gwenn agreed with her physician that an immediate reduction in her nighttime basal rate would be wise.

need at the next visit, and who to contact for various information. Know the particular high and low test results that you should report by phone to your doctor or nurse. Fill out Box 9.9 with your physician's help for when to seek medical help after your pump start. Keep all follow-up appointments even if you feel you are doing well. If you do not have glucagon and ketone testing materials on hand, ask your physician for a prescription for these. Be sure that those around you know how and when to administer glucagon.

Backup Resources

When you first start on a pump, you want 24-hour telephone access to your physician or health care team and to your insulin pump manufacturer (24-hour phone contact is on the back of each pump.) to deal with any unanticipated problems. Know who to call and which red flag situations, such as extremely high or low blood sugars, site problems (itching, infection), and emergencies require a call. Do not hesitate to call if you have problems. The earlier a problem can be resolved, the better.

For Follow-up, Know:

- Who to contact if problems with the pump or blood sugar control occur
- When to call for help

Follow up technical problems (alarms, unclear messages, etc.) with the pump company. Have your pump handy when you call.

Insulin Adjustments Are Often Needed Shortly After A Pump Start

As you and your doctor work out better ways to deliver insulin from your pump, your blood sugar may at first seem to be more stable than it was on injections. If your prior readings were mostly high or frequently went up and down, an excess release of stress hormones makes you less sensitive to insulin. When control suddenly improves on a pump, insulin starts to work better. New pumpers also often improve their diet when they start on a pump and this results in more effective insulin use.

Be careful! A sudden improvement in your control over 2 or 3 days may increase your insulin sensitivity. If lows suddenly begin, a further reduction in your basals and boluses will be needed. Do NOT get discouraged if low begin when you start. Realize you need to stop them but that an additional reduction in your basals or boluses will take care of this. Lower them, paying attention to your basal/bolus balance, if you are confident and comfortable doing this, or call your doctor right away.

Keep glucose tablets handy and know how many carbs you may need to treat a low. Do not panic or stop your pump because of lows. Instead, be prepared to reduce your basal rates and raise your carb factor number to lower carb boluses.

If you have been experiencing frequent lows or have little obvious pattern to your readings prior to your pump start, your physician may opt to be conservative about your starting basal and boluses doses. Here, instead of having improved control after starting on a pump, you may find you are experiencing frequent high readings. Again, do not become discouraged about your pump. It is not at fault and a series of gradual increase in your doses will improve your control.

Your starting basal rates and boluses will likely need to be changed at least once or twice during the first couple of weeks. Under most circumstances, a small change will be needed and then wait a couple of days to see if you are stable at that level.

Your goal is to stay between 70 and 120 mg/dl (3.9 and 6.7 mmol) before meals and between 140 and 180 mg/dl (7.8 and 10 mmol) after meals at least 75% of the time. Your target range may differ according to the values you and your health provider agree on. Set realistic goals, pace yourself, and celebrate small steps as you move toward a good match between goals and your new self-management routine.

For the best control, check your blood sugar at least 7 times a day and anytime you may be going low or high. Use a continuous monitoring device if you have access to one. As your physician and health care team give you more responsibility in adjusting your basals and boluses, make these adjustments gradually after adequate testing to meet the goals they recommend.

Tips On Pumping

Test Often: For the quickest path to optimum readings when starting on a pump, check your blood sugar at least 7 times a day or use a continuous monitoring device if possible. As your physician and health care team give you more responsibility in adjusting your basals and boluses, make adjustments only after adequate testing. Adjust your doses gradually to the level recommended by your physician and health care team.

Lows: Your symptoms of a low blood sugar may be less noticeable because of the more gradual drop often experienced on a pump. Monitor frequently to catch any drop in blood sugar before it becomes serious.

9.11 Going Off Your Pump

Situations like water skiing, river rafting, or pump failure may necessitate going off a pump for various lengths of time. These suggestions help maintain control when going off a pump for various lengths of time. Less insulin than the amounts below may be needed if you will be more active. Carefully discuss how to do this with your physician.

Time off pump:	Try this:
Less than 1 hour	Nothing if BG is OK. Bolus or inject rapid insulin before detaching if your BG is already high or carbs will be eaten.
1 to 5 hours	Cover 80% of the basal during your time off the pump with a bolus prior to disconnecting or an injection of rapid insulin. Cover carbs eaten during your time off the pump by reconnecting and bolusing or with an injection.
More than 5 hours or overnight	Use a bolus before disconnecting or an injection of rapid insulin to cover meal carbs plus the next 4 hours of basal insulin. Every 4 to 5 hours, replace the basal insulin with an injection of rapid insulin and cover any meal carbs as needed. For overnight basal coverage, an alternative to injecting rapid insulin every 4 to 5 hours is to take NPH equal to the next 12 hours of basal insulin at bedtime.
Longer than a day	Determine your average TDD from your pump history. Give 1/2 of the average TDD in one or two injections of Lantus per day. Use injections of rapid insulin as needed to cover carb and correction doses.

Check Your Eyes: If you have existing eye damage from diabetes, arrange regular follow-up after you go on a pump with your ophthalmologist. When control is rapidly improved, existing retinopathy can worsen due to a rise in VEGF levels. This will improve after about a year, but your ophthalmologist will need to check for any unexpected eye changes during the transition period.

Change Sites In The Morning: Change your reservoir and infusion set in the morning whenever possible. This ensures that any problem that may occur after a set change will be detected with normal daytime blood sugar tests, rather than worsening over several hours during sleep. If you change an infusion set near bedtime, set a timer to wake you four hours later and check your blood sugar to verify it is working.

Disconnect From Your Infusion Site: Always remove your infusion set or detach your infusion line before attempting to free a clogged infusion line, remove your reservoir from your pump, or prime the infusion line to avoid accidentally infusing yourself with a large dose of insulin.

People are very creative in where they wear their pumps and use a range of clothing, cases and carriers, including backpacks for kids, sleep and sports clothing with specially designed pockets, cases strapped around the waist, thigh, or calf, and pouches attached to a bra or garter belt. Pumpers wear their pumps from head to foot! This list is compiled from a larger one by Barb Chafe of Insulin Pumpers Canada™ with input from pumpers all over the world!

• Upside down to keep bubbles out of the tubing

• On the inside of your clothing with only the pump clip showing

• Clipped on bathrobes

• In bicycle shorts that are then worn under pants, skirts and dress

• In a regular or sports bra in the front middle

• Clipped onto the back of a bra

• Clipped onto a bra under the arm

• In a little baby sock against the skin to prevent sweating

• Clipped onto a garter belt clipped to underwear

• In a garter

• In a pocket sewn inside a bathing suit

• In a leather gun holster

• Clipped to your belt - front or back

• Clipped to your waistband - front or back

• Slipped in a pocket with a hole in the backside of the pocket to hide the tubing

• Inside pump cases like the Waist-It, Round About, Thigh Thing, Clip-N-Go, Tag-A-Long, or Leg Thing

• In a vest with pockets for electronic gadgets

• In little pockets sewn on the inside of favorite jammies or on clothing

• In matching pockets sewn on the outside of clothing so that the pump is easily accessible with the tubing threaded through the back of the pocket.

• Slipped under a pillow at night

• Pinned or clipped to bedsheets

• Strapped to the headboard of the bed

• Carried in a fanny pack

• On a backpack strap

• Strapped on the arm with the tubing neatly wrapped up and out of the way   Continued on next page

9.12b Where To Wear Your Pump - continued

• Velcroed or baby pinned in homemade products

• In Calvin Klein body slimmers under other clothing

• In the pocket of tennis shorts worn under other clothing

• Hanging from a collar

• Hanging in a pouch attached to a strap around the neck (useful when trying on clothes at a store)

• In your boot

• Slipped into the top of a sock with the tubing running down the leg

• Hanging inside or outside of anything from a carabiner (mountain-climbing clip) in combination with a key ring and case

• Strapped to a thigh or calf with elastobandage

• In a Sports Pak

• In a Frio pump wallet for extreme cold or heat

• In a cell phone case

• In a change purse

• In a shelf bra sewn into the top of a camisole

• In Tubi-Grip, a stretchy wrap that can be put around an arm or leg (available at home health stores)

• Clipped to panties or briefs

• In a money belt

• Hanging from your ear, don't know why, but someone has done it

Beware Of Highs: A high blood sugar may be your first sign that your pump has stopped delivering insulin. When a high is unexpected, there may be a problem with the infusion site or pump. If basal and bolus delivery has become disrupted, the situation can become serious quickly. If your blood sugar is above 300 mg/dl (16.6 mmol) once or above 250 mg/dl (13.9 mmol) for two tests in a row without a clear reason, check for the presence of ketones and take an injection to lower your blood sugar. Keep in mind that your correction doses in this situation will need to be larger than normal because little or no basal is being delivered and ketones create resistance to insulin. Replace the pump reservoir and infusion set, using a fresh bottle of insulin if available. Check your blood sugar in two hours to ensure you have solved the problem. If your blood sugar remains high, call your physician for advice.

Recognize Ketoacidosis Quickly: When insulin flow is interrupted by a leak, clog, displaced infusion set, or removal of the pump, ketones may start rising in the blood within 5 hours.

If an infusion set becomes displaced near bedtime, the rise in the blood sugar will not be detected for several hours. If the person wakes up in the morning and does not recognize the cause of their high reading, they may further delay treatment if they go to work or school without the supplies they need to correct the problem. If a blood sugar is very high at bedtime but the tiredness it creates stop you from testing before you go to sleep. Giving a bolus will have no effect if there is a delivery problem. Always test when tired and inject insulin by pen or syringe to lower any unexplained high blood sugar.

Never go to sleep when a high blood sugar may be the cause for your tiredness. Test your blood sugar and ketones and take an injection to lower the blood sugar if ketones are present. If moderate or large amounts of ketones are present, more insulin than normal will be needed to lower the blood sugar. Change your reservoir and infusion site and set an alarm to awaken you in two hours to monitor your progress.

Get Regular A1c Tests: Your A1c level every three to six months to evaluate your overall control. The A1c test provides an average of the last several weeks' blood sugar readings. It reflects your blood sugar control over the last four to six weeks and provides good guidance about your need to increase (or occasionally to decrease) overall insulin use.

Check Your Clock: Especially if you use more than one basal rate a day, be sure your pump's time is set correctly. Basal rate changes depend on having the correct time, and like having the correct date and time in your meter, the value of your data depends on having the correct time. Just think if your physician's download or review shows lots of high readings at 9 a.m. when they actually happen at 9 p.m. or 1 a.m.! Periodically check your pump clock to ensure it stays timely.

A pump is only as good as the technique and knowledge of the person using it. Learn all you can and practice until your technique is excellent.

If you can't change your fate, change your attitude.

Amy Tan

9.13 Control Numbers You Want To Know

You and your doctor will set and test these numbers to ensure optimum control on your pump. Record your current numbers for a convenient record.

1. **My TDD:** My total daily insulin dose = _____ units

2. **My basal rates:**

   _____ am/pm _____ u/h   _____ am/pm _____ u/h

   _____ am/pm _____ u/h   _____ am/pm _____ u/h

   _____ am/pm _____ u/h   _____ am/pm _____ u/h

   My total basal = _____ units a day   My basal makes up _____ % of my TDD.

3. **My carb factor:** 1 unit of insulin covers _____ grams of carb.

4. **My correction factor:** 1 unit of insulin drops my BG _____ mg/dl (or mmol)

   My correction boluses make up _____ % of my TDD.

5. **My carb equivalent:** 1 gram of carb raises my BG ____ mg/dl (or mmol)

6. **My duration of insulin action:**
   A smart pump shows how much BOB (Bolus on Board) is still left to work. This calculation depends on an accurate action time for your insulin.

   My duration of insulin action = ____ hrs ____ min

7. **My target ranges**

   _____ before meals   _____ after meals   _____ bedtime

Nine tenths of wisdom is being wise in time.

Theodore Roosevelt

Overview For Finding Your Best Doses

The next four chapters show how to set up basal and bolus doses when first starting on a pump or when you have a major control problem and want a fresh start. As shown below, the TDD is found first. From this, the starting basal rates and carb and correction factors are determined. These starting values are then tested and readjusted until they keep your blood sugar in the range you want.

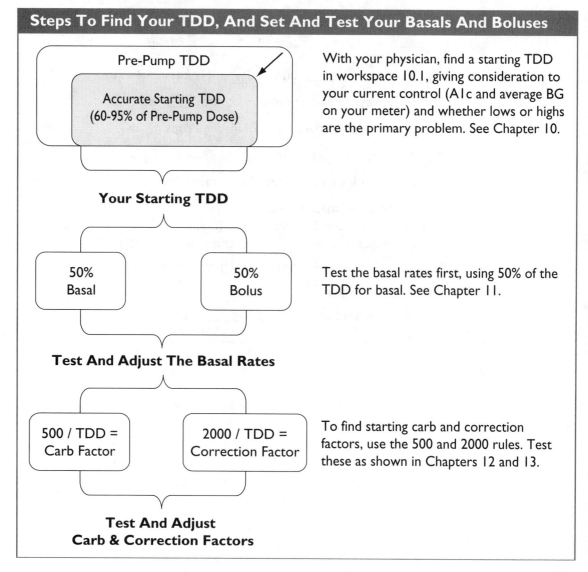

Steps To Find Your TDD, And Set And Test Your Basals And Boluses

Pre-Pump TDD

Accurate Starting TDD
(60-95% of Pre-Pump Dose)

With your physician, find a starting TDD in workspace 10.1, giving consideration to your current control (A1c and average BG on your meter) and whether lows or highs are the primary problem. See Chapter 10.

Your Starting TDD

50%
Basal

50%
Bolus

Test the basal rates first, using 50% of the TDD for basal. See Chapter 11.

Test And Adjust The Basal Rates

500 / TDD =
Carb Factor

2000 / TDD =
Correction Factor

To find starting carb and correction factors, use the 500 and 2000 rules. Test these as shown in Chapters 12 and 13.

**Test And Adjust
Carb & Correction Factors**

Find Your Starting TDD, Basals And Boluses

For New Pump Start Or Major Control Problem

Your TDD or total daily dose of insulin on injections usually needs to be reduced when you start on a pump. To find a starting TDD, your current TDD on injections is determined and compared to a TDD for someone of your weight who has a normal sensitivity to insulin. Averaging these two values and taking into consideration your current control provides a safe starting TDD. From this new TDD, you can closely estimate your starting basals and boluses.

You may want to consider calculating a new TDD if you begin to have major control problems after wearing your pump for awhile. Here, a fresh TDD can be estimated from the current average TDD on your pump and your current control.

In this chapter, you will learn

- How to determine a starting TDD for switching from injections to a pump

- How to determine a new TDD to fix major control problems on a pump

- Based on your TDD, how to determine starting basals and boluses

Be patient and persistent when you make the changes you need to improve your control. Optimum readings do not occur automatically just because you are on a pump. Like a computer, a pump becomes a valuable tool once it is properly programmed and understood. The steps required to improve your control are outlined in this chapter and the next three chapters, as well as in the Optimal Control Checklist on pages 12 and 13. Read or skim this information before you begin taking the steps to find your own optimum doses.

Will Your TDD Change When You Start On A Pump?

For those with Type 1 diabetes, a reduction of 5 to 12 units a day in the TDD is usually required. In contrast, with Type 2 diabetes the TDD sometimes has to be cut as much as 50 percent within the first few days of pump use.[59,60] Your physician will help you find a starting TDD based on your current TDD, your weight, and your level of control. Consideration is given to recent A1c results, the average blood glucose on your meter, and the frequency and severity of low blood sugars. The starting TDD is usually 5% to 25% lower than the total used for injections, but this also depends on how well your current injected doses control your blood sugar.

If on injections you require larger insulin doses than those typically given for someone of your weight, a larger reduction in your TDD may be needed as you start on a pump. A growing teen with high levels of growth hormone or an adult with Type 2 diabetes and significant insulin resistance may find that a TDD of 90 units a day on injections needs to drop rapidly to 50 or 60 units a day once they start on a pump.

Not everyone needs to lower their TDD. Someone in excellent control on MDI may find their total insulin requirement remains the same or drops only slightly. Someone whose readings are consistently above 200 mg/dl (11.1 mmol) on injections, may need the same or a higher TDD on a pump to improve control.

Find Your Starting TDD

For A New Pump Start

Workspace 10.1 is one of one of the most important parts of this book. Though it may at first appear complicated, it provides a clear way to estimate an accurate starting TDD. One TDD is determined from your weight in Box A and a second TDD from your actual insulin doses in Box B. These values are then used in Box C to find a starting TDD. There is no foolproof way to select a perfect starting TDD, so the guidelines in this chapter cannot be exact. For safety, monitor at least 6 to 8 times a day after your start and use phone or email access to your health care team until you determine your correct TDD, basals, and boluses.

Use your current weight (Not the weight listed on your driver's licence!) in Box A of Workspace 10.1 to estimate a TDD for someone of your weight who is moderately active and has an average sensitivity to insulin. Next, enter your typical average doses, including correction doses, that you give at each time of day into Box B, then add them up to find your current average TDD on injections.

Once an ideal TDD for someone of your weight and your current TDD are found in Box A and B, an estimated TDD is derived in Box C. Usually A will be greater than B. If A is greater than B, A and B are added together and multiplied by 0.45 on the left side of Box C to obtain 90% of the average of the two. This provides a safe starting TDD. However, if your current TDD (current injected doses) in Box A is less than that based on your weight in Box B, a safer estimate is derived on the right side of Box C by using 90% of your current TDD on injections. This ensures extra protection against lows for those who are sensitive to insulin.

Some modification of the TDD found in C may be needed. For instance, if A is less than B but you have a high A1c above 8.5% or 9% because your current insu-

10.1 Find Your Starting TDD From Your Weight, Current Doses, And Current Control

1. In A, find your weight on the left and circle the average TDD for this weight on the right.
2. In B, calculate your current TDD on injections.
3. In C, compare A and B to obtain a reduced starting TDD.
4. In D, adjust the result in C upward or downward as required based on your recent control.
   Consider a recent A1c, the average blood sugar on your meter, and the frequency of lows.

A. TDD By Weight

For this weight	an average TDD in	
in lbs(kg)	adults[1] is	children[2] is
40 (18)	-	5.0 u/day
60 (27)	-	7.5 u/day
80 (36)	20 u/day	10.0 u/day
100 (45)	25 u/day	12.5 u/day
120 (54)	30 u/day	-
140 (64)	35 u/day	-
160 (73)	40 u/day	-
180 (82)	45 u/day	-
200 (91)	50 u/day	-

B. Current TDD

1. Write down typical doses given at each time of day over the last week.
2. Add together to find your current average TDD.

Insulin	Rapid*	Long	*Rapid = carb + correction
Breakfast	_____ u	_____ u	
Lunch	_____ u	_____ u	
Dinner	_____ u	_____ u	Total = Current TDD ↓
Bedtime	_____ u	_____ u	
Totals	_____ u +	_____ u =	_____ u/day

C. Is the TDD in A less than or greater than B?

A is greater than B:

Suggests excess insulin or some insulin resistance. Add A and B and multiply by 0.45 to obtain 90% of the average as your starting TDD:

TDD from A = _____ u/day

TDD from B = _____ u/day

A + B = _____ u/day

x 0.45

TDD = _____ u/day

A is less than B:

Suggests you are sensitive to insulin. Multiply A times 0.9 to obtain 90% of A as your starting TDD:

TDD from A = _____ u/day

x 0.9

TDD = _____ u/day

D. Your Starting TDD

Consider raising the TDD found in C for a recent high A1c or a high average blood sugar on your meter or lowering it if lows have been frequent or you plan to start a diet or exercise program.

TDD from C of _____ u/day modified to Starting TDD of _____ u/day

---

[1] An average adult dose ranges from 0.23 to 0.32 unit/lb/day (0.5 to 0.7 unit/kg/day). We use 0.25 u/lb/day.
[2] The average pediatric dose ranges from 0.09 to 0.23 unit/lb/day (0.2 to 0.5 unit/kg/day). We use 0.125 u/lb/day here.

lin doses are too low, your TDD from C may need to be increased. Frequent high readings may also indicate that the TDD needs to be increased. However, the TDD may need to be lowered below the estimate from C if frequent lows are a problem. Discuss these control issues with your physician and make these modifications, if needed, in Box D.

Carefully discuss how to change your current insulin dosage with your physician before you start on a pump. Your physician will help you determine a starting TDD based on your results in Workspace 10.1, while taking into account your current control. Your starting TDD, along with the basal rates and boluses that are derived from it, will need to be tested and adjusted to fit your needs.

When Already On A Pump

Let's say you are already on a pump but are having frequent high readings. If you test at least four times a day and take correction boluses for these highs, the TDD listed in your pump can safely

be used in Table 10.4 (or Table 10.6 or 10.7 if one of these better fits your basal need) to obtain a more appropriate average basal rate and new carb and correction factors.

If blood sugars are mostly high but monitoring is infrequent, raise your TDD by 5% and increase monitoring to at least four times a day. If lows are the major problem, lower your TDD by 5 to 10%. Table 10.2 shows new TDDs that are 5% and 10% above and below your current TDD.

10.3 The Total Daily Dose (TDD) Of Insulin Table

A quick way to estimate your TDD is to take your weight in pounds and divide it by 4. How much insulin a person really needs varies from this, determined by diabetes type, weight, level of fitness and stress. Typical TDDs are shown below for people who weigh 100 to 200 pounds at different levels of fitness and while undergoing puberty, pregnancy, or an infection. The "moderately active" line is used to determine the adult doses in Box B in Workout 10.1.

Compare your current TDD to that of someone else who has a similar variable that affects their insulin requirement. For instance, a moderately active person who weighs 160 lbs. will have a TDD that is close to 40 units a day. If you weigh 160 lbs. but use only 30 units a day, this suggests that you are very sensitive to insulin, that you may still be producing some insulin of your own, or that you are not taking enough insulin to keep your blood sugar down. On the other hand, if you use 60 units a day, you may be resistant to insulin, eating too much, exercising too little, or using too much insulin.

Variables to Consider	100 lbs (45 kg) TDD units	120 lbs (55 kg) TDD units	140 lbs (64 kg) TDD units	160 lbs (73 kg) TDD units	180 lbs (82 kg) TDD units	200 lbs (91 kg) TDD units
New start Type 2*	5-11	6-14	6-16	7-18	8-20	9-23
New start Type 1*	13-18	16-22	19-26	22-29	25-33	27-36
Physically fit	20	24	29	33	37	41
Moderately active	25	30	35	40	45	50
Sedentary or adolescent	30	37	44	50	56	62
Moderate stress or 2nd trimester preg.**	36	43	51	58	66	73
Greater stress or 3rd trimester preg.**	40	49	57	65	74	82
Severe stress	45	55	64	73	82	91
Infection, DKA, or steroid medication	50-90	60-108	70-126	80-144	90-162	100-180

* Starting doses are designed for safety. Higher starting doses may be needed for someone who has very high blood sugars, an infection, or is an adolescent.

** Pregnancy doses are for Type 1 or Type 2. Those with Type 1.5 or Type 2 diabetes may require greatly varying amounts of insulin depending on how resistant they are to insulin and how much internal insulin production they retain.

Adapted from a presentation by Lois Jovanovic, M.D., at the 2002 annual meeting of the American Association of Clinical Endocrinologists, and from N.S. Pierce: Diabetes and Exercise, Br J Sports Med: 161-173, 1999.

Compare Your TDD

Table 10.3 shows typical TDDs in children, adolescents, and adults with different types of diabetes in different health situations. In this table you can compare your TDD to the TDD of others who live with variables that affect their insulin requirement.

For instance, a moderately active person who weighs 160 lbs. will have a TDD close to 40 units a day. If you weigh 160 lbs. but use only 30 units a day, this suggests that you are sensitive to insulin, or that you may still be producing some insulin of your own, or that you are not taking enough insulin to keep your blood sugar down. On the other hand, if you use 60 units a day, you may have some resistance to insulin, or eat too much, exercise too little, or use too much insulin.

Find Your Starting Basals And Boluses

Once a starting TDD is determined, use this number to find starting basal rates and boluses. Table 10.4 and Tables 10.6 and 10.7 provide a rapid way to use the starting TDD to find starting values for your average basal rate, carb factor, and correction factor. The tables are set up for 40%, 50%, and 60% of the TDD used for basal delivery. To begin pumping, most people will use half of their TDD as basal as outlined in Table 10.4. If your estimated starting TDD is accurate, the starting doses in this table will provide reasonable control and a good place from which to begin testing your doses.

Tables 10.6 and 10.7 differ from Table 10.4 in how much of the TDD is given as basal. A basal percentage closer to 40% as shown in Table 10.6 may work better for some children and adults who are physically fit and for those who eat a high carb diet. These people require more bolus insulin. Prior to puberty, when growth and activity make a child's carb intake higher than an adult relative to their weight, children may require more than half of their TDD in carb boluses. Within the first five years after diagnosis, children often retain some of their own insulin production, and this tends to reduce basal insulin requirements. Lower basal rates may work for adults within the first five years of diagnosis, as well as for thin adults, and for those who are more fit and active.

A higher basal percentage of around 60% often works better for teens who have high levels of circulating hormones, those who have insulin resistance, those who want to reduce after meal spikes in their blood sugar, and those who are on a low carb diet. This may include many adults, many teens, and most of those with Type 2 diabetes, as well as those who are overweight and less active. Table 10.7 provides appropriate basal rates and boluses for those who use about 60% of their TDD as basal.

Both the percentage of insulin used for basal delivery and the percentage of carbs in the diet affect how much bolus insulin is required to cover carbs and to lower high readings. As more of the TDD is used for basal delivery, the carb and correction factor numbers usually need to be larger to make the boluses smaller. Basal insulin delivery usually makes up between 40% and 60% of the TDD, although there are occasional exceptions, while carb and correction boluses make up the remainder.[57] Tables 10.4, 10.6, and 10.7 use different rules, listed at the bottom of each table, to calculate carb and correction factors.

122

10.4 50% Basal And 50% Bolus

Once a starting TDD is determined, find your value in column one and look across that row for close estimates of your starting basal rate, carb factor, and correction factor.

Starting TDD[1] =	Day's Basal[2]	Average Basal[3]	Carb Factor[4] 1u covers:	Corr. Factor[5] 1u lowers BG:
18 units	9 units	0.38 u/hr	28 grams	111 mg/dl (6.1 mmol)
22 units	11 units	0.46 u/hr	23 grams	91 mg/dl (5.0 mmol)
26 units	13 units	0.54 u/hr	19 grams	77 mg/dl (4.2 mmol)
30 units	15 units	0.63 u/hr	17 grams	67 mg/dl (3.7 mmol)
35 units	18 units	0.75 u/hr	14 grams	56 mg/dl (3.1 mmol)
40 units	20 units	0.83 u/hr	12 grams	50 mg/dl (2.8 mmol)
45 units	23 units	0.96 u/hr	11 grams	45 mg/dl (2.4 mmol)
50 units	25 units	1.04 u/hr	10 grams	38 mg/dl (2.2 mmol)
60 units	30 units	1.25 u/hr	8 grams	33 mg/dl (1.8 mmol)
70 units	35 units	1.46 u/hr	7 grams	29 mg/dl (1.5 mmol)
80 units	40 units	1.67 u/hr	6 grams	25 mg/dl (1.3 mmol)
90 units	45 units	1.88 u/hr	6 grams	22 mg/dl (1.2 mmol)
100 units	50 units	2.08 u/hr	5 grams	20 mg/dl (1.1 mmol)

[1] Calculate the starting TDD on page 117.
[2] Day's basal is 50% of the TDD
[3] Avg Basal = day's basal/24 hrs

[4] Carb Factor = 500/TDD
[5] Correction Factor = 2000/TDD in mg/dl or 110/TDD in mmol

Workspace 10.9 shows how to do the calculations in Table 10.4 to give a better understanding of how these tables are created.

Periodically Check Your Basal/Bolus Balance

One beauty of a pump is that it allows you to adjust your basals and boluses to fit your needs. As you make these periodic changes, however, you may end up over time throwing off your basal/bolus balance. Make sure you are maintaining your basal/bolus balance, that is, that your basal rates for the day make up 40% to 60% of your TDD (or occasionally more), with the rest given primarily as carb boluses. Use Table 10.4, 10.6, or 10.7, depending on which basal percentage works best for you. Adjust if needed to return to a better basal percentage. These tables should be referred to whenever you encounter a control issue and need a fresh starting point to regain control.

Whenever a new basal rate, carb factor, or correction factor is entered into your pump, test the new setting for accuracy to minimize glucose exposure and variability. Then check your pump history a week or so later to ensure your basals and boluses remain balanced. Keep a record of the changes you make so if the new settings do not improve

10.5 Common Basal Percentages	
40%	Kids and adults who are fit, people on high carb diets, occasionally those in first 5 years after diagnosis when some insulin production is retained
50%	Most people
60% or more	Some adults, many teens, most people with insulin resistance, people on low carb diets, people using durgs like Symlin

your control or disrupt your balance, you may return to your earlier settings or ask your health professionals for their advice. Learning comes from trying, and since diabetes control is never totally stable, you want to be able to adjust for better control when required.

With experience, begin to make basal and bolus changes on your own with your physician's approval. Test and reset them as shown in the next three chapters. Before beginning your tests, make sure you have an accurate duration of insulin action set in your pump. This step is critical to having your carb and correction factors work, and to avoid insulin stacking when boluses overlap. See pages 43-48 for directions.

Change Your TDD To Solve A Major Control Issue

Control problems are usually managed with small adjustments in basal rates or boluses. These routine adjustments are made by recognizing the patterns in your readings or with direct testing of your basals and boluses. Both methods are described later in the book.

When a fresh start is needed for a major control problem, the best way may be to change your current TDD and start with new basal rates and carb and correction factors derived from this TDD. Blood sugar problems like a high A1c level, frequent highs, or frequent lows strongly suggest that your current TDD needs to change.

The guidelines for when to change your TDD are simple:

Lower your TDD: When you have frequent lows

Raise your TDD: When your A1c is over 8% or you have frequent high readings

Always stop frequent or severe lows first when trying to regain control. Reduce your current TDD until most lows are eliminated, with the goal of having only 2 or 3 readings below 70 mg/dl (3.9 mmol) each week and none below 50 mg/dl (2.8 mmol). Once this is done, you will be able to raise specific basals or carb boluses to correct patterns of high readings.

For a major control problem, increase or decrease your TDD and use Table 10.4 to recalculate new basal and bolus doses. Keep the basal/bolus percentage at 50% at this

10.6 40% Basal And 60% Bolus

Once a starting TDD is determined, find your value in column one and look across that row for close estimates of your starting basal rate, carb factor, and correction factor.

Starting TDD[1] =	Day's Basal[2]	Average Basal[3]	Carb Factor[4] 1u covers:	Corr. Factor[5] 1u lowers BG:
18 units	7 units	0.30 u/hr	25 grams	100 mg/d (5.5 mmol)l
22 units	9 units	0.37 u/hr	20 grams	82 mg/dl (4.5 mmol)
26 units	10 units	0.43 u/hr	17 grams	69 mg/dl (3.8 mmol)
30 units	12 units	0.50 u/hr	15 grams	60 mg/dl (3.3 mmol)
35 units	14 units	0.58 u/hr	13 grams	51 mg/dl (2.9 mmol)
40 units	16 units	0.67 u/hr	11 grams	45 mg/dl (2.5 mmol)
45 units	18 units	0.75 u/hr	10 grams	40 mg/dl (2.2 mmol)
50 units	20 units	0.83 u/hr	9 grams	36 mg/dl (2.0 mmol)
60 units	24 units	1.00 u/hr	8 grams	30 mg/dl (1.6 mmol)
70 units	28 units	1.17 u/hr	6 grams	26 mg/dl (1.4 mmol)
80 units	32 units	1.33 u/hr	6 grams	23 mg/dl (1.3 mmol)
90 units	36 units	1.50 u/hr	5 grams	20 mg/dl (1.1 mmol)
100 units	40 units	1.67 u/hr	5 grams	18 mg/dl (1.0 mmol)

[1] Calculate the starting TDD on page 117.

[2] Day's basal is 40% of the TDD

[3] Avg Basal = day's basal/24 hrs

[4] Carb Factor = 450/TDD

[5] Correction Factor = 1800/TDD in mg/dl or 100/TDD in mmol

point until it becomes clearer what doses you require through testing. This will generally improve your overall control dramatically. For a few mild lows, such as going below 70 mg/dl (3.9 mmol), use Table 10.2 to reduce your TDD by 5%. For frequent or severe lows, such as readings below 50 mg/dl (2.8 mmol), you may want to reduce the TDD by 10% or more. Similarly, for occasional highs, increase your TDD by 5%. Increase by 10% if highs are frequent or severe. Alternatively, if you're having highs, keep the same TDD and redistribute your correction boluses into higher basal rates or carb boluses.

If you are already on a pump, resetting your TDD is even easier. Most pumps will find your average TDD over the last 2 to 30 days. Use your pump to average your TDD over the last 14 days, raise or lower your current average TDD by 5% or 10% using Table 10.2, and use this new TDD in Table 10.4 to calculate more appropriate basal rates and carb and correction factors.

10.7 60% Basal And 40% Bolus

Once a starting TDD is determined, find your value in column one and look across that row for close estimates of your starting basal rate, carb factor, and correction factor.

Starting TDD[1] =	Day's Basal[2]	Average Basal[3]	Carb Factor[4] 1u covers:	Corr. Factor[5] 1u lowers BG:
18 units	11 units	0.45 u/hr	31 grams	122 mg/dl (6.7 mmol)
22 units	13 units	0.55 u/hr	25 grams	100 mg/dl (5.5 mmol)
26 units	16 units	0.65 u/hr	21 grams	85 mg/dl (4.6 mmol)
30 units	18 units	0.75 u/hr	18 grams	73 mg/dl (4.0 mmol)
35 units	21 units	0.88 u/hr	16 grams	63 mg/dl (3.4 mmol)
40 units	24 units	1.00 u/hr	14 grams	55 mg/dl (3.0 mmol)
45 units	27 units	1.13 u/hr	12 grams	49 mg/dl (2.7 mmol)
50 units	30 units	1.25 u/hr	11 grams	44 mg/dl (2.4 mmol)
60 units	36 units	1.50 u/hr	9 grams	37 mg/dl (2.0 mmol)
70 units	42 units	1.75 u/hr	8 grams	31 mg/dl (1.7 mmol)
80 units	48 units	2.00 u/hr	7 grams	28 mg/dl (1.5 mmol)
90 units	54 units	2.25 u/hr	6 grams	24 mg/dl (1.3 mmol)
100 units	60 units	2.50 u/hr	6 grams	22 mg/dl (1.2 mmol)

[1] Calculate the starting TDD on page 117.
[2] Day's basal is 60% of the TDD
[3] Avg Basal = day's basal/24 hrs
[4] Carb Factor = 550/TDD
[5] Correction Factor = 2200/TDD in mg/dl or 120/TDD in mmol

If you are on a pump and have recently had too many highs, but have been testing at least 4 times a day and taking correction boluses to bring down these highs, the average TDD from your pump will closely approximate your actual TDD need. This TDD includes the correction boluses you have been taking to bring down your high readings. In this situation, you may only need to take your current average TDD from your pump that includes these correction doses and use it in Table 10.4 as your new TDD to calculate more appropriate basal rates and carb and correction factors.

Ask your physician to help you raise or lower your TDD depending on whether the primary problem is frequent highs or frequent lows. Your physician can help you safely distribute your current TDD into basal rates and boluses. At first, try to keep the basal/bolus balance close to 50/50%. A higher or lower basal percentage may eventually work, but start with an even balance and adjust by the results you find in your basal testing.

Normally, the TDD remains relatively steady from day to day. Major changes in activity or hormone level, like preparing to run a marathon, monthly menses for women, or turning dirt for a spring garden, may necessitate a rapid adjustment in your TDD, basal and bolus doses. If your weight, activity, or stress level changes substantially, as may occur between the normal school year and summer vacation for students, or a change in employment, you will require a different TDD and different basals and boluses for these changes.

10.8 Circumstances That Change Your TDD			
Circumstance		**Change in TDD**	
		Less	**More**
Change in fitness, activity, exercise -	More	✓	
	Less		✓
Change in weight -	More		✓
	Less	✓	
Change of weather or season -	Colder		✓
	Warmer	✓	
Significant change in altitude -	Higher	✓	
	Lower		✓

Your TDD is correctly set when
1) *you test at least 4 times a day and your 14-day average on your meter is 150 mg/dl or less,*
2) *you use less than 8% of your TDD for correction boluses, and*
3) *you have few low blood sugars.*

You can't steal second base with one foot on first.

Anon.

10.9 How To Find Basals And Boluses From Your TDD

After calculating a starting TDD in Table 10.1. your average basal rate and carb and correction factors can be determined below.

1. Find Your Average Hourly Basal Rate

To find your average basal rate per hour, take your TDD from Table 10.1, divide by 2 to find you total basal for the day, then divide by 24 hours to find your avg. hour rate.

_____ u/day / 2 = _____ u/day / 24 hrs = _____ units/hr
New TDD · · · · · · · · · · · · · · · · Basal u/day · · · · · · · · · · · · · · · · Avg. basal per hr

My average hourly basal = _____ units/hr

Basal doses usually make up 40% to 60% (0.40 to 0.60) of the TDD.

2. Find Your Carb Factor

Find your Carb Factor with the 500 Rule:

500 * / _____ = _____ grams of carb covered by 1 unit
· · · · · · · · New TDD

1 unit will cover _____ grams of carb for me

Example: 500 / 25 units = 20 grams of carb per unit

Carb boluses usually make up 35% to 55% (0.35 to 0.55) of the TDD.

* The numbers 450 and 550 can also be used here. The larger this number is, the safer (smaller) a carb bolus becomes.

3. Find Your Correction Factor

Find your Correction Factor with the 2000 Rule:

2000 ** / _____ u/day = _____ mg/dl per unit
· · · · · · · · · · · New TDD

1 unit will decrease my blood glucose by _____ mg/dl.

Example: 2000 / 25 units = 80 mg/dl per unit

Correction boluses usually make up no more than 8% to 10% (0.08 to 0.10) of the TDD.

** The numbers 1800 and 2200 can also be used here. The larger this number is, the safer (smaller) a correction bolus becomes.

Select And Test Your Basal Rates

Once you select a starting TDD, this total insulin for the day is distributed into basals and boluses so your pump can best mimic a normal pancreas. The first step is to select one or more basal rates that keep your blood sugar from rising or falling when you are not eating.

This chapter discusses

- How to find your total basal and average hourly basal
- Why basal rates may need to vary through the day
- How to select and test your basal rates
- How to adjust basal rates
- When to use temporary and alternate basal rates
- How to use a continuous monitor to test basal rates

Your physician will suggest a starting basal rate or rates to meet your needs. Some people start a single basal rate for the entire day. This rate may then be increased or decreased, or split into more than one rate as indicated by basal testing.

Among experienced pumpers, only 9% use one basal rate for the day and another 14% are on two basal rates a day.[72] Most pumpers are on three or more basal rates a day. Variable basals work better for those who have a Dawn Phenomenon or whose insulin sensitivity varies due to changes in activity, stress, or other variables during the day. For instance, some pumpers find they need a lower basal rate during the night, such as between 9 or 10 p.m. to 1 or 2 a.m. because they are more sensitive to insulin just after midnight.

Optimal basal rates let you:

- wake up in the morning with a great reading
- skip meals without encountering lows or highs
- eat meals later than usual without worrying about loss of control
- use boluses to cover carbs precisely and lower high blood sugars safely

129

Select And Test Your Basal Rates

Most people will use half of their new starting TDD from the previous chapter for their basal rate as shown in Table 10.4. If a single basal rate is desired to start, half of the TDD can be evenly divided over 24 hours. Use Table 10.6 or 10.7 if your physician wants you to start with basal rates closer to 40% or 60% of your TDD, respectively.

After choosing starting basal rates, test them for accuracy. Basal rates will be correctly set when they keep the blood sugar level or allow it to fall no more than 30 mg/dl (1.7 mmol) during sleep or when a meal is skipped. Ideally, the blood sugar does not rise when no food is eaten, although a rise of up to 30 mg/dl (1.7 mmol) is acceptable for someone who lives alone or has hypoglycemia unawareness. Follow the 30 Rule in testing the basal rate or rates.

The 30 Rule

Optimal basal rates keep your glucose from rising or falling more than 30 mg/dl (1.7 mmol) during sleep or over a 5 hour period when no food is eaten.

New basal rates are always tested within the first few days of use and a second test is conducted to verify a basal profile that appears to work in an initial test. Once the control provided by a particular basal profile is satisfactory, it needs to be retested only when control deteriorates or there are indications it may be too high or too low.

Basal Testing

When switching from injections to a pump, basal testing can begin 30 hours after the last injection of Lantus (glargine) or Levemir (detemir) or 24 hours after the last injection of NPH. If you are already on a pump and are changing the basal rate, testing can begin five hours after new rates have been entered. See Table 9.2 for how to taper off injected insulin for a pump start.

Basal testing is broken into three segments for convenience: overnight, breakfast to midafternoon, and midafternoon to bedtime. The overnight basal is the most critical one to set as this is the only insulin controlling your blood sugar through the night. Figure 11.1 shows when to test the blood sugar for each basal test. Specific steps for testing are given in Workspace 11.2.

Overnight Basal Test

The overnight basal test is done first to reduce the risk of nighttime lows and morning highs. Night basal rates are adjusted until you can consistently sleep soundly and wake up with readings in your target range. Repeat any successful basal test at least once to verify your results. Young children often go to bed early and are sensitive to insulin. For them, basal testing can begin at 10 p.m. with additional tests at 12 a.m., 2 a.m., 4 a.m., and upon waking.

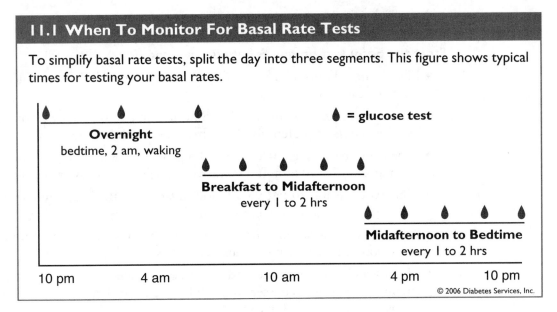

11.1 When To Monitor For Basal Rate Tests

To simplify basal rate tests, split the day into three segments. This figure shows typical times for testing your basal rates.

🌢 = glucose test

Overnight
bedtime, 2 am, waking

Breakfast to Midafternoon
every 1 to 2 hrs

Midafternoon to Bedtime
every 1 to 2 hrs

10 pm   4 am   10 am   4 pm   10 pm

© 2006 Diabetes Services, Inc.

Daytime Basal Tests

Daytime testing is split into two 6 to 8 hour segments done on different days. These tests require that you skip a meal and eat another meal earlier or later on the day of the test. Repeat the test until your adjusted basal rates keep your blood sugar relatively flat on two consecutive tests. Those who work odd hours, a night shift, or varied shifts will need to individualize testing times to fit their schedule.

Children may do well on daytime testing broken into three segments. Try morning segment (skip breakfast and snack), afternoon (skip lunch) and evening (skip dinner).

Most people can use the same basal rate they wake up with to begin the breakfast to midafternoon test. However, if you require a higher basal rate in the early morning hours to offset a Dawn Phenomenon, this higher rate often needs to be lowered at some point during the morning hours, usually between 9 a.m. and 11 a.m. If you use more than one basal rate overnight, you might start with a rate halfway between the lowest and highest rates used during the night for the late morning and afternoon period.

On another day, test the midafternoon to bedtime period. Start the test six to eight hours before you usually go to bed and at least three hours after your last meal and five hours after your last bolus. Fast during the test and then enjoy a snack or late dinner near bedtime when the test is finished. Repeat any successful basal test at least once to verify your results. With experience, you will be able to test and make basal changes as needed. Be sure to consult with your physician if you are uncertain what your test results mean.

Basal Testing Steps

Start the basal test on any otherwise average day

- Five or more hours after your last carb or correction bolus and at least three hours after any carb intake.
- When you can skip eating for 6 to 8 hours (unless you go low). You may snack on *small amounts* of protein foods, such as nuts or cheese, during the test.
- When your blood sugar is 100 to 150 mg/dl (5.6 - 8.3 mmol)★, or between 120 and 180 mg/dl (6.7 - 10 mmol) if you have hypoglycemia unawareness or a fear of lows.
- When you are able to test your blood sugar often. Be sure to test at any time you feel you may be low or excessively high.
- When no low blood sugar has occurred in the previous 12 to 24 hours as this may cause you to be either more sensitive or less sensitive to insulin.
- When stress, recent exercise, and illness are not affecting your blood sugar. Avoid strenuous or prolonged exercise for 24 to 36 hours before the test begins, unless this is routine activity for you.

★ If the starting blood sugar is less than 100 mg/dl (5.6 mmol) or low blood sugar symptoms are present, end the test.

Write down and graph your test results in Workspace 11.2. Watch for any rise or fall in blood sugar from the starting reading. Plot the change in your blood sugar on the graph. Again, your goal is to rise or fall no more than 30 mg/dl (1.7 mmol) over this 6 to 8 hour period. If your blood sugar goes below 70 mg/dl (3.9 mmol), stop the test and correct the low. Plot your readings on the graph and refer to Table 11.3 if any basal adjustment is needed. See Example 11.4 for guidance.

How To Adjust Basal Rates

Your basal rate may be too high if:

- you have low blood sugars during the night or before breakfast
- your blood sugar drops when you skip a meal
- you have frequent lows
- you become more active, less stressed, or you start a diet to lose weight

Your basal rate may be too low if:

- your blood sugar rises when you skip a meal
- you have frequent highs
- you need frequent correction boluses to bring down high blood sugars
- you become less active, more stressed, gain weight

11.2 Test Your Basal Rates

1. Start your basal test:
   - at least 5 hours after your last bolus and at least 3 hours after your last carb intake
   - when your starting BG is reasonable, such as between 100 and 150 (5.6 to 8.3 mmol)
   - on a day when there has been no unusual strenuous activity, moderate or severe hypoglycemia, or stress.

2. Monitor your glucose every 1-2 hours (or at 0, 4, and 8 hours for an overnight basal test).

3. Record times, BGs, and change from starting BG in mg/dl or mmol.

4. Plot the change in your BG.

5. If your glucose level rises or falls more than 30 mg/dl (1.7 mmol), refer to Table 11.4 for how much to change your basal.

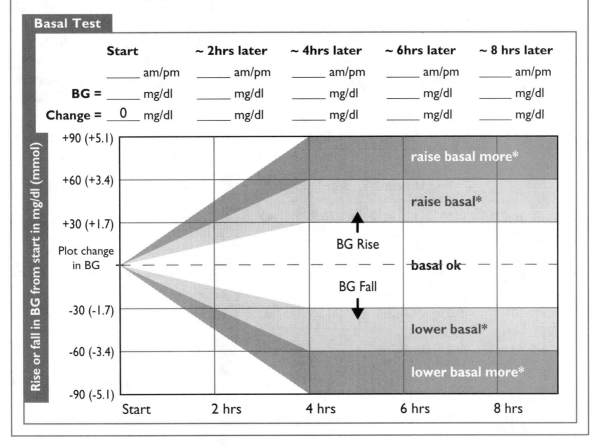

If your blood sugar falls more than 30 mg/dl (1.7 mmol) during a basal test, discuss with your physician how much to lower your basal rates. Lower the basal rate at least 4 to 8 hours before the time at which the low occurred. Change your basal rates by 5% to 10% (usually 0.05 or 0.1 units per hour) unless frequent high or low blood sugars clearly indicate that a larger change is needed. If your blood sugar falls rapidly, you will need a larger reduction in your basal rates, while a smaller basal reduction may work for a slow drop. Table 11.3 provides a convenient guide for how much total basal reduction may be needed based on your TDD and how far your blood sugar falls during the test.

If your blood sugar rises more than 30 mg/dl (1.7 mmol) during a test, take a correction bolus and adjust using Table 11.3. If your glucose rises rapidly, you will need a larger basal increase. If the rise is slow, a smaller basal increase may work. Raise the basal rate at least 4 to 8 hours before the time at which the high reading occurred, then retest. Factors like a Dawn Phenomenon in Type 1 diabetes or a cyclic rise in insulin resistance during the early morning hours with Type 2 may require a higher basal rate in the early morning hours.

When To Change The Basal Rate

The timing of basal changes is often as important as how much it is changed. Basal delivery is far "slower" than boluses even though the same insulin is being used. Boluses given in units are delivered over a minute or so, whereas basals are usually increased by only about a tenth of a unit an hour, and the first tenth unit is not completely delivered

11.3 How Much To Change Your Basal Rates From Your Basal Test

The suggested basal changes below are less than may be needed. This avoids raising and lowering basal rates in an endless search for "ideal" rates. If a 0.5 unit basal reduction is needed, you might lower your basal by 0.1 u/hr for 5 hrs between 2 and 7 hrs before the low reading occurs.

mg/dl (mmol)	For this fall in blood sugar,				For this rise in blood sugar,			
	-100 (5.5)	-80 (-6.1)	-60 (-3.3)	-40 (-2.2)	+40 (+2.2)	+60 (+3.3)	+80 (+6.1)	+100 (+5.5)
and this TDD	lower basal by a TOTAL of				raise basal by a TOTAL of			
20 u	-0.5 u	-0.3 u	-0.1 u	retest	retest	+0.1 u	+0.3 u	+0.5 u
30 u	-0.8 u	-0.5 u	-0.2 u	retest	retest	+0.2 u	+0.5 u	+0.8 u
40 u	-1.2 u	-0.8 u	-0.4 u	retest	retest	+0.4 u	+1.8 u	+1.2 u
50 u	-1.5 u	-1.0 u	-0.5 u	retest	retest	+0.5 u	+1.0 u	+1.5 u
60 u	-1.9 u	-1.3 u	-0.7 u	-0.1 u	+0.1 u	+0.7 u	+1.3 u	+1.9 u
80 u	-2.6 u	-1.8 u	-1.0 u	-0.2 u	+0.2 u	+1.0 u	+1.8 u	+2.6 u
100 u	-3.2 u	-2.3 u	-1.3 u	-0.3 u	+0.3 u	+1.3 u	+2.3 u	+3.2 u

Chris's current average TDD is 60 units a day. He uses a single basal rate through the day of 1.3 u/hr. His bedtime reading of 116 mg/dl (6.4 mmol) was almost 6 hours after an early light dinner at 4:15 p.m. When he tested at 1:47 a.m., his reading had risen 23 mg/dl (1.3 mmol), still well within his target of rising or falling no more than 30 mg/dl (1.7 mmol). But when he woke up that morning he had risen 60 mg/dl.

Basal Test

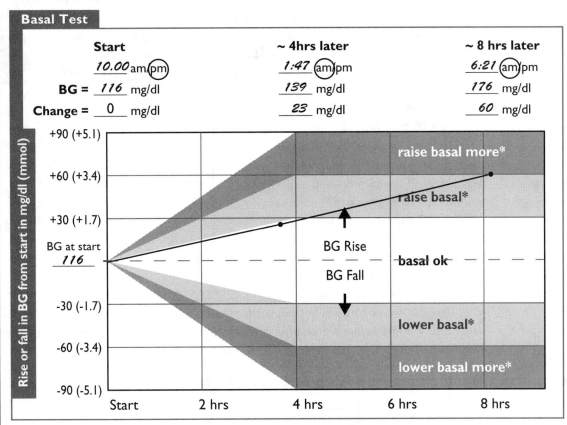

	Start	~ 4hrs later	~ 8 hrs later
	10.00 am (pm)	1:47 (am) pm	6:21 (am) pm
BG =	116 mg/dl	139 mg/dl	176 mg/dl
Change =	0 mg/dl	23 mg/dl	60 mg/dl

Chris realized that he needed to raise his basal rate before 1 a.m. when this rise had already begun. From Table 11.4, a blood sugar rise of about 60 mg/dl (3.3 mmol) during a basal test for someone whose TDD is 60 units requires that the basal rate be raised by at total of 0.7 u/hr, or by 0.1 u/hr over 7 hours during the night. Chris decided to raise his basal rate from 1.3 u/hr to 1.4 u/hr between 10 p.m. through 5 a.m. On a followup basal test the next week, his blood sugar still rose by 36 mg/dl (2.0 mmol) overnight. He had seen a consistent tendency for his blood sugar to rise overnight, so he felt confident about raising his basal rate by another 0.1 u/hr over 5 hours. This rate worked well and kept his blood sugar flat during the night.

until the end of the hour. For this reason, basal rate changes have to be made 4 to 8 hours before you will see their effect.

Basal Testing With A Continuous Monitor

A continuous monitor greatly simplifies basal testing. To start, wait for at least 5 hours after your last bolus and three hours after any food intake. A starting blood sugar between 100 and 140 mg/dl (5.6 to 7.8 mmol) is ideal. Write down the start time and your starting blood sugar, then watch how it changes over the next 6 to 8 hours.

If awake, write down some of these readings to better track your trends. Overnight monitoring will show any high and low readings that you may be unaware of.

If your blood sugar stays flat, keep the current basal rates. If the blood sugar rises or falls more than 30 mg/dl (1.7 mmol) overnight or during any 5 to 8 hour period during the day, raise or lower the basal rates using Table 11.3. If the blood sugar

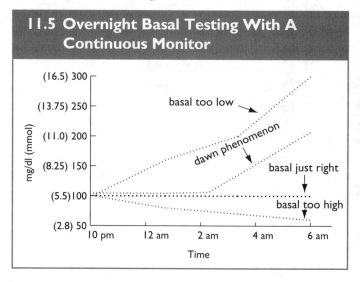

11.5 Overnight Basal Testing With A Continuous Monitor

is at first flat but at some point begins to rise or fall, raise or lower your basal rate *at least 2 to 4 hours before the change begins*. Discuss these adjustments in your basal rates with your health care provider before implementing them.

Temporary Basal Rates And Alternate Basal Profiles

Pumps offer two complementary types of basal delivery.

Temporary basal rates are used for periods when you know from experience that you will need more or less basal insulin. A higher temporary basal might be used when you are under more stress or for other reasons need more insulin. A temporary basal reduction may be needed for exercise or at night after a long day of activity to prevent a night low. Use of a temporary basal rate is also convenient for testing higher or lower basal rates to see how they perform before you program them as your regular basal rates.

11.6 First Things First

For great control, set your overnight basal rates first so that they keep your glucose flat overnight. Once you can wake up with a normal blood sugar, test and adjust your daytime basal rates. Once this is done, you are ready to start testing and fine-tuning your carb and correction boluses.

Alternate basal profiles are complete 24-hour basal rate profiles you can switch back and forth between whenever that profile is needed. Most pumps allow at least four different basal profiles to be set up and some pumps allow these changes to be scheduled on a regular basis for different days of the week.

A single basal profile may work well when weekdays and weekends are similar in activity and stress. When activity or stress differ significantly between weekends and weekdays, an alternate basal profile may be needed for the weekend. People who are significantly more or less active on one or both days of the weekends often set up an alternate profile for use on weekends.

Many women may want to set up an alternate basal profile to manage the higher insulin need they encounter around the time of their period. Some women find they

> ### 11.7 Clever Pump Tricks
>
> #### Use Alternate Basal Profiles For Basal Testing
>
> An alternate basal profile provides an easy way to test new basal rates. If you think your current basal rates are causing high or low readings, enter your current basal rates into your pump as a new basal profile. After modifying these rates, usually in 0.05 or 0.1 u/hr increments, in a way that you think will improve your readings, switch to this profile and test it out. If it improves the situation, keep it. If it does not, modify it further. Meanwhile, your original rates remain available if you need them.

need three basal profiles: their usual profile, a higher premenstrual profile, and a lower-than-normal profile for the couple of days during or after their period when they are more sensitive to insulin. Each alternate basal profile should be tested to ensure it works well.

Tips On Testing Basal Rates

- Select appropriate starting basal rates with your health care provider's help.

- Select and test the overnight basal first so that you can sleep through the night without going low and wake up with a blood sugar within your target range.

- Monitor often if you suspect your blood sugar is likely to fall during a test.

- If your eating, activity, or stress are significantly different on weekends, an alternate basal profile may be needed for this time. If you need a different profile during the week, be sure to switch between different profiles at the same times each week.

- As a starting basal percentage, 50% of the TDD works well for most people. Check your total basal dose periodically to be sure it makes up an appropriate percentage (usually 40% to 60%) of your TDD.

- When needed, change basal rates by 0.05 or 0.1 units per hour unless frequent high or low blood sugars clearly indicate a larger change is needed.

Never assume a basal rate is correct from one test. Always test twice.

Quick Check: Do your basal insulin doses make up 40% to 60% of your TDD?

11.8 Are You Getting Everything You Can Out Of Your Pump?

People choose pumps for convenience, a greater sense of control, and an improved quality of life, but they often fail to get the most out of this marvelous device. If you have worn a pump for a while, look through this checklist to see if you use all the features that might help your control:

Wearing a pump, can you depend on your insulin delivery?	Yes / No
Do your infusion sets work well for you? That is, no irritation, rashes, discomfort, or unexplained highs?	Yes / No
Do you encounter random unexplained periods of high blood sugars that disappear when you change your infusion site? (May indicate that your current infusion set is not the best choice.)	Yes / No
Do you trust the bolus recommendations your pump gives you? Do you often increae or decrease these recommended boluses or ignore then? (Indicates that your pump settings need to change.)	Yes / No
Have you entered an accurate carb factor, correction factor, and duration of insulin action into your pump so it can recommend accurate boluses?	Yes / No
Do you enter all your blood sugar readings into your pump, even when they are near or below your target range, to obtain accurate bolus recommendations?	Yes / No
Do you count carbs correctly?	Yes / No
If you sometimes forget meal boluses, have you set bolus reminders to help you remember?	Yes / No
Do you use temporary basal rates? (Easy to do and helps in many situations, such as when activity changes or you become ill.)	Yes / No
When a control problem appears, do you quickly readjust your TDD and basals or boluses, and review your carb counting to correct it?	Yes / No
Do you regularly review your average TDD, basal/bolus balance, and the percentage of your TDD being used for correction boluses (usually less than 8% of the TDD) to improve your insulin use?	Yes / No
Is your meter accurate, easy to use, and can you easily transmit test results to your pump?	Yes / No
Do you have an easy way to carry your meter(if separate), lancing device, and strips?	Yes / No
Is your pump easy to carry with you and is wearing it comfortable and unobtrusive? Do you have carrying cases or clothing that protect your pump and help you wear it during sports, water activities, formal occasions, and sleep? (Many pump cases and accessories are available – visit www.diabetesnet.com/ishop/.)	Yes / No
Does your record system, logbook, charts, or PDA allow you to record glucose results, carbs, insulin doses, stress, and activity clearly? (Helps you identify the sources for control problems.)	Yes / No

Select And Test Your Carb Factor

"How much insulin do I take to cover a bagel, a plate of pasta, or a bowl of fruit?" Your answers to these questions determine half your control each day. The more carbohydrate in a meal, the larger the carb bolus you need.

This chapter shows how to

- Select your starting carb factor and test it
- Time boluses and choose bolus types
- Reduce or skip carb boluses

Carb counting or a consistent carb intake is critical to good control and makes life easier on a pump. To match carbs with accurate boluses, you need to know your carb factor or how many grams of carbohydrate one unit of insulin will cover for you. An appropriate carb factor combined with accurate carb counting lets you cover any number of carbs with well-matched boluses. With this calculation, you can vary how many carbs you eat without losing control.

Most people need one unit of insulin for somewhere between 5 and 25 grams of carbohydrate. Someone in good control on a small daily TDD will use a larger number for their carb factor, while someone who requires a large TDD will use a smaller carb factor number. Carb factors outside this range certainly occur. Someone who weighs less, eats healthy, and is physically active may need only one unit for every 30 grams. A growing teen, on the other hand, may need one unit for every 3 or 4 grams, while a person with Type 2 diabetes and severe insulin resistance may use one unit for every 2 grams.

Three things are required to cover carbs well:

1. **Accurate Basal Rates:** If your basal rates are set too high, a correction bolus that might otherwise be appropriate will make your glucose go low. If your basal rates are too low, appropriate correction boluses will be too small to bring high readings down. Always test your basal rates first before testing your correction factor.

2. **Accurate Carb Counting:** Your pump requires an accurate carb count to determine the size of the carb bolus required to cover the carbs eaten.

139

3. An Accurate Carb Factor: This is needed to determine the size of the carb bolus. With this and an accurate carb count your pump can determine an accurate carb bolus.

After eating carbs, the blood sugar starts to rise within 5 to 10 minutes and reaches a peak at about 70 minutes later. The rise in blood sugar reflects how quickly glucose from digesting carbs reaches the blood stream. This rise totals no more than 40 to 60 mg/dl (2.2 to 3.3 mmol) above the starting blood sugar in people who do not have diabetes.

Compared to most carbs, a "rapid" insulin is slow to act. It only starts to work to lower the blood sugar 15 to 20 minutes after it is given, and only half of its glucose-lowering action is seen two hours later, with about 90% of its action gone after five hours. Better control of the postmeal blood sugar occurs when carb boluses are given at least 20 minutes before eating begins.

An accurate carb factor allows your pump to determine boluses

12.1 The 500 Rule*		
If Your TDD is:	**Your Carb Factor is:**	**Bolus Per 10 g of Carb**
15 units	33 grams	0.3 units
20	25	0.4
25	20	0.5
30	17	0.6
35	14	0.7
40	13	0.8
45	11	0.9
50	10	1.0
55	9	1.1
60	8	1.3
70	7	1.4
80	6	1.7
90	5	2.0
100	5	2.0

*500 √ TDD = # of grams of carb covered by 1 unit. 450, 550, and 600 can also be used. The larger this number, the safer (smaller) a carb bolus becomes.

that keep postmeal readings reasonable. To determine a carb bolus for a particular meal, divide the number of carbs you plan to eat by your carb factor. For instance, if you plan to eat 70 grams of carb and use one unit of insulin for every 10 grams, you would take 7 units to cover these carbs.

A smart pump does this calculation automatically. After entering your carb factor into your pump, simply enter how many carbs you want to eat and a precise carb bolus is calculated. This suggested bolus can be adjusted as needed for activity or other factors. Be as consistent as possible in the number of carbs you eat and timing of meals until you find an accurate carb factor.

Your carb factor may differ slightly at different meals during the day, but this difference should be small when the basal rates are appropriately set. Assuming that up to 8% of the TDD may be needed for correction boluses, carb boluses usually make up between 32% and 52% of your TDD.

When boluses are given for meals or snacks more often than every 4 or 5 hours, BOB from the previous bolus will still be active when a new bolus is given. Smart pumps alert you to this BOB and some pumps will automatically reduce a carb bolus when there is BOB still active. (See the discussion of BOB on pages 48-50 for use and exceptions.)

Select A Starting Carb Factor

Someone who uses 25 units of total insulin per day will find that a unit of insulin covers more carbs, around 20 grams, than someone who uses 100 units of insulin per day. A unit of insulin for the second person will cover only about 5 grams of carb. The person who uses 100 units of insulin a day will need a carb bolus four times as large as the first person will need.

When your basal rate makes up about 50% of your TDD, a starting carb factor can be estimated from Table 10.4 or by dividing the number 500 by your TDD which is the 500 Rule.[73] The numbers 450, 500, and 550 are common numbers used to find starting carb factors. A smaller number like 450 gives larger carb boluses, while using 550 gives smaller and safer carb boluses.

If your basal rate is closer to 40% of your TDD, use Table 10.6 to find your TDD and read across to find a starting carb factor. This table uses 450 which, as noted, is more aggressive but which is usually needed when the basal rate makes up about 40% of the TDD. If your basal rate is closer to 60% of your TDD, use Table 10.7 which uses 550. This less aggressive number is used when basal rates make up a greater percentage of the TDD to give smaller carb boluses.

If you have too many highs or lows after giving carb boluses, your carb factor may not be the right one for you. Incorrect basal rates can also cause this. Reexamine whether your TDD is correct, and pay special attention to retesting your basal rates.

If your carb count is correct, a smart pump can use your carb factor to recommend the carb bolus you need to bring your blood sugar back to your target 3 to 5 hours later. If this does not consistently occur on a smart pump, your carb factor is incorrect, carb counting is inaccurate, or another problem exists.

Test Your Carb Factor

As soon as the basal rates have been tested and a starting carb factor has been selected with your physician's help, its accuracy is validated through testing, using Workspace 12.2. Make sure you already have set and tested your basal rates so that they keep your blood sugar flat when you are not eating. A correct carb factor returns your blood sugar to within 30 mg/dl (1.7 mmol) of your starting blood sugar 3 to 5 hours later.

Test your carb factor when:

- You have not had a low blood sugar in the last 8 hours
- Your premeal blood sugar is between 70 and 150 mg/dl (3.9 to 8.3 mmol)
- You can count exactly the carbs you will eat
- You have little or no active BOB working

Follow these steps to test your carb factor:

- Eat enough carbs to challenge your carb factor and find if it really works. Eat about half your weight in pounds (or an amount equal to your weight in kilograms) in grams of carb. For example, someone who weighs 160 lbs. would eat about 80 grams of carb.

- Avoid unusual foods and excess fat and protein

- Enter the grams of carb into your pump and take the carb bolus the pump recommends 20 minutes before eating

- Finish the meal within 20 minutes

- Test your blood sugar hourly for the next 5 hours (more often if you may go low).

Your carb factor is correct when your blood sugar starts at your target before a meal, rises about 40 to 80 mg/dl (2.2 to 4.4 mmol) 2 hours later and ends up within 30 mg/dl (1.7 mmol) of your starting value 4 to 5 hours later. Once a carb factor appears to be correct, repeat the test to verify it. See Example 12.4 for guidance.

Your carb factor number may be too small and carb bolus too large if your premeal blood sugar starts in a normal range but often goes low within 5 hours. Check your basal rates also, as too much basal will cause the same problem.

Your carb factor number may be too large and carb bolus too small if your premeal blood sugar starts in a normal range but is often above normal 4 to 5 hours later. Check the basal rates also, as too little basal may cause the same problem.

The glucose level usually rises 40 to 80 mg/dl (2.2 to 4.4 mmol) above its start at one to two hours after a meal. If it rises less than 40 mg/dl (2.2 mmol) at one hour, a low blood sugar is more likely. If you have a low blood sugar in the next five hours, your carb bolus was too large and your carb factor number is too small. Eat carbs to correct the low and raise your carb factor before the next test.

If your blood sugar rises more than 80 mg/dl (4.4 mmol), enter the reading into your pump to see if it suggests that you take a correction bolus. If no bolus is recommended, continue the test for another hour to see if the reading comes down. If at any point your pump recommends that a correction bolus be given for a blood sugar, you may want to stop the test and take the correction bolus. If this happens, the carb bolus was likely too small and your carb factor number may need to be lowered.

After a meal, if your blood sugar often goes low:

- shortly after carb boluses, a large increase in the carb factor may be needed, or

- three or four hours after carb boluses, a small increase in the carb factor may work.

For instance, if lows occur an hour or two after you eat and you use 1 unit for each 12 grams of carb, next time try 1 unit for each 14 or 15 grams. If lows happen three hours after carb boluses, you might try 1 unit for each 13 grams. Figure 12.3 shows how appropriate the carb bolus was depending on where your blood sugar ends up after a meal.

12.2 Test Your Carb Factor

Start to test your carb factor when:

1. You have not had a low blood sugar or symptoms of one in the last 8 hours.

2. Your blood sugar is between 90 to 150 mg/dl (5.0 to 8.3 mmol) before a meal.

3. You have not eaten in the last 3 hours or given yourself a bolus in the past 5 hours.

4. You are able to count the carbs accurately in your meal.

Enter the exact number of carbs you will eat in your pump and take the bolus it recommends. Bolus 15 to 20 minutes before the meal if possible.

Test each hour for 4 to 5 hrs and plot your results below

© 2006 Diabetes Services, Inc.

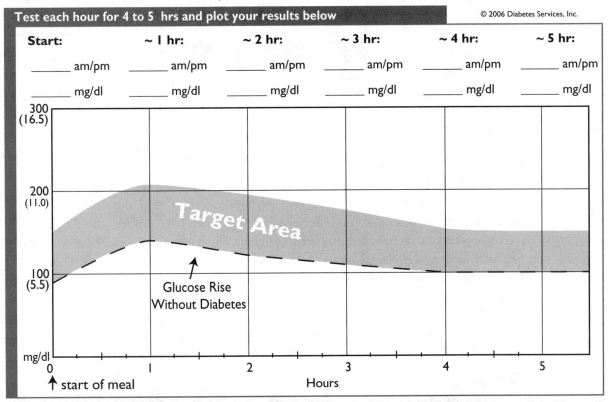

Start:	**~ 1 hr:**	**~ 2 hr:**	**~ 3 hr:**	**~ 4 hr:**	**~ 5 hr:**
_____ am/pm	_____ am/pm	_____ am/pm	_____ am/pm	_____ am/pm	_____ am/pm
_____ mg/dl	_____ mg/dl	_____ mg/dl	_____ mg/dl	_____ mg/dl	_____ mg/dl

At 4 to 5 hours after this carb bolus, is your blood sugar:

More than 30 mg/dl (1.7 mmol) below your start?	**Within 30 mg/dl (1.7 mmol) of your start?**	**More than 30 mg/dl (1.7 mmol) above your start?**
Eat carbs to raise your BG. Retest later using a larger carb factor. For example, if it was 1u/12 grams use 1u/13 grams	Your carb factor works. Retest to verify.	Take a correction bolus. Retest later using a smaller carb factor. For example, if it was 1u/12 grams use 1u/11 grams

143

If the blood sugar often stays high after meals with a particular carb factor, the carb factor number can be decreased to increase carb boluses. Subtract 1 or 2 from the carb factor so that, for example, instead of 1 unit for every

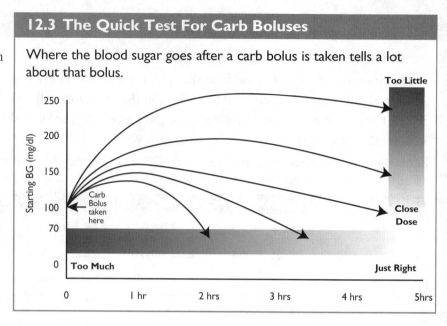

12.3 The Quick Test For Carb Boluses

Where the blood sugar goes after a carb bolus is taken tells a lot about that bolus.

Starting BG (mg/dl)

250
200
150
100
70
0

Carb Bolus taken here

Too Little

Close Dose

Too Much

Just Right

0   1 hr   2 hrs   3 hrs   4 hrs   5hrs

12 grams of carb, you would use 1 unit for every 11 or 10 grams. Test the new carb factor before reducing it further.

If different carb factors are required during the day, most smart pumps allow you to set different factors for different times. For example, one unit of insulin may not cover as many grams of carb at breakfast compared to other meals. This is often caused by a reduced sensitivity to insulin at breakfast from rising levels of growth hormone, cortisol, and free fatty acids in the blood during the early morning hours, commonly called a Dawn Phenomenon. One carb factor may be needed for breakfast and a higher one for lunch, dinner, and snacks eaten later in the day. Carb factors will usually differ by only 1 to 3 grams through the day (may be more for carb factors above 20). A large change in the carb factors at different times of the day suggests that the basal rates may not be correctly set. If you need a lot more insulin for carbs eaten at breakfast, retest your overnight basal rates.

Example

On Thursday, Elaine was busy at work and did not get a chance to take a lunch until 2 p.m. This was over six hours after her last bolus at breakfast, so she thought it would be a good time to test her carb bolus. She had recently tested her basal rates and knew her basal kept her blood sugar level when she was not eating. On Tuesday, she had undercovered a linguine and clam dish at a nearby restaurant and had gotten an exact carb count of 72 grams in the meantime for the portion she wanted to eat.

With a carb factor of one unit for every 18 grams, she took a 4 unit bolus for these carbs. Her starting blood sugar was 132 mg/dl (7.3 mmol), but she took no correction bolus in case her blood sugar fell. Testing hourly, her reading rose only 35 mg/dl (1.9 mmol) at 3:10 p.m., was about level at 141 mg/dl (7.8 mmol) at 4:05 p.m., had fallen a bit to 111 mg/dl (6.2 mmol) after 3 hours, and was going low at 76 mg/dl

12.4 Example: Elaine Tests Her Carb Factor

Elaine plans to eat 72 grams of carbs. She uses one unit of insulin for every 18 grams of carb.

$$\frac{\text{grams of carb}}{\text{carb factor}} = \frac{72 \text{ g}}{18} = 4 \text{ units as her carb bolus}$$

Elaine took 4.0 units as a carb bolus with these glucose test results:

Test each hour for 4 to 5 hrs and plot your results below

© 2006 Diabetes Services, Inc.

Start:	~ 1 hr:	~ 2 hr:	~ 3 hr:	~ 4 hr:	~ 5 hr:
2:00 am/(pm)	3:10 am/(pm)	4:05 am/(pm)	5:00 am/(pm)	6:07 am/(pm)	- am/pm
132 mg/dl	167 mg/dl	141 mg/dl	111 mg/dl	76 mg/dl	— mg/dl

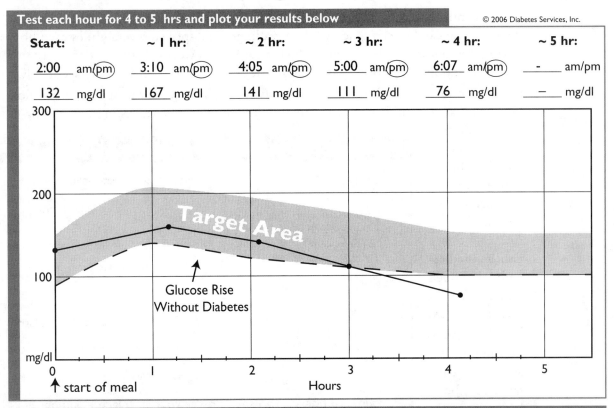

At 4 to 5 hours after this carb bolus, is your blood sugar:

More than 30 mg/dl below your start?	Within 30 mg/dl of your start?	More than 30 mg/dl above your start?
Eat carbs to raise your BG. Retest later using a larger carb factor. For example, if it was 1u/12 grams use 1u/13 grams	Your carb factor works. Retest to verify.	Take a correction bolus. Retest later using a smaller carb factor. For example, if it was 1u/12 grams use 1u/11 grams

After 4 hours, Elaine had fallen more than 30 mg/dl below her start. She ate carbs to raise her glucose, retested later using 1 unit for every 19 grams of carb. This carb factor worked well.

145

(4.2 mmol) after 4 hours. She had been having frequent mild lows after meals, but was unsure whether to raise her correction factor from 1 unit for every 18 grams to one for 19 or one for 20 grams. After calling her doctor's office, the nurse called back to say her doctor suggested trying one for 20 to lessen the risk of lows until she could do further testing on another day.

Testing Your Carb Factor With A Continuous Monitor

A continuous monitor makes it easy to test your carb factor. How carbs affect your glucose can be seen quickly when readings are displayed several times each hour during the four to five hours over which a carb bolus works. With practice, you can use a continuous monitor to judge the impact of your carb boluses quite accurately.

A continuous monitor lets you identify foods that have a low or high glycemic index so that you can better match them with appropriate changes in bolus timing or amounts. You can even see whether the glucose from foods enters your bloodstream in the fashion predicted by the food's ranking in a glycemic index.

Continuous monitoring allows you to tailor carb boluses to specific meals and identify individual

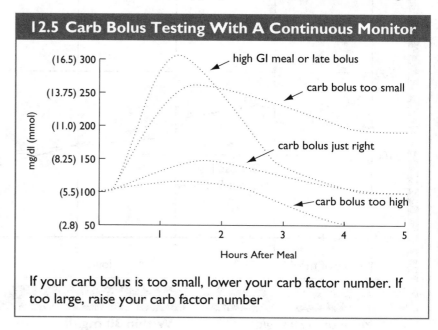

12.5 Carb Bolus Testing With A Continuous Monitor

high GI meal or late bolus

carb bolus too small

carb bolus just right

carb bolus too high

mg/dl (mmol)

(16.5) 300
(13.75) 250
(11.0) 200
(8.25) 150
(5.5) 100
(2.8) 50

1   2   3   4   5
Hours After Meal

If your carb bolus is too small, lower your carb factor number. If too large, raise your carb factor number

food effects. You can see whether potato chips or a meat pizza, for example, cause your glucose to rise farther or longer than predicted by their carb content.

Importance Of Bolus Timing For Control

When a carb bolus is given can have a great impact on postmeal readings. Although it is convenient to give carb boluses just before eating, this often leads to postmeal spiking. A carb bolus can be given just before meals that have only a small number of carbs, but for meals that contain larger amounts of carb or foods with a high glycemic index, the carb bolus has to be taken 15 to 20 minutes before eating to prevent the blood sugar from spiking an hour or two later.

12.6 How Much Insulin Did You Miss In Your Last Carb Bolus?

When you have a high blood sugar 4 to 5 hours after a carb bolus, this table estimates how many units you were short in that bolus.

1. Find your TDD on the left.
2. Look across to find the column nearest your blood sugar.
3. The value you find shows about how many units you were short in your last bolus.

Your TDD (units/day)	Your Blood Sugar in mg/dl (mmol)							
	140 (8)	180 (10)	220 (12)	260 (14)	300 (17)	340 (19)	380 (21)	420 (23)
20 u	-0.4 u	-0.8 u	-1.2 u	-1.6 u	-2.0 u	-2.4 u	-2.8 u	-3.2 u
30 u	-0.3 u	-1.2 u	-1.8 u	-2.4 u	-3.0 u	-3.5 u	-4.1 u	-4.6 u
40 u	-0.8 u	-1.6 u	-2.4 u	-3.2 u	-4.0 u	-4.8 u	-5.6 u	-6.4 u
50 u	-1.0 u	-2.0 u	-3.0 u	-4.0 u	-5.0 u	-6.0 u	-7.0 u	-8.0 u
60 u	-1.2 u	-2.4 u	-3.6 u	-4.8 u	-6.1 u	-7.3 u	-8.5 u	-9.7 u
70 u	-1.4 u	-2.8 u	-4.1 u	-5.5 u	-6.9 u	-8.3 u	-9.7 u	-11.0 u
80 u	-1.6 u	-3.2 u	-4.8 u	-6.4 u	-8.0 u	-9.6 u	-11.2 u	-12.8 u
100 u	-2.0 u	-4.0 u	-6.0 u	-8.0 u	-10.0 u	-12.0 u	-14.0 u	-16.0 u

How much your blood sugar changes from before a meal to one or two hours afterward tells you how well the bolus you took and its timing match the carbs in a meal. The American Diabetes Association recommends that the postmeal blood sugar go no higher than 180 mg/dl (10 mmol) two hours after eating. The European Diabetes Policy Group recommends that postmeal blood sugars in Type 2 diabetes go no higher than 165 mg/dl (8.9 mmol) to prevent diabetes complications like retinopathy. It is also their opinion that a postmeal reading go no higher than 135 mg/dl (7.5 mmol) to prevent heart attacks and strokes.[74]

If you are not already meeting these goals, try matching the types and quantities of carbs you eat with boluses that match them and that are taken early enough to improve your postmeal readings. You can also change the quantity or type of carbs eaten, or try a medication like Symlin to reduce postmeal spiking.

Of course, bolus early before meals only when your blood sugar is not low and you are certain you will eat on time. Eating must not be delayed longer than expected once a bolus is given. Be realistic about how likely you are to be distracted from eating. When the timing of a meal is uncertain, it is usually better to wait to bolus until the food arrives or take a partial bolus now and the rest when your food arrives. See Textbox 12.9.

If the blood sugar is low before a meal, have some fast carbs right away and cover the carbs in the meal with a slightly reduced bolus. Fast carbs should raise the blood sugar before this bolus begins to work unless your BOB

at the time is excessive. Enter the low reading into your pump and let it calculate the bolus you need. Again, do not delay eating in this situation.

The more carbs you eat and the higher your reading, the earlier you want to bolus.

Combination And Extended Boluses

Not every bolus needs to be given before a meal to have the best effect. Most carbs are digested and turned into glucose within an hour or two of eating. However, low glycemic carbs break down more slowly because of the type of carb or fat or quantity of protein they contain. Some meals may be eaten over an extended time period, such as a brunch, cocktail party or holiday celebration where food is eaten in small amounts over several hours. Extended boluses also work well when gastroparesis has slowed the digestive process.

Pumps offer two types of boluses that slow bolus delivery to better match situations like these. One is an **extended or square wave bolus**, which delivers a bolus over an extended period of time, such as 5 units over an hour and a half. The other is called a **combination or dual wave bolus**, which gives part of the bolus right away and the rest over a period of time, such as 60% of the bolus now and the remaining 40% delivered over the next two hours.

Experiment with combination and extended boluses until you find an approach that works for the foods you eat. Keep a record of the ratio and duration you use for particular foods so that you can rely on the same pattern in the future when you need it. Many pumps can be programmed to remember particular doses, such as for pizza or other foods when you eat them again.

12.8 If Your Carb Factor Does Not Work

If your carb factor usually works but you experience a high or low reading after a particular meal, consider:

- Did you count the carbs carefully?
- Did you take your carb bolus soon enough?
- Do the carbs in this meal have an unusually high or low glycemic index?
- Did the meal contain more fat or protein than usual that slowed digestion or caused an unusual rise in a reading?
- Was your pre-meal activity more or less than usual?
- Did you have a recent low blood sugar?

When a slower bolus is used, verify that it is working by checking your blood sugar one and two hours after eating. Your reading should not go low nor rise more than 40 to 80 mg/dl (2.2 to 4.4 mmol) from where it started.

Situations Where A Carb Bolus May Need To Change

An accurate carb count is the major factor but not the only factor in determining bolus size. For instance, if you will be more active after a meal, a smaller carb bolus will be needed than the one recommended by your pump. If you are experiencing pain, your meal bolus will likely need to be raised. Keep your current circumstances in mind each time you bolus.

A carb bolus might not be given at all:

- when a meal or snack has few carbs,
- when carbs are eaten to raise a low blood sugar,
- when the carbs are needed to cover exercise or increased activity, or
- when you are unsure you can keep food down due to nausea or vomiting.

Smart pumps provide a recommended carb bolus each time you enter the grams of carb you plan to eat. However, certain circumstances will affect your final dose decision and cause you to reduce or eliminate a bolus. Here are some to consider:

Hypoglycemia

When you have a low blood sugar, you want to eat enough carbs to return your blood sugar to normal. No bolus is taken for the carbs you eat to treat a low. If a bolus were given for these carbs, your blood sugar would simply go low again!

> **12.9 Clever Pump Tricks**
>
> **Uncertain Timing Of Restaurant Meals**
>
> When eating out, you may not know exactly when your meal will arrive nor its exact carb content. You may want to lead a meal like this with a partial carb bolus, taking perhaps half of the total bolus you anticipate needing for the meal. Take the remainder in a second bolus once your food arrives and its true carb content can be accurately determined.
>
> Splitting a carb bolus in two allows your insulin level to start rising for the meal, yet reduces the risk of a low blood sugar. Keep fast-acting carbs handy in your purse or pocket in case your blood sugar drops more than you expect before the meal arrives. Before giving the first bolus, check to see how much BOB is active!

A smart pump can recommend an appropriate bolus reduction to balance carbs eaten, your current blood sugar, and any BOB. For instance, if your blood sugar is 50 mg/dl (2.8 mmol), you need enough free carbs (carbs you don't cover with a bolus) to raise your blood sugar to normal. For most adults, one gram of carbohydrate raises the blood sugar about 4 mg/dl (.22 mmol), so for a blood sugar of 50 mg/dl (2.8 mmol), 15 grams of carb times 4 mg/dl (.22 mmol) per gram will raise the blood sugar to 110 mg/dl (6.1 mmol).

If any BOB is present at the time of the low, the number of unused units can be multiplied by the carb factor to calculate the additional grams of carbohydrate that will be needed to offset the remaining BOB. Of course, if you consume more carbs than you need to raise your blood sugar to your target, these extra carbs should be covered with a bolus to avoid a high blood sugar later.

Exercise And Activity

For planned exercise or hard work after a meal, the normal carb bolus may need to be reduced. Chapter 23 on exercise describes how to adjust bolus and basal doses for various activities.

Bedtime

If your pump is set up well, you don't have to eat a bedtime snack. If you want to eat one, reduce the bolus for the snack to prevent night lows. Pumps allow different carb factors to be set at different times of day. Increase the carb factor number a couple of hours before your normal bedtime to reduce bedtime boluses. This can help avoid night lows and ensure that you wake up in the morning with a reading near your target range.

Tips On Carb Coverage

- Test your carb factor only after you have correctly set and tested your basal insulin. If your factor differs at different times of day, be sure to test each one.

- Count or estimate all carbs as closely as possible before determining a meal bolus.

- Before taking any carb bolus suggested by your pump, adjust it as needed for any planned activity or other circumstances.

- The correct carb factor determines a bolus that returns the blood sugar to within 30 mg/dl (1.7 mmol) of the starting blood sugar 5 hours after eating.

One half of what we eat enables us to live, the other half enables the doctor to live.

Anon.

Select & Test Your Correction Factor

Even with appropriate basal rates and carb boluses, you will need correction boluses from time to time. When your blood sugar is high, you want to bring it back to your target range without going low. To do this, you need to know your correction factor or how far your blood sugar drops for each unit of bolus insulin. An accurate correction bolus will bring a high reading back to your target range about 5 hours later.

This chapter shows how to

- Select a starting correction factor
- Test this correction factor
- Reset doses when correction boluses are more than 8% of the TDD
- Combine a correction bolus and carb bolus
- Test your duration of insulin action

An appropriate correction bolus speeds the fall from a high blood sugar and reduces glucose exposure without causing a low. A rapid insulin takes 4 to 5 hours to completely bring a high blood sugar down once it is given. This time may be slower than many people would like, but patience prevents taking too much insulin and causing unnecessary lows. If a faster reduction in the blood sugar is desired, carb and correction boluses can be combined as described later in this chapter, or a Super Bolus can be given as discussed on page 56.

The best way to treat a high is to prevent it.
The second best way is to not overtreat it.

Four pump settings are required to bring high readings down safely:

1. **Accurate Basal Rates:** If your basal rates are set too high, a correction bolus that might otherwise be appropriate will make your glucose go low. If your basal rates are too low, appropriate correction boluses will be too small to bring high readings down. Always test your basal rates first before testing your correction factor.

2. **An Accurate Duration Of Insulin Action:** Your pump requires an accurate duration of insulin action to determine how much insulin remains from recent carb and correction boluses. With this, the pump can determine the BOB or active bolus insulin to calculate an accurate correction bolus.

3. **Blood Sugar Targets:** The pump subtracts the target blood sugar from the current high reading to accurately determine a correction bolus.

4. **An Accurate Correction Factor:** This is needed to determine the size of the correction bolus to bring a high reading down to the target.

Once you enter a correction factor into your pump, and your basal rates, blood sugar targets, and duration of insulin action are also accurately set, the pump can calculate an appropriate correction bolus for a high reading at any time of the day. Consult with your health provider about the values for these pump settings to start with.

Select A Starting Correction Factor

Someone who uses 25 units of total insulin per day will find their blood sugar drops farther per unit, around 80 mg/dl (4.4 mmol), than someone who uses 100 units of insulin per day. The second person's blood sugar will drop only about 20 points (1.1 mmol) per unit. To lower the same high blood sugar, the person who uses 100 units of insulin a day will need a bolus four times as large as the first person will need.

When your basal rate makes up about 50% of your TDD, a starting correction factor can be estimated from Table 10.4 or by dividing the number 2000 by your TDD.[75] For those who use millimoles, the 2000 Rule can be conveniently replaced with an 110 Rule for millimoles. The numbers 1800, 2000, and 2200 are the most commonly used numbers for finding a correction factor as shown in Table 13.1. A smaller number like 1800 gives more bolus insulin when lowering a high reading.

If your basal rate is 40% of your TDD, use Table 10.6 to find your TDD and read across to find your correction factor. This table uses 1800 which, as noted, is more aggressive but which is usually needed when the basal rate makes up about 40% of the TDD. If your basal rate is closer to 60% of your TDD, use Table 10.7 which uses 2200. This less aggressive number is used when basal rates make up a greater percentage of the TDD for smaller correction boluses.

If you often have highs or lows after giving correction boluses, your correction factor may not be the right one for you. Also keep in mind that incorrect basal rates or DIA can also cause this. Reexamine whether your TDD is correct, and pay special attention to retesting your basal rates and ensuring that your duration of insulin action is appropriate.

A smart pump uses your correction factor, target range, duration of insulin action, BOB, and current blood sugar to recommend how much correction bolus is needed to bring your blood sugar back to your target about 5 hours later. If this does not consistently occur on a smart pump, one or more of these settings in your pump is incorrect or another problem exists.

A Smart Pump Helps Prevent Overcorrection

If you miss a carb bolus and find you have a high blood sugar 2 hours later, enter the high into your pump and take the correction bolus recommended. Do NOT enter the carbs you ate 2 hours ago and do NOT take a carb bolus to cover them. These carbs have already had their effect and only the high blood sugar needs to be treated.

If a blood sugar is 200 or 400 mg/dl (11 mmol or 22 mmol) a couple of hours after a meal because it was already that high before the meal, a correction bolus may not be needed now for this high reading because the previous correction bolus is already at work. The BOB feature on your pump will let you know whether any additional correction bolus is needed. For example, if your reading is 250 mg/dl (13.9 mmol) two hours after a meal but it had been 225 mg/dl (12.5 mmol) before the meal, and you took a combined carb and correction bolus, your blood sugar may come down from the action of this combined bolus in another 2 to 3 hours.

After a meal, the blood sugar rises 40 to 60 mg/dl (2.2 mmol to 3.3 mmol) in people without diabetes. In the last example, it had risen only 25 mg/dl (1.4 mmol) in 2 hours because the correction bolus had already begun to work. This suggests that no additional insulin will be needed despite the temporary elevation in the two-hour reading. A smart pump will let you know this.

13.1 Correction Factor For mg/dl and mmol			
TDD: Total Daily Insulin Dose	**1 Unit Lowers BG by**		
	40% basal 1800 Rule (100 Rule):	**50% basal** 2000 Rule (110 Rule):	**60% basal** 2200 Rule (120 Rule):
15 units	120 (6.7)	133 (7.3)	147 (8.0)
20	90 (5.0)	100 (5.5)	110 (6.0)
25	72 (4.0)	80 (4.4)	88 (4.8)
30	60 (3.3)	67 (3.6)	73 (4.0)
35	51 (2.9)	57 (3.1)	63 (3.4)
40	45 (2.5)	50 (2.8)	55 (3.0)
45	40 (2.2)	44 (2.4)	49 (2.7)
50	36 (2.0)	40 (2.2)	44 (2.4)
55	33 (1.8)	36 (2.0)	40 (2.1)
60	30 (1.7)	33 (1.8)	37 (2.0)
70	26 (1.4)	29 (1.6)	31 (1.7)
80	23 (1.3)	25 (1.3)	28 (1.5)
90	20 (1.1)	22 (1.2)	24 (1.3)
100	18 (1.0)	20 (1.1)	22 (1.2)

1800, 2000, or 2200 divided by your TDD = how far your BG will fall in mg/dl for different basal percentages of the TDD (100, 110, and 120 are used for mmol). 2200 provides less risk for lows, while 1800 may provide tighter control.

© 2006 Diabetes Services, Inc.

Steps For Testing

Test your correction factor to ensure it safely brings high blood sugars back into your target range. Keep in mind that the accuracy of your starting correction factor will only be as good as the accuracy of your TDD.

Follow these steps for testing:

- Start the test when your blood sugar is over 200 mg/dl (11.1 mmol), it has been at least 3 hours since you last ate, and at least 5 hours since your last bolus
- Do not eat for 5 hours unless your blood sugar goes low
- Test at least once each hour
- Repeat the test until a correction factor consistently brings your blood sugar within 30 mg/dl (1.7 mmol) of your target by 5 hours without going low

Test Your Correction Factor

Use Workspace 13.3 to test your correction factor. Plot your readings to see whether your blood sugar is returning to target. Adjust and retest your factor as needed until your correction factor will consistently bring your blood sugar to target. Follow a successful test with another test to confirm it. Use Example 13.5 as your guide.

You can also determine your correction factor from your own experience. On three or four occasions when you have a high reading but no BOB, do not eat for 5 hours after you have taken a correction bolus. Test every hour or two. Then divide how many mg/dl (or mmol) you dropped during this period by the number of units you took to correct the high reading. Take the average of these results on different occasions and use it as your correction factor.

Testing Your Correction Factor With A Continuous Monitor

A continuous monitor makes it easy to test your correction factor. How a correction bolus affects your glucose can be clearly seen with readings displayed several times each hour during the four to five hours over which it works. With practice, you can use a continuous monitor to judge the impact of correction boluses quite accurately. It is also easier to identify what causes each high reading.

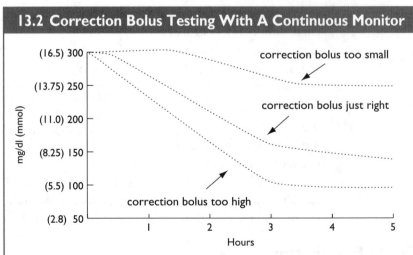

13.2 Correction Bolus Testing With A Continuous Monitor

correction bolus too small

correction bolus just right

correction bolus too high

mg/dl (mmol)

(16.5) 300
(13.75) 250
(11.0) 200
(8.25) 150
(5.5) 100
(2.8) 50

1   2   3   4   5
Hours

If your correction bolus is too small, lower your correction factor number. If too large, raise your correction factor number.

154

13.3 Test Your Correction Factor

1. Start the test when your blood sugar is 200 mg/dl (11.1 mmol) or higher, it has been 5 hrs or more since your last bolus, 3 or more hrs since you last ate, and you can wait 4 to 5 hours to eat.
2. Take the correction bolus your pump recommends.
3. Monitor each hour or more often if you appear to be dropping quickly.

Check your blood sugar hourly for 4 to 5 hrs and enter/plot your results here.

Start:	~ 1 hr later:	~ 2hrs later:	~ 3 hrs later:	~ 4 hrs later:	~ 5 hrs later:
_____ am/pm	_____ am/pm	_____ am/pm	_____ am/pm	_____ am/pm	_____ am/pm
_____ mg/dl	_____ mg/dl	_____ mg/dl	_____ mg/dl	_____ mg/dl	_____ mg/dl

Day: ____ / ____ / ____
Correction Factor:
1u / _____ mg/dl
Bolus: _____ u

Suggested Target Area

130

70

Hours

After 5 hours, is your blood sugar:

Over 30 mg/dl below target?	Within 30 mg/dl of target?	Over 30 mg/dl above target?
Treat the low. Retest with a larger correction factor. For example, if it was 1u for 50 mg/dl, try 1 u for 55 mg/dl.	Your correction factor appears to work. Retest to verify.	Correct the high. Retest with a smaller correction factor. For example, if it was 1u for 50 mg/dl, try 1 u for 45 mg/dl.

Adjust Your Doses If Correction Boluses Make Up Over 8% Of Your TDD

Correction boluses are intended to correct high readings that occur occasionally, not to be used several times a day to correct high readings. When several correction boluses are required each day, your basal rates or carb boluses are too low.

Many pumps track how much bolus insulin is used for correction boluses. (See your pump manual for how to access this information.) Correction boluses should make up no more than about 8% of your TDD over a few days' time.

When over 8% of your TDD is needed for correction boluses for several days, work the excess into your basal rates or carb boluses. Look in your charts or logbook for the times of the day when correction boluses are typically given. Compare the total insulin you use each day for basal rates and carb boluses. If one is significantly less than the other, move your excess correction bolus amount into this area. If the basal and carb bolus totals are similar, add half of the excess correction amount to each. Alternately, if blood sugars are highest at one time of the day, add some or all of the excess to the carb bolus and basal rates prior to this period. For example, if highs typically occur before breakfast, the night basal probably needs to be raised. If dinner readings are usually high, raise your afternoon basal rate or increase the carb bolus at lunch.

If you often require correction boluses to lower high readings that are caused when you overtreat lows, a lower TDD may be more appropriate. Here, excess insulin along with overtreating the lows is the main problem. By reducing the TDD and the number of lows, many highs and the need for correction boluses will also disappear.

Use Table 13.4 to check whether you are using too much insulin to bring down highs. The average amount of insulin used for correction boluses should make up no more than 8% of the TDD over a 7 day period. To check how you are doing, find your current average TDD for the last 7 days in the left column, and compare your current daily correction bolus total with the 8% maximum figure for this total in the right column.

13.4 Keep Correction Boluses Less Than 8%	
If Your TDD is:	**Correction boluses should make up no more than:**
10 u	0.8 u/day
20 u	1.6 u/day
30 u	2.4 u/day
40 u	3.2 u/day
50 u	4.0 u/day
60 u	4.8 u/day
70 u	5.6 u/day
80 u	6.4 u/day
90 u	7.2 u/day
100 u	8.0 u/day

Combine Carb And Correction Boluses

When a reading is high before a meal, one way to bring it down quickly is to combine your correction bolus with a carb bolus for the meal. Put your blood sugar

13.5 Example: Elaine Tests Her Correction Factor

Elaine tested her basal rates recently and knew they kept her blood sugar level when she was not eating. On Tuesday at noon, she had a pasta dish at a restaurant and underestimated how many carbs she ate. At 5 p.m. when she had a chance to check her blood sugar, her reading was 328 mg/dl (18 mmol). It had been 5 hours since her last bolus and she was able to skip dinner that evening, so she decided it would be a good time to test her correction factor. Her correction factor is 1 unit for every 50 mg/dl (2.8 mmol) above her target of 100 mg/dl (5.6 mmol), so she gave a correction bolus of 4.6 units to lower her blood sugar 228 mg/dl (12.7 mmol).

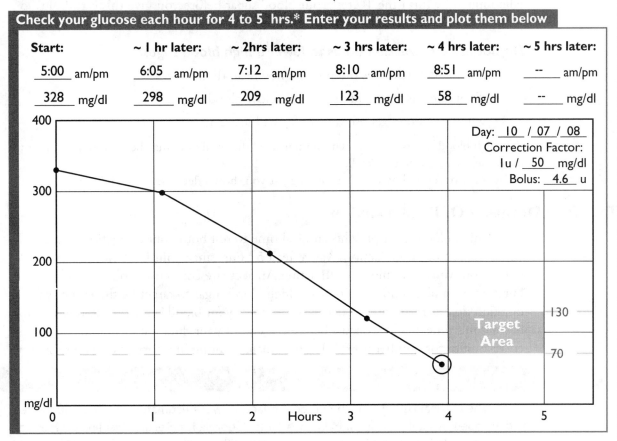

Check your glucose each hour for 4 to 5 hrs.* Enter your results and plot them below

Start:	**~ 1 hr later:**	**~ 2hrs later:**	**~ 3 hrs later:**	**~ 4 hrs later:**	**~ 5 hrs later:**
5:00 am/pm	6:05 am/pm	7:12 am/pm	8:10 am/pm	8:51 am/pm	-- am/pm
328 mg/dl	298 mg/dl	209 mg/dl	123 mg/dl	58 mg/dl	-- mg/dl

Day: 10 / 07 / 08
Correction Factor:
1u / 50 mg/dl
Bolus: 4.6 u

Elaine checked her blood sugar each hour. She had already gone low at 58 mg/dl (3.2 mmol) less than 4 hours later. After treating the low, she decided to raise her correction factor to 1 unit for each 55 mg/dl (3.1 mmol) and retest on another day.

reading and how many carbs you will eat into your pump, and let the pump recommend a combined carb and correction bolus minus any BOB. Take this combined bolus, but wait to eat until your blood sugar is below 150 mg/dl (8.3 mmol) to reduce glucose exposure or the time spent at an elevated reading.

Just remember to eat at the planned time to avoid a low blood sugar. Set an alarm so that you do not delay eating any longer than planned, especially if you take a walk while waiting. Recheck your blood sugar within an hour to determine its effect or, if wearing a continuous monitor, watch your trend line.

Delayed eating can cause severe hypoglycemia, so do not use this method if you have hypoglycemia unawareness or frequent lows. Here, it is safer to take only the correction bolus to allow for a partial drop in your blood sugar, and then give the carb bolus 15 to 20 minutes before eating, even though your blood sugar will not have fallen much by this time. Retest your blood sugar before you give this carb bolus so your pump can accurately calculate a new carb bolus with the BOB.

Do not use a correction bolus to lower a high blood sugar:

- if your high readings often come down on their own ★
- if you are having frequent or severe low blood sugars +
- when pending exercise or activity will lower it

★ If high blood sugars come down on their own, the basal rates may be set too high or a carb factor number may be too small.

+ Frequent or severe low blood sugars suggest you should decrease your TDD immediately.

Test Your Duration Of Insulin Action

A high blood sugar presents an ideal time to test both your correction factor and your duration of insulin action. Wait at least 5 hours since your last bolus to start this test so you won't have much BOB acting. An accurate correction bolus and a correct duration of insulin action will return a high blood sugar to target by the end of your duration time period with no excess lowering of your blood sugar during the 2 hours beyond this time. If a low occurs before the end of your duration of insulin action, your correction factor number is probably too small, resulting in a correction bolus that is too

---

13.6 The Original 1500 Rule

The original rule by which correction factors were estimated was the 1500 Rule developed by Paul Davidson, M.D. in Atlanta, Georgia for Regular Insulin.[78, 79] He created this rule based on his clinical experience with people having diabetes. With rapid insulin now used by most pumpers, we find that the numbers 1800 and 2000[80] work better because of the difference in action times. In 2003, Dr. Davidson reviewed the insulin settings actually used by his pumpers and found that for those who were in very good control, the number 1716 was their average numerator or number into which their TDD was divided to provide a good correction factor. He then revised his 1500 Rule to a 1700 Rule. We prefer to use a 2000 Rule because we find that it works well and is also more cautious, giving a slightly smaller number of units for correction boluses when readings are high.

large (or the basal rate may be too high). If a low occurs after the end of your duration of insulin action, either the duration is too short (usually at least 4.5 to 6 hours is appropriate) or the basal rate may be too high and needs retesting. Test the basal rate first to ensure it is accurate before testing your correction bolus. See pages 43-47 for more information on the DIA.

Tips On Correction Doses

• An accurate correction bolus should lower a high blood sugar to within 30 mg/dl (1.7 mmol) of your target blood sugar after five hours.

• If you use more than one correction factor for the day, they will usually be close in number to each other through the day. If they vary quite a bit, retest your basal rates to be sure they have been correctly set.

• Be careful, though, when correcting high readings at bedtime. Consider use of a larger correction factor near bedtime to reduce the size of correction boluses and lessen the risk of night lows. Consider setting an alarm for 2 a.m. to check your blood sugar or use a continuous monitor.

• If your correction factor differs significantly from the amount predicted in Tables 10.4, 10.6, and 10.7, your TDD or your basal rates may be incorrect. Retest to ensure this is not the case.

• Certain situations require correction boluses that are larger than usual. An extremely high blood sugar, ketoacidosis, an infection, use of prednisone, or an injection of cortisone can cause insulin resistance and make your blood sugar difficult to bring down. Take the correction bolus recommended by your pump or your correction bolus scale, but don't be surprised if it doesn't bring you down to target. Call your physician for advice in this situation.

• If an unexpected high reading occurs, consider whether you have a problem in insulin delivery or your insulin is bad. If in doubt, always use an insulin injection from a new bottle of insulin, then change your infusion set and reservoir.

• Loss of weight and increased activity will lower the TDD, causing the blood sugar to fall farther per unit of insulin. This means you will need to raise your correction factor.

• If high readings often fail to drop to your target after correction boluses, lower your correction factor number, usually by 5 mg/dl (0.3 mmol), to increase make your correction boluses larger.

• If high readings often go low after correction boluses, raise your correction factor number, usually by 5 mg/dl (0.3 mmol), to make your correction boluses smaller.

Your correction factor should bring a high reading down to target over about 5 hours.

13.7 Wait To Eat When You Are High

When a BG is high before a meal, how soon you eat determines your exposure to glucose. For highs, take a bolus that includes carb and correction coverage, then wait to eat, if possible, until your blood sugar comes down to lessen glucose exposure.

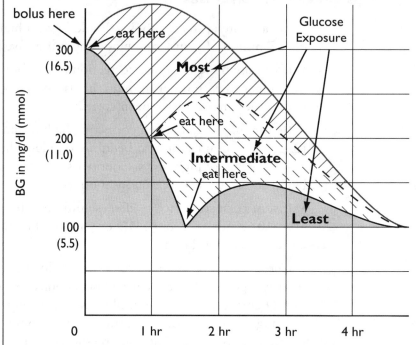

Caution: Delayed eating is the most common cause of severe hypoglycemia. Do not delay eating, even when high, if you may become distracted and not eat. It may help to set a timer to remind yourself to eat, but do not ignore it!

Quick Check: Do your correction boluses make up less than 8% of your TDD?

A stumble may prevent a fall.

Fuller Thomas

Lifestyle Issues In Control

When blood sugars are out of control with high or low readings at the same time each day, a solution is usually easy to track down and apply through insulin adjustments. On the other hand, truly erratic blood sugars with readings that stray out of target range at various times of the day have little pattern.

Lifestyle issues, such as pain, stress, skipping meal boluses, taking boluses too late, overeating, or not monitoring can all contribute to a loss of control. Work to avoid mismatches between insulin need and insulin delivery by dealing with these habits and lifestyle issues first.

This chapter addresses these lifestyle issues

- Inaccurate carb counting
- Carb boluses taken late or not at all
- Eating types or amounts of foods that create control problems
- Overtreating lows and fear of lows
- Erratic schedules
- Other circumstances

Issues related to natural causes, habits, or a lack of habit can all impact your readings. Some circumstances may be straightforward and clearly indicate that habits or insulin doses need to change, while others take time to figure out. Some require a periodic adjustment in your doses while others necessitate immediate and large changes in basal and bolus doses.

A little detective work and some patience will often uncover the likely sources for out-of-control blood sugars. This chapter deals with frequently encountered lifestyle issues that can impact your control. Assess lifestyle-related issues by answering the questions in Table 14.1 and try the suggestions below to minimize these issues.

Carb Counting Errors

About half of the insulin you need each day is used to cover meals and snacks. Variety in types of foods, amounts eaten, or meal times make establishing accurate boluses harder to achieve. Any mismatch between carbs and carb boluses will cause readings to stray outside your target range, especially if your carb factor is not yet accurate or your carb counting is not yet precise. If basal testing shows your basal rates are good but your blood sugar becomes erratic when you eat, you are probably not matching carbs with carb boluses well. Not knowing how many carbs are in typical food servings, not learning how to measure carbs, and eating out frequently can all create problems.

When a blood sugar goes high after a meal, many people think, "I shouldn't have eaten so much." This may be an accurate assessment of the problem, but a different approach is to think, "Next time I'll take enough insulin to cover those carbs!" Skimping on insulin only makes the effects of overeating worse. Many people eat a relatively small number of foods over and over again. As you learn the carb counts in these foods, the more exact your carb boluses for these foods will become. It is important to make carb intake consistent and to cover carbs with appropriate boluses.

Refresh your carb counting skills and adjust your boluses or diet as needed based on the records you keep. Start by testing before, two hours after, and four hours after meals. Record your results for a week or two to find how high or low blood sugars may relate to particular meals. Mark meals that need refiguring so that you can take a better matched bolus for them next time. Table 14.2 provides a way to estimate how many carbs you did not bolus for when your reading goes high after a meal.

14.2 How Many Carbs Were Not Covered?

When you have a high reading before a meal or at bedtime, this table estimates how many carbs in the previous meal were not covered by a bolus.

1. Find your glucose reading on the left.
2. Look under your weight to find the approximate carbs not covered.

Number Of Carbs Not Covered

Glucose Reading	100 lbs (45 kg)	150 lbs (68 kg)	200 lbs (91 kg)
140 mg/dl (2.2 mmol)	8	10	13
180 mg/dl (4.4 mmol)	16	20	27
220 mg/dl (6.6 mmol)	24	30	40
260 mg/dl (8.8 mmol)	32	40	53
300 mg/dl (11.0 mmol)	40	50	67
340 mg/dl (13.2 mmol)	48	60	80
380 mg/dl (15.4 mmol)	56	70	93
420 mg/dl (17.6 mmol)	64	80	107

This table assumes that your control is generally good, that your basal rates keep your blood sugar flat when you do not eat, and that you have not had a recent low blood sugar.

© 2006 Diabetes Services, Inc.

Carb Counting Tips

- Review how to count carbs with your dietitian or diabetes educator and review Chapter 7 on carb counting. Use a carb database in your pump or PDA, food labels, books, measuring cups and spoons, a calculator and gram scale to improve your accuracy.

- Count your carbs carefully for awhile. Eat meals with the same amount of carb at the same time each day until you see a pattern developing and adjust your basals or carb boluses to stabilize your readings. Vary carbs only after you establish good control.

- If you eat out often, try eating a favorite meal at the same restaurant several times until you learn how to best cover it. Test before, two hours after and four hours after eating. A few tries will reveal the size of the carb bolus you need for that meal.

- *The Guide To Healthy Restaurant Eating, Eat Out, Eat Right*, and *Calorie King's Guide To Calories, Fat, and Carbohydrates* listed on page 76 are very handy books to have for eating out. They list foods available in fast food and chain restaurants and tell how many grams of carbohydrate per portion they contain. You may need to verify their values as they affect you, but they make a good place to start.

Late Or Missed Carb Boluses

Most carbs raise the blood sugar far more quickly than "rapid" insulin can lower it. Giving boluses after eating almost always creates extreme spikes in the blood sugar an hour or two later unless a medication like Symlin is used to delay absorption of these carbs. Delayed boluses are sometimes necessary, such as if a child refuses to eat what the parent serves or when an adult has gastroparesis that delays food absorption. Taking boluses as you begin to eat is the most convenient timing and is better than taking them afterward for avoiding spikes. However, in most cases, control is greatly improved by giving boluses at least 15 to 20 minutes before eating when the blood sugar is in your target range.

If your pump history shows your TDD to be erratic from day to day or that relatively little insulin is being used to cover carbs, this suggests that forgetfulness may be an issue. If it is, use the excellent built-in reminders in your pump that will alarm if a bolus is not given at a certain time of day. As an alternative, set a reminder in your pump to alarm at the time of day when you usually eat. If you cannot remember if you gave a bolus, check your pump history to see when the last bolus was given.

If you are forgetting boluses, slow down. Enjoy eating and feel better by covering the food you eat with appropriate boluses. With diabetes, it makes sense to bolus for every carb you eat, just as your pancreas would do if it still produced insulin. Be sure to take the time to bolus, even if only a small amount, for every meal or snack you eat. If anger about having diabetes is causing you to skip boluses, this only makes you and those around you miserable, and you pay the ultimate price.

Unusual Food Effects

Some foods have unexpected effects on the blood sugar. For example, candies or foods sweetened with sorbitol may send the blood sugar higher than expected. Chips and fried foods often raise blood sugar readings more than their carb count would indicate because the type of fat in them creates resistance to insulin for a few hours.

Research has shown that pizza can raise the sugar higher, later and longer than the carb content suggests it should,[71] confirming the experience many people have had with it. A pizza that is lower in fat, such as a vegetarian one, or some particular brands of pizza often do not raise the blood sugar as high. Pasta may have a lingering effect on the blood sugar and cause a high as much as eight hours later. Pasta and pizza can even cause a low if the meal bolus peaks ahead of the digesting carbohydrate. Try a combo or dual wave bolus to match this digestion action. Look for any unusual rise or lingering low in your blood sugar when you eat foods such as these, and adjust your carb boluses or food choices appropriately.

Other Food And Carb Bolus Tips

- Write down all the foods you eat on your charts, not just the carbs. Record brand names and quantities if you think a particular food has an unwanted effect on your blood sugar. Compare your readings after eating these foods to those after other meals with similar carb amounts to see whether there may be a difference.

- If you suspect a particular food, even cheese or meat, is affecting your blood sugar, experiment by omitting it or eating less to see if your readings improve.

- Experiment with combination or dual wave boluses to see if they allow you to keep your blood sugar on target when you eat foods that cause your blood sugar to rise later than expected.

- Make an appointment with your dietitian, diabetes educator, or physician to sort problems out. Bring a three-day food diary to show some of your results.

Fear Of Lows

Hypophobia or excessive fear of lows may lead to underdosing. This can cause harm when basals and boluses are underdosed so much that highs become common. Someone who is afraid of lows may not fully realize the effect this fear is having. One pumper calls it being "gun shy". He had gotten into the habit of avoiding carb and correction boluses that would bring him to target, partly because he felt he was too busy at his competitive, exacting job to keep track of his blood sugars. As a result, his A1c hovered around 9% until he had a hemorrhage in one eye. He finally realized it was time to improve his control, bring down his A1c, and reduce his risk for eye and other complications. His began to test more often and learned to fully utilize the BOB feature in his pump. This allowed him to bring his A1c down into the upper 6% range with no serious hypoglycemia.

Erratic Schedules

If your work or school schedule is erratic or you eat or exercise irregularly, the source of ups and downs in your blood sugar readings is not hard to find. Perhaps you have started a new job, added exercise to an already jumbled schedule, or changed your meal or sleep times. A variable lifestyle can challenge anyone's management skills.

A consistent lifestyle makes it easier to set appropriate insulin doses. Try to create a more stable lifestyle. If this improves your control, you can gradually reintroduce variability as you master how to adjust your insulin doses for it. You can handle changes better once you have a baseline of more consistent blood sugar readings. A flexible lifestyle requires frequent testing, consistent recording of variables that affect the blood sugar, and appropriate basal and bolus adjustments. If regulating your lifestyle is not possible, take the steps to learn how to adjust your basals and boluses to match your lifestyle. A continuous monitor can do wonders in situations like this, although it does add some extra tasks to your day.

Schedule Tips

- Keep good records and routinely review them when your control is not optimum.
- Record your blood sugar results, carb intake, insulin doses, and the timing for each. Make notes on your charts about stress, exercise, pain, sleep, or work that may affect your readings. This is vital to cope with a variable lifestyle and make reasonable adjustments. Improvements are usually evident within a week or two.
- Keep regular mealtimes. Monitor before and two hours and four hours after meals.
- When possible, eat meals with the same number of carbs at the same time of day while you are smoothing out your life.
- Exercise at regular times. Note whether the type, amount, or timing of your exercise affects your blood sugar. Make notes on how to avoid lows after exercise.
- If you work an overnight shift, discuss with your doctor how to change your basals and boluses to match the change in schedule.
- If you work a rotating shift, seek help from your physician. You may want to use a single basal rate for the entire day for better control. Ask if you can work the same shift until your basal rate(s) and boluses have been correctly set.

Other Circumstances

Other internal and environmental circumstances can cause control problems and require a change in TDD, basals or boluses.

Menses

Women often find their blood sugar rises for a few days before their menstrual period begins. Some women need large adjustments in basal rate and bolus doses during these few days to avoid high readings, while others need only a small insulin adjustment or none at all. If you need a monthly basal change, set up an alternate basal profile to use for this time each month. The extra insulin may lessen premenstrual symptoms as well as improve blood sugar control. Increased insulin need may show up gradually but can return to normal quickly once the period begins, so it is important to reduce basal and bolus doses quickly when this occurs.

For most women, the required insulin adjustments are consistent from month to month. For some women, the required insulin dose adjustments will vary from one period to the next, especially if their period is irregular. Since it occurs monthly, it pays to be aware of the adjustment needed. Each woman needs to figure out her own pattern and be prepared to make these adjustments to stay in good control.

Illness

An illness places stress on the body and causes resistance to insulin. Bacterial infections like pneumonia, strep throat, an impacted wisdom tooth, a bladder infection, or a sinus infection can cause the need for insulin to double or triple as inflammatory particles like tumor necrosis factor and cytokines are released. A higher temporary basal profile and higher bolus doses are required to counteract this physical stress. Once an antibiotic is started, the increased need for basal and bolus doses will gradually return to normal over a few days as insulin sensitivity returns to normal.

Short viral illnesses like a cold or flu usually have a milder effect on the blood sugar. Control during these illnesses can be achieved with the use of additional correction boluses as needed. Raising the basal rates may or may not be needed. Viral illnesses that last longer, like hepatitis and mononucleosis, and periods of high fever during an illness are more likely to require increased basal and bolus doses.

Illnesses that cause vomiting or diarrhea may keep you from eating. If this occurs, carb boluses are not needed, but usual basal delivery is needed, along with any correction boluses required for high readings. Always drink plenty of liquids during illnesses of this type. Dehydration can be very serious if you don't drink enough to compensate for fever, diarrhea, or vomiting. If a low occurs when the stomach is unsettled, a half can of regular clear soda often works well or a half dose of glucagon can be given.

Frequent blood sugar testing is needed to determine how much extra insulin you require to speed your path back to better control so that your body will heal sooner. Call your health care professional for guidance any time you become ill and are unsure how to bring your readings under control. Be sure to test your blood sugar more often or have someone else test it during any illness.

Illnesses and ketoacidosis can be strikingly similar. The symptoms of ketoacidosis caused by an infusion site problem or bad insulin are nearly identical to those caused by a flu or food poisoning, and can easily masquerade as a viral or other illness. Check blood sugar and ketone levels at the start of an illness, frequently during its course, and at the first sign of nausea. If you take insulin for a high reading before going to sleep, always set an alarm and test two hours later to ensure your blood sugar is coming down. The presence of moderate or large levels of ketones in the urine or blood suggests that "an illness" may actually be a failure in insulin delivery. Presence of ketones will require that larger than normal correction boluses by injection or by pump once the delivery problem is resolved. Do not fall asleep before getting assistance if ketoacidosis is making you tired. See Chapter 19 for more information on ketoacidosis.

Stress

Stress caused by a specific problem, such as a friend or relative's extended illness, the death of a family member or friend, or problems at work or in a relationship can have dramatic effects on blood sugar control. Chronic stress, especially at low, persistent levels, is often hard to recognize due to its long-term nature. It may be difficult to tell exactly when it is affecting your blood sugar.

Fight-or-flight hormones help you remain alert and active during stress but they also raise your resistance to insulin. In addition, they cause extra glucose to be produced and released into the blood. High blood sugars, in turn, magnify emotional reactions and cause more stress hormones to be released. Elevated blood sugars cause depression and irritability that further impair the ability to deal with the stress at hand.

During stressful events, sleep may be lost, exercise and other calming activities put aside, and comfort foods high in sugar and fat eaten more often. Controlling the blood sugar during stress becomes difficult not only because glucose-raising hormones are released but because the order of daily life becomes disrupted.

The challenge of caring for diabetes can cause additional stress and frustration. During your first attempts at blood sugar control, you may become frustrated when improvements are slow in coming. Later on, readings that jump outside your target range can produce the stress response again.

Stress that is intermittent may be treated with correction boluses as needed since its effect is unpredictable from day to day. If you anticipate a limited period of stress, such as a day of tension-filled business meetings, check your blood sugar more often and take correction boluses as needed or use a temporary basal rate. If you encounter a longer period of stress, such as occurs when a family member is in the hospital, consider raising both your meal boluses and using a higher temporary basal profile to improve your control. Maintaining or increasing exercise during stress can lessen its impact significantly.

Feeling like a totally different person on vacation is often a good indication of the amount of stress you are under in your day-to-day life, especially if your blood sugar becomes easier to control. Listen to your family and friends who may see your stress before you do and alert you to the need to make changes or seek treatment.

Pain

Physical pain is often not recognized as the major player in blood sugar control that it is. When the body hurts, inflammatory particles like tumor necrosis factor and cytokines are released, causing pain but also making the body more resistant to insulin. A higher temporary basal profile and increased bolus insulin must be given in the presence of pain, whether caused by a chronic problem like arthritis, or a short-term situation like an illness, or an accident. The more pain, the more insulin you need for good control.

With care, pain can often be eliminated or greatly reduced. Talk with your physician about strategies to reduce pain and about how to adjust basals and boluses for episodes when pain may be more pronounced.

Steroids

Steroids like prednisone are often prescribed for poison ivy, allergic reactions to medications, and illnesses such as lupus, asthma, or arthritis. When a steroid medication is required, this can cause your need for insulin to rise dramatically. Larger boluses and a higher temporary basal rate will be required.

Oral steroids increase insulin requirements while they are being used and for a few days after they have been tapered off. When a short course of steroids is tapered off gradually over a few days, the need for extra insulin gradually disappears some three to five days after the last pill is taken. Test your blood sugar often during this time to raise your doses quickly in response to the rapid rise in blood sugar and to lower them slowly as the steroid medication is being tapered off.

When steroids are injected to curb a system-wide allergic reaction or directly into a joint to treat arthritis or injury, a large increase in insulin doses will be needed for at least three to five days. Gradually reduce insulin doses as the injection wears off. Newer injectable steroids remain active for longer periods and can raise insulin requirements dramatically for one to three weeks after being placed into a joint.

Any time you require injected or oral steroids, notify your diabetes team for guidance on the insulin adjustments that will be needed.

Over-The-Counter Products

Some over-the-counter vitamins and herbs can raise or lower the blood sugar dramatically. Products with ephedra, a form of speed, can lead to unexpected high blood sugars. The FDA removed ephedra from sale as a weight loss product after a number of deaths were reported, but it still may be sold for weight loss under other names, such as ma huang, Bringham tea, squaw tea, yellow horse, horsetail, sea grape, and others.

Chinese herbal products sold to treat diabetes often contain chlorpropamide, an old prescription medication called Diabenese that increases beta cell production of insulin. This diabetes medication can cause hypoglycemia in people with Type 2 diabetes who have residual beta cell activity. Be careful what you take and be watchful for unexpected effects on your blood sugar when you add any new supplement or herbal product.

Thyroid Disease

Thyroid disease is common in people with Type 1 and Type 2 diabetes for different reasons. Type 2 and thyroid disease become more prevalent as people age. Thyroid disease affects one of every 10 women over the age of 65. Thyroid disease is more common with Type 1 diabetes because it can also be caused by an autoimmune disorder.

In early stages of thyroid disease, excess thyroid hormone release may occur before the hormone level gradually falls below normal. The blood sugar may go higher when the thyroid is overactive and then go low as the thyroid becomes underactive. Because the transition into thyroid disease occurs gradually over weeks or months, it takes time to identify the thyroid as the source for the blood sugar problems it creates.

If your blood sugar control seems to have changed and you have thyroid symptoms such as nervousness, tiredness, sleeping difficulties, or are feeling hotter or colder than usual, have your thyroid checked. If you have a low thyroid level and are placed on thyroid medications, you will probably need to raise your basal rates and boluses slightly, especially if your insulin doses have been lowered gradually while your thyroid level decreased. If your thyroid is overactive and you receive radioactive iodine or medication or if you undergo surgery to reduce the excess thyroid production, you may need to lower your basal and bolus doses. Rely on your health professionals to advise you during these transition periods.

Gastroparesis

Gastroparesis is a partial paralysis of the intestine's normal peristaltic or wavelike motion after high glucose levels have damaged the nerves that control it. This damage often slows the absorption of food after meals. A low blood sugar may occur an hour or two after a meal bolus is given because the insulin acts before the food is absorbed. The blood sugar may then climb high over the next six to eight hours as delayed absorption occurs while little of the insulin from the meal bolus is left to cover it.

Symptoms that suggest the presence of gastroparesis include mild stomach pain, feeling full immediately after eating or for prolonged periods, excessive gas, bloating, nausea, and vomiting. Gastroparesis is a form of autonomic neuropathy and is often accompanied by other damage to the autonomic nerves, such as loss of constriction of the pupils to light, loss of variability in the heart rate, and the inability of the blood vessels to constrict when going from lying in bed to standing. Symptoms that suggest autonomic neuropathy include light-headedness when first standing up, a heart rate that does not rise appropriately when exercising, sweating after eating, and impotence.

Fortunately, simple tests can determine whether gastroparesis may be a source for erratic blood sugar control. One test involves lying down for a few minutes, checking the blood pressure, and then rechecking it after standing up. A drop of more than 20 points in the upper blood pressure number or more than 10 points in the lower blood pressure number upon standing suggests autonomic neuropathy.

Another way to detect autonomic neuropathy involves a standard EKG test. If the QTc interval, which measures how long it takes the heart muscle to lose its electrical charge after a heart beat, is longer than 0.44 seconds, autonomic neuropathy is likely. Other tests measure the heart rate variability seen after deep breathing or a Valsalva maneuver, or blood pressure variability while wearing a Holter monitor during daily activities over 24 hours.

Gastroparesis does change the TDD as much as it does the type and timing of carb boluses or basal rates. Someone who has gastroparesis may benefit from a higher than normal daytime basal rate, perhaps as high as 70% of the TDD, along with reduced boluses. These settings help balance the slowed digestion of carbs. A good alternative to raising the basal rate is to spread carb boluses over several hours using extended or combination boluses. This allows the bolus to match carb digestion more precisely. The time delay required for boluses can be determined from experience.

Gastroparesis symptoms may be reduced by acidophilus capsules or culture, yogurt with live culture, or by eating small meals that contain low glycemic index carbs which provide a more consistent rate of digestion. Several prescription medications are available to treat gastroparesis and stabilize digestion. Consult your physician if you believe gastroparesis may be contributing to your control problems.

Be kind, for everyone you meet is fighting a hard battle.

Plato

Control Tools And Tips

Everyone eventually faces a gradual or sudden loss of their hard-won control. Basal and bolus settings that once worked may need to be adjusted to accommodate a change in diet, activity, stress, weather, or other factors. A smart pump simplifies the complex math required to calculate accurate boluses, yet a pump cannot do all the thinking nor prevent every control problem. You still need to know how to anticipate and solve problems to keep your blood sugars where you want them.

This chapter describes how to

- Make easy and safe insulin adjustments
- Use records to spot patterns
- Use pattern management for specific control problems
- Reduce high glucose exposure and variability
- Use Symlin or GLP-1 inhibitors to lower postmeal blood sugar

Exactly what is affecting your control can be hard to identify, even for those who live a relatively steady lifestyle. If your blood sugar rises or becomes erratic, be sure to consider any lifestyle issue discussed in the previous chapter that may be contributing, such as inaccurate carb counts, boluses not taken soon enough before meals, stress, or pain.

Even when lifestyle issues are at work, high or low blood sugars show that your pump settings are no longer ideal. Many pumpers spend weeks or years in poor control because they do not stop and realize they need to adjust their doses. They may have become accustomed to poor control, not noticed their blood sugar has worsened, or not know how to change their pump settings to correct a problem.

If you are not yet confident about changing your pump settings, discuss any control issue with a diabetes expert who can assist you, teach you, and get you back on track quickly. Do not keep doing the same things you've always done and expect different results. When you are open to help and ask for it, solutions come your way. Allow diabetes professionals to help you and learn better management skills from these encounters. Table 15.1 lists ten steps to take that can improve your control.

For Major Control Problems, Adjust Your TDD

Major control problems, such as a high A1c or frequent or severe lows, are best dealt with by raising or lowering your average TDD and then using this new TDD to determine new basal rates and carb and correction factors. Table 15.2 lists control problems that may be similar to your own and provides suggestions for how to adjust your TDD for them. Choose one of the quick adjustments recommended and try it for the problem you are having. More specific adjustments for problem patterns are covered in Chapters 18 and 20.

Adjust your current TDD by increasing or decreasing it based on your A1c and whether the major problem you are having is too many highs or too many lows. Raise your TDD if you have too many highs and lower it if lows are the primary problem. Always try to get rid of lows first by appropriate reductions in your doses, then go after the highs. Your revised TDD can be used to estimate more appropriate basal rates, carb factor, and correction factor from Table 10.4, 10.6 or 10.7.

If lows are your main problem, don't wait until your next clinic visit to lower your basals or boluses. Frequent or severe lows need to be dealt with immediately to avoid serious consequences. Unless caused by an obvious problem, such as bolusing for a meal but not eating, frequent lows indicate that your TDD needs to be lowered. If you have frequent, mild lows, a 5% reduction in your TDD will help. For frequent or severe lows, a reduction of 10% or more may solve the problem. Remember that lows include not only low readings on your meter but all lows that you treated based on your symptoms, whether a test was done at the time or not. (Another reason to keep good records!) Be sure to let your doctor know about all your lows, whether you tested to confirm it or not.

15.1 Ten Steps To Successful Control
1. Keep detailed records to make solutions easier to find.
2. Review records regularly and pay special attention to problems that repeat.
3. Spot problems early before they get big.
4. Work on one problem at a time.
5. Keep making changes until control improves.
6. Learn from the things that did not work.
7. Know yourself. Recognize stressors and adjust your insulin to compensate.
8. Ask your doctor or diabetes educator for ideas if you run out of them.
9. Do not expect perfection. Just get more of your readings right.
10. Keep improving and celebrate successes!

When both highs and lows are happening, many pumpers have difficulty deciding whether their problem stems from too little or too much insulin.

To decide, look at:

1. Your A1c

2. How often you have lows (both on your meter and those you treat but do not test for) and highs each week

15.2 You Have A Control Problem When....

Lows	Make Quick Adjustments:
You go lower than 70 mg/dl (3.8 mmol) more than once every other day.	Lower your TDD by 5%.*
Your readings often fall below 50 mg/dl (2.7 mmol).	Lower your TDD by 10%.*
Highs	
Your A1c is above 7.5%.	Raise your TDD (basals or boluses) by the amounts suggested in Table 15.3.
Your glucose is often above 140 mg/dl (7.8 mmol) before eating.	Raise your basal by 5%.*
Your glucose often rises more than 80 mg/dl (4.4 mmol) above its start at 2 hours after eating.	Raise your carb bolus by 5%*, take bolus earlier, or lower amount of carb.
Your readings are often above 200 mg/dl (11.1 mmol).	Raise your TDD and basals by 10%.
The average glucose on your meter is above 170 mg/dl (9.4 mmol).	Raise your TDD by 5%.*
When the amount of insulin used for correction boluses averages more than 8% of your TDD.	Shift any amount of correction bolus above 8% into basals or boluses.
You have sudden unexplained highs.	Check infusion set/site and insulin.
Erratic Readings	
Your blood sugars seem to follow no pattern.	Lower your TDD, count carbs accurately, check your insulin and infusion site.
Your TDD is not consistent from day to day.	Live a more consistent lifestyle and be sure to take a bolus for every bite.

To lower your TDD, check your basal/bolus balance and reduce both if they are about equal or the one that is largest if they are not equal. To raise your TDD, check your basal bolus/balance and increase both if they are about equal, or the smallest if they are not equal.

*See Table 10.2

3. Whether lows lead to highs or highs lead to lows. Compare each week how many readings are below 70 mg/dl (3.9 mmol) and above 180 or 200 mg/dl (10 or 11 mmol).

4. Specific patterns in your readings

Ask your family and friends to share their observations on your control and insulin doses. Get regular A1c tests at your doctor's office or with one of today's accurate at-home A1c kits. If your A1c is above 8% and you have few lows, you certainly require

15.3 How Much To Raise Your TDD When Your A1c Is High

Work first to eliminate any frequent or severe lows. Once this is done, this table provides a safe guide to how much to increase your current TDD to bring you about half way toward an A1c of 6.5% when a recent A1c is found to be high. Find your current TDD and your approximate average plasma glucose level and A1c. Move down and to the right and this is the amount to add to your current TDD

Approx. Avg Plasma Glucose mg/dl (mmol)	A1c	Total Daily Dose (TDD)								
		20	25	30	35	40	50	60	80	100
170 (9.5)	7%	0.4 u	0.5 u	0.6 u	0.7 u	0.8 u	1.0 u	1.2 u	1.6 u	2.0 u
205 (11.5)	8%	1.1 u	1.4 u	1.7 u	1.9 u	2.2 u	2.8 u	3.3 u	4.4 u	5.5 u
240 (13.5)	9%	1.8 u	2.3 u	2.7 u	3.2 u	3.6 u	4.5 u	5.4 u	7.2 u	9.0 u
275 (15.5)	10%	2.5 u	3.1 u	3.8 u	4.4 u	5.0 u	6.3 u	7.5 u	10 u	13 u
310 (17.5)	11%	3.2 u	4.0 u	4.8 u	5.6 u	6.4 u	8.0 u	9.6 u	13 u	16 u
345 (19.5)	12%	3.9 u	4.9 u	5.85 u	6.8 u	7.8 u	9.8 u	12 u	15 u	20 u

Thanks to Mark Crandall for his contributions to this table.

a higher TDD for your current lifestyle. Make any lifestyle changes that are needed, such as to stop drinking regular sodas, or go ahead and increase your TDD.

With infrequent lows, and an elevated A1c or a high average glucose on your meter, use Table 15.3 to quickly estimate how much to raise your TDD. These suggested increases in TDD provide about half of the total increase in insulin you will likely need. Of course, an increase would not be as large if you also decide to lower your carb intake or increase exercise. Monitor your progress toward improved control by writing down on a calendar the 7 or 14 day average glucose from your meter each week, along with how many glucose tests were done.

If you have many high readings in the upper 100's and low 200's mg/dl (10 to 12 mmol) but rarely have a low, a 5% increase in your TDD is appropriate (see Table 10.2). On the other hand, if your readings are often in the high 200's and 300's mg/dl (15 to 17 mmol) a 10% or greater rise in your TDD will be needed. If you are concerned that a 10% increase may be too much, raise your TDD by 5% and give this a few days to see how your blood sugar responds. If your readings remain high, increase your TDD again.

However, if both highs and lows are common, get rid of the lows first. If many lows are followed by highs, lower your TDD by at least 5% and review what you eat to treat these lows.

Monitor your glucose variability by checking your standard deviation over the past week with software or one of the new meters that does this. Your SD should be less than half of your average blood sugar. For example, for an average blood sugar of 170 mg/dl (9.4 mmol), the SD should be less than 85 mg/dl (4.7 mmol). Keep a record:

My last A1c was ____% on ___/___/___

My A1c target is ____%

My average meter blood glucose is ____mg/dl on ___/___/___

My average meter target is ____mg/dl with a SD target of ____mg/dl

Check Your Basal/Bolus Balance

Once you have a new TDD, most pumpers will want to give half this total dose for the day in their basal rates and the other half as carb and correction boluses. Correction boluses should generally average less than 8% of the TDD when control is optimum and sufficient testing is done each day.

Some people, such as those eat a high carb diet and are very physically active may find that a lower basal percentage around 40% may work better. Others, such as those who are insulin resistant or those on a low carb diet, may find that a basal percentage of 60% or higher works better for them. Make sure you maintain your basal/bolus balance, that is, that your basal rates for the day should make up 40% to 65% of the TDD, with the rest given primarily as carb boluses, using Table 10.4, 10.6, or 10.7, depending on which basal percentage works best for you. These tables should be your guide any time you encounter control issues and need a fresh starting point to regain control.

Use Pattern Management For Smaller Adjustments

A change in TDD is the best way to treat major control problems. Once a lower or higher TDD begins to provide better control, make smaller basal or bolus adjustments to fine tune your readings through pattern management.

Correct control problem early, when solutions are easier to find!

To identify patterns, find the time of day when lows or highs tend to be most problematic. Work toward getting 5 out of 7 of your readings into your target range at each time of day over a week's time. Chapters 18 and 20 provide information on how to find and correct problem patterns.

The patterns in your readings can be found from records such as:

- *Smart Charts* that show blood sugars in a graphical format (plus details on carbs, insulin doses, stress, and activity),
- an enhanced logbook that has a pattern log at the bottom, or
- the memory in your meter or pump downloaded to a software program or to a written record using Worksheet 15.5).

The goal of pattern management is to determine at what period of the day an insulin change may be needed: breakfast to lunch, lunch to dinner, dinner to bed, or bed to breakfast. If a problem often occurs at one period of the day, work on this first by tweaking a particular basal rate or carb bolus.

Evaluate your control regularly to prevent small problems from becoming big ones. Choose one day of the week, such as Saturday or Sunday, to look at the last week's readings, and one time of the month, such as the 1st or the 15th, to review the last month's readings.

Find The Patterns In Your Meter

> ## 15.4 Checklist For Pattern Control
>
> 1. What is your target blood sugar before and after meals, and at bedtime?
>
> 2. Are you testing at least 4 to 6 times a day or using a continuous glucose monitor?
>
> 3. Do you record your blood sugar readings, carbs, boluses, and exercise?
>
> 4. Do you routinely look for patterns in your test results?
>
> 5. When a problem pattern appears, do you know how to adjust your basals or boluses, or make a lifestyle change that will correct it?
>
> 6. Have you tried adjusting your basal or bolus insulin doses, and did this adjustment solve the problem? If not, you may need to let a professional help you.

If you do not regularly write down your blood sugar readings, you can quickly find patterns in your readings from your meter's memory. Make copies of Table 15.5, then hit your meter's recall button and write down each blood sugar and the time and date each test was taken for at least the last seven days. Add any details you remember about particular highs or lows. Transfer this list to an enhanced logbook (see page 98) or *Smart Chart*. Then assess the last week's readings by completing these steps:

1. Select a target range for your blood sugar before each meal, at bedtime, and in the middle of the night.

2. Circle or mark all readings that are above or below your target ranges. Use one color or symbol for all readings above your target range and another for all readings below it.

3. To identify successes and problems in your patterns, use the bottom of the enhanced logbook on page 98 or Table 15.6 to add up how many readings are within, above, and below your target range at each time of day.

Correct unwanted patterns by adjusting insulin doses or changing the quantity of carbs eaten. For instance, high readings in the late afternoon may be caused by an inadequate basal delivery for several hours or by a lunch bolus that is too small. Test the afternoon basal rate first and adjust it upward if the test reveals it is too low. You may also need to change your carb choices or your carb factor at lunch.

15.5 Meter Download Sheet

1. Make sure the time and date in your meter is correctly set!

2. Record the blood sugars and averages from your meter in the form below.

3. Transfer them to Smart Charts or a logbook to look for patterns by time of day.

Record Blood Sugars

Downloaded ___ /___ / ___   14 Day Avg. = _____ mg/dl   ___ # of tests

at _____ am/pm   30 Day Avg. = _____ mg/dl   ___ # of tests

Date	Time	Blood Sugar
___ / ___ / ___	_____ am/pm	_____ mg/dl (mmol)
___ / ___ / ___	_____ am/pm	_____ mg/dl (mmol)
___ / ___ / ___	_____ am/pm	_____ mg/dl (mmol)
___ / ___ / ___	_____ am/pm	_____ mg/dl (mmol)
___ / ___ / ___	_____ am/pm	_____ mg/dl (mmol)
___ / ___ / ___	_____ am/pm	_____ mg/dl (mmol)
___ / ___ / ___	_____ am/pm	_____ mg/dl (mmol)
___ / ___ / ___	_____ am/pm	_____ mg/dl (mmol)
___ / ___ / ___	_____ am/pm	_____ mg/dl (mmol)
___ / ___ / ___	_____ am/pm	_____ mg/dl (mmol)
___ / ___ / ___	_____ am/pm	_____ mg/dl (mmol)
___ / ___ / ___	_____ am/pm	_____ mg/dl (mmol)
___ / ___ / ___	_____ am/pm	_____ mg/dl (mmol)
___ / ___ / ___	_____ am/pm	_____ mg/dl (mmol)
___ / ___ / ___	_____ am/pm	_____ mg/dl (mmol)
___ / ___ / ___	_____ am/pm	_____ mg/dl (mmol)
___ / ___ / ___	_____ am/pm	_____ mg/dl (mmol)
___ / ___ / ___	_____ am/pm	_____ mg/dl (mmol)
___ / ___ / ___	_____ am/pm	_____ mg/dl (mmol)
___ / ___ / ___	_____ am/pm	_____ mg/dl (mmol)

To correct unwanted patterns, consider:

1. a change in basal or bolus doses,

2. an increase or decrease in carb intake,

3. different types of carbs,

4. stress reduction,

5. or better adjustments for exercise or activity.

If your readings are relatively steady and usually within or close to your target range, smaller changes at specific times will be needed in your basal rates or boluses.

A carb factor might be changed by one point, a correction factor by two to five points, or a basal rate by 0.05 to 0.1 u/hr.

To improve your readings, always start with the smallest change in your doses that seems likely to help. Develop a plan and ask your doctor for assistance if you are not sure your approach makes sense. Keep in mind that mistakes may be made anytime you change insulin doses, but that the errors you make can also be educational. Making small changes usually lets you learn with greater safety.

15.6 Are Your Readings In Your Target Range?			
Mark how many of your blood sugars were below, within, and above your target range over the last week.			
My Target Range at:	**Below**	**In Target**	**Above**
Breakfast _____ to _____ mg/dl			
Lunch _____ to _____ mg/dl			
Dinner _____ to _____ mg/dl			
Bedtime _____ to _____ mg/dl			
2 am _____ to _____ mg/dl			

You may not discover your best doses until you test and adjust your doses several times with the help of your physician and health care team. Keep new settings for at least three to seven days before deciding whether they are ones you want to adopt. Do not fall asleep at the wheel and assume that any new doses will always be better.

Be sure to write down causes for all unusual highs or lows and all suspected lows at the time they happen, rather than trying to remember these specifics a week later. When you review your weekly charts or logbook to find patterns of high or low readings, check your notes for explanations for unusual high and low readings.

You want to be able to easily identify common patterns that are likely to appear in your readings. Common unwanted patterns are reviewed in Table 15.7 and in more

15.7 Some Patterns And Some Solutions

Pattern	Solution
Severe lows	Reduce bolus (or occasionally basal) insulin
Frequent lows	Reduce basal and/or boluses to lower TDD
Frequent Highs	Increase basal and/or boluses to raise TDD
Highs that follow lows	Treat lows with fewer fast carbs
Lows that follow highs	Reduce corr. factor for boluses at that time
Regular highs or lows at a particular time of day, such as high blood sugars when you wake up	Adjust basal and/or bolus
High or low blood sugars following a particular food, such as pizza or cereal	Recheck carb count, adjust bolus for that particular food, or try a different type of bolus (square wave, etc)
High or low readings after eating out	Refigure carb count and note where meal was eaten and record corrected carb count
Fall or rise in blood sugar with exercise	Try faster acting carb, adjust basal rates, or eat larger or smaller snacks
Difference between weekend and workday blood sugars	Use alternate basal rates and/or carb boluses for weekends and keep a record of what works
Stress, pain, medications affect your blood sugar	Recognize need for better coverage of these factors and increase insulin accordingly

detail in Chapters 18 and 20. Once you identify out-of-control readings and which ones form a pattern, use this information to improve your control. Good records and a systematic approach make control easier to achieve. Rewards are usually seen quickly, making it easier to continue.

Be neither bashful nor foolish about raising and lowering your doses!

Ways To Reduce Excess Glucose Exposure And Variability

High and erratic blood sugars are the major causes of complications and both must be reduced to improve health. Improving control means reducing excess glucose exposure as measured by an A1c or your average blood sugar from a meter, as well as excess glucose variability measured by your standard deviation or SD. Some meters and most software programs that download meters will show your SD.

The lower your standard deviation, the more stable your readings. A preliminary recommendation for a someone with Type 1 diabetes is to keep the standard deviation below 65 mg/dl (3.5 mmol) or to keep it less than half of the average blood sugar.

Currently the European Diabetes Policy Group recommends that postmeal blood sugars go no higher in Type 2 diabetes than 165 mg/dl (8.9 mmol) to prevent diabetes complications like retinopathy, and no higher than 135 mg/dl (7.5 mmol) to prevent heart attacks and strokes.[74] At times, your own blood sugar will certainly go higher than these values, but keep them in mind as goals to gradually work toward.

A pump has major advantages in the quest for better control. Unlike injections, a pump creates no depot of long-acting insulin under the skin where absorption may vary from changes in temperature or activity. The injection site stays in place for three days rather than being switched to a different location with different absorption characteristics several times a day. Only one rapid insulin is used with no mixing of different types of insulin. Insulin stacking is avoided through tracking of BOB. Precise delivery minimizes variations in insulin activity. Pumps have features like calculators, reminders, alarms, and suggested doses that make life easier and lead to better control.

The suggestions below provide ways to reduce glucose exposure and variability. Some are better for lowering the average blood sugar while others lessen variability.

Test Often Or Use A Continuous Monitor

Frequent testing provides the numbers needed to successfully lower your A1c. A study of 378 pumpers by Dr. Paul Davidson and Dr. Bruce Bode at their clinic in Atlanta showed that testing four tests a day brings the average A1c below 7% and six tests a day brings the average A1c down to the current recommended goal of 6.5%. Figure 15.8 shows a large, self-reported study of A1c values from 10,378 pumpers. Here, it took four to five tests a day to get an A1c of 7%.

Frequent monitoring is required for optimal control. Test before and two hours after meals, at

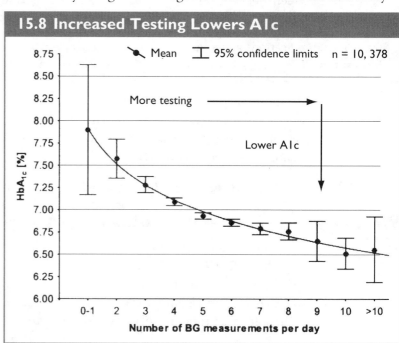

15.8 Increased Testing Lowers A1c

(Chart: Mean with 95% confidence limits, n = 10, 378. Y-axis: HbA1c [%], ranging 6.00 to 8.75. X-axis: Number of BG measurements per day, from 0-1 to >10. "More testing" arrow pointing right, "Lower A1c" arrow pointing down.)

bedtime, and occasionally at 2:00 a.m. on a day-to-day basis to know your blood sugar level, to identify what affects it, and to speed corrections. Regular testing reveals the larger picture of patterns in your readings and enables appropriate adjustments to be made. Knowing your blood sugars and patterns allows you to adjust carb amounts, bolus size and timing, basal rates, activity, stress, and other things that affect your control.

The more readings, the better your ability to make adjustments that improve your control. A continuous monitor provides the ideal tool for improved control, showing short-term blood sugar trends that help avoid many lows and highs. Action can be taken to correct the blood sugar before a problem becomes acute, making it easier to keep readings in an acceptable range. Continuous monitors lower both the A1c and the SD.

Use Symlin Or A GLP-1 Inhibitor To Lower Postmeal Spikes

Symlin When beta cells are destroyed by antibodies in Type 1 or Type 1.5 diabetes, the body actually loses two hormones, insulin and amylin, that are produced by the beta cells. Normally co-secreted with insulin in smaller amounts, amylin production is lost by the time destruction of beta cells is complete in Type 1 diabetes, while in Type 2 diabetes, its production tends to fall over time. Insulin was the first of the two to be discovered in 1922 because it is so critical to survival. However, amylin also plays an important role in glucose regulation. Like insulin, amylin appears to be released in small amounts all the time, with levels rising sharply at mealtime.

Amylin works by slowing digestion of foods and by suppressing an abnormal release of glucagon that causes glucose to be released by the liver. This occurs in many people with diabetes after meals. Amylin uses both of these actions to reduce glucose spiking after meals.

Use of Symlin, a modified form of amylin, can dramatically improve blood sugar control and reduce glucose variability in anyone whose insulin production is limited. When prescribed and given as an injection before meals, postmeal blood sugars become easier to control. Symlin decreases glucagon secretion, decreases appetite, delays gastric emptying and reduces sleepiness after eating. Less hunger is experienced after meals, enabling many people who are overweight to lose significant amounts of weight, yet normal weight individuals lose none. Symlin is undergoing studies seeking approval by the FDA as a weight loss drug.

However, Symlin may cause severe low blood sugars if carb boluses are not lowered on start day and during the first few days of Symlin use. If carb boluses are not reduced, up to 30% of users experience severe hypoglycemia within about 3 hours of eating. To lessen the risk of hypoglycemia, smaller starting doses of Symlin are gradually increased over time. As soon as Symlin is started, carb boluses are reduced by 30% to 50%. Then doses are adjusted based on pre and postmeal glucose results once a final Symlin dose is reached. Basal rates may also need to be lowered, especially if current basal doses make up more then 50% of the TDD. If weight loss occurs in someone who is overweight, both carb boluses and basal rates will need to be lowered as weight comes down.

Because Symlin is injected by a standard syringe, dosing is flexible. How much to use depends on what it is used for. For weight loss, maximum doses are usually best, while lower doses often work when the goal is to normalize after-meal blood sugars. The manufacturer recommends starting with 2.5 units and increasing to 5 units, then 7.5 units, and 10 units before each meal if no nausea is encountered for three days. For weight loss, the dose may occasionally need to go higher. An alternate way to increase is to start with 2 units before two or three meals a day and increase by 1 unit per meal every three days as long as nausea is not present.

If your goal is to reduce postmeal spiking and glucose variability, raise the Symlin dose by one unit every three days until you reach a dose where most of your postmeal blood sugar readings rise no more than 40 to 60 mg/dl (2.2 to 3.3 mmol) above where they started. The idea is to take enough to have good postmeal control (less variability) without overly delaying the normal rise in glucose after a meal (less problem correcting a low reading). Keep raising the Symlin or increasing meal boluses until postmeal readings are consistently less than 60 mg/dl (3.3 mmol) higher than the premeal readings.

The correct doses of Symlin and insulin will keep most postmeal readings from rising much while causing few lows. In many Type 1s, only 2 to 6 units taken two or three times a day before meals are required to do this. Symlin is usually taken just before meals that contain at least 250 calories or 30 grams of carbohydrate. If a dose is missed, wait until the next meal to take the regular scheduled dose.

The reduction in glucose spiking after meals can be striking at larger doses, with flat trend lines sometimes seen on a continuous monitor. If a large carb meal is consumed, however, the rise in the blood sugar may be seen several hours later, such as a high reading at breakfast the next morning after a large carb intake at dinner.

On a pump, the delay in digestion caused by Symlin often requires use of combo (some now, the rest over time) or extended boluses to match the slower rise in glucose after meals. If a blood sugar is low before a meal, raise it before taking Symlin. Reduce the meal bolus and give it as an extended bolus. If Symlin doses are missed for more than two or three days, do not restart with full doses. Instead, restart at a lower dose and build up to lessen the risk of hypoglycemia.

Excess doses are easy to spot by a feeling of fullness or nausea after the dose is given. Vomiting and diarrhea may also occur. If any side effects occur, lower the dose by one unit for a few days. Increase the dose again after there is no fullness or nausea for at least three days.

Symlin and the GLP-1 inhibitors discussed below will delay the digestion of all food, including the carbs you use to raise a low blood sugar. If a low occurs, use glucose tablets if available and chew them as long as possible to allow more glucose to be absorbed directly into the bloodstream. Be patient, as the rise in your glucose will also be slower because of Symlin. Likewise when lowering a high reading with insulin, it will take longer when food is still being absorbed.

Even though Symlin affects the blood sugar, it does nothing to control it. Your carb boluses and basal rates must still be adjusted to match the carb amounts and types that you eat. Once an effective dose of Symlin is found, adjust your boluses and basal rates as needed and be prepared to readjust periodically if you are losing weight.

> ## 15.10 Frustration
>
> Everyone who tries to improve control encounters frustration at times. Remember:
>
> - You are able to change your insulin doses, carb intake, and activity to improve your control.
> - Success will not come with every decision, but every decision improves your chances for learning and success.
> - Diabetes control is not the only important matter in your life.
> - Take a break when you need one and come back to the challenge refreshed.

GLP-1 Inhibitors One GLP-1 inhibitor, called Byetta, has received FDA approval and is currently available as a prescription for people with Type 2 diabetes who are not on insulin. Like Symlin, it is injected and slows food absorption. The GLP-1 inhibitors also stimulate insulin production and restore first phase insulin secretion. This combination decreases postmeal blood sugar and improves control. Whether they may delay progression of Type 2 diabetes is not yet known. They have multiple sites of action in the body and it will take time to be sure there are no unwanted long-term effects. Research has shown that people on Byetta eat about 20% less and often lose weight. Because of the similarity in action between GLP-1 inhibitors and Symlin, similar adjustments in pump doses would be required.

Count Carbs And Match Every Carb With A Bolus

A personalized carb factor and use of BOB improves the accuracy of carb bolus calculations, but accurate carb counting is required for this to work to lower the A1c and SD. The use of accurate carb counting can lower the A1c by 0.8% compared to simply guessing the size of a bolus needed to cover a meal.[76]

Most pumpers underestimate carbs. One study showed that pumpers underestimated the carbs in their meals by 30%. After attending a class in carb counting, they still underestimated carbs, but by only 17%.[77] To get the most out of your pump, enter into it exactly how many carbs you eat at each meal or snack so that it can give you a bolus to match the carbs well. Every snack or meal requires a bolus unless it is raising a low or balancing exercise. (Some smart pumps do not adjust active insulin or BOB for carbs. See page 48.)

Correct and timely carb boluses reduce postmeal spiking and eliminate the need to chase high readings. Some people find that eating fewer carbs at breakfast when insulin resistance may be higher helps their control. Carb intake can also be spread through the day using smaller meals plus snacks. Having fewer postmeal spikes and the highs and lows that go with them is a great way to reduce glucose variability.

Eat Healthy

If you eat foods high in calories, fat, and sugar, blood sugar control becomes more difficult. A healthy and balanced diet protects your health, reduces the need for insulin, and improves your A1c. It is not necessary to be a food purist. Instead, get rid of poor food choices one at a time and gradually select healthier foods – vegetables, fruits, and whole grains – that ease your path toward optimum control. Eat more fiber and lower glycemic index carbs to reduce spiking of the blood sugar after meals. Select foods that rank 60 or less on the glycemic index and, if you eat those that rank higher, eat only small amounts.

Take A Combined Bolus Early For Highs Before A Meal

When a premeal reading shows that your blood sugar is high, as often as possible take a combined carb and correction bolus and wait until your blood sugar has come down below 150 mg/dl (8.3 mmol) before eating as described in Fig. 13.7. Waiting to eat is not always possible or convenient, but it does lessen glucose exposure and avoids spiking to an even higher reading. If you can't wait to eat, choose a meal with fewer carbs or save the carbs to eat at the end of the meal.

Avoid Overtreating Lows

When you treat all lows with the exact number of carbs required to come back to target, you eliminate the highs caused by overtreatment. Use bolus tipping (see Textbox 5.5) on your pump or use a pump that tells you how many carbs you need when you are low.

Summary

Many of the ways to reduce glucose exposure also reduce variability. When you put the suggestions in this chapter into action, not only will you decrease the amount of time you stay at high blood sugar levels but you will also stabilize your blood sugar.

A good scare is worth more than good advice.

Edgar Watson Howe

Solutions For Lows

Mild lows may be annoying or embarrassing but a severe one can become frightening or dangerous. Most organs are able to switch from glucose to fat or protein for fuel during a low blood sugar, but the brain and nervous system cannot, depending instead on glucose as their source for fuel. Deprived of sufficient glucose, thinking and coordination become impaired and behavior changes.

This chapter discusses these aspects of hypoglycemia

- Symptoms
- Causes
- Treatment
- What the person with diabetes can do
- How others can help
- Prevention
- Hypoglycemia and driving

Even with a smart pump and extensive training, the most conscientious person with diabetes cannot prevent all lows. Testing your blood sugar frequently improves your chances of detecting a low in an early stage when symptoms are minimal. On a smart pump, bolus tipping (see Table 5.5) provides a way to identify a carb deficit before the blood sugar goes low and allows hypoglycemia to be prevented. A continuous monitor reveals blood sugar trends that, if paid attention to, can forewarn before a low actually occurs and alarms to warn of a low. Prevention or early treatment prevents mental confusion and minimizes release of stress hormones that cause the blood sugar to spike afterward.

If lows last too long or occur too often, the brain, nerve cells, heart, and blood vessels may suffer. Frequent lows impair short-term memory, especially for names and words, although this can be largely reversed by avoiding lows. Never accept a low blood sugar as harmless. Letting lows linger adds to the harm, so treat them quickly. On the other hand, avoid developing an obsessive fear of lows as this makes the goal of good control impossible. Realize that today's technology combined with an understanding of how to use insulin will allow you to master your control. Although some lows may be necessary as you strive to reduce glucose exposure, the risk lessens as you gain experience and as continuous monitors becomes more widely available.

Symptoms

Hypoglycemia symptoms vary from person to person and from event to event, depending on how often lows occur and how low the blood sugar falls. Symptoms usually start when the blood sugar goes below 55 or 65 mg/dl (3.1 to 3.6 mmol), although some people feel symptomatic at 90 mg/dl (5 mmol) and others will drop to 40 mg/dl (2.2 mmol) before any symptoms appear. Some symptoms are caused by release of stress hormones while others are caused when too little glucose reaches the brain and nervous system:

<table>
<tr><td>16.1 Clever Pump Tricks</td></tr>
<tr><td>Check Short Term Basal Versus Bolus

When a low blood sugar occurs, you want to know whether your basal or your bolus insulin caused the problem. One way to "measure" the relative effect of each is to add up all the bolus insulin taken in the previous 5 hours and compare this to the amount of basal insulin you have received during this time. Suspect the insulin (basal or bolus) that was a higher dosage during this time.</td></tr>
</table>

Symptoms Caused By Stress Hormone Release (~65 mg/dl or 3.6 mmol):

Sweating, shaking, irritability, fast heart rate, hunger, feeling amped or nervous, resisting help, tingling of the lips or fingers, nausea, vomiting

Symptoms Caused By A Lack Of Glucose In The Brain (~55 mg/dl or 3 mmol):

Confusion, poor concentration, mental dullness, blurred vision, sudden tiredness, headache, frequent sighing, inability to form words, silliness, yawning, seizure, coma

During a low blood sugar, you may shake, sweat, and feel disoriented, or you may feel rather normal. Symptoms become harder to recognize during exercise, or when someone is involved in a project, concentrating on something, drinking, or driving. Symptoms can be harder to recognize on a pump because the blood sugar may fall more gradually with fewer symptoms, but a slower fall also allows more time to recognize and respond to the low.

Even if you feel normal during a low, those around you will often notice changes in your personality or capabilities. A willingness to test is particularly important under these conditions. Be sure to check your blood sugar any time you suspect a low blood sugar or anyone around you suspects you are having one. When someone asks you to check your blood sugar, do so immediately and willingly. Refusing to do so is common since irritability and stubbornness occur early in the low. Always agree to test.

Nighttime Symptoms

Over half of all severe hypoglycemia occurs during sleep when symptoms are least likely to be recognized. Unrecognized night lows are the most common cause of hypoglycemia unawareness. The symptoms below are specific for night lows. If any of these wakes you up, check your blood sugar immediately or eat quick carbs and then test. Always keep fast-acting glucose close to your bed within easy reach.

Symptoms during the night:

- nightmares
- waking up very alert and finding it hard to go back to sleep
- waking with a fast pulse or heart rate
- waking up with your night clothes, sheets, or pillow damp with sweat
- waking up with a feeling that something isn't right

Symptoms the next morning that suggest a low occurred during the night:

- waking up "foggy-headed" or with a headache
- having an unusually high blood sugar after breakfast or before lunch
- having a small amount of ketones but no glucose in the morning urine
- a temporary loss of memory for words or names
- feeling worn out

Wearing a continuous monitor with an alarm for a low blood sugar or testing in the middle of sleep does wonders to identify and correct night lows. Any time that night lows occur, review causes and change your carb intake, insulin doses, or exercise to prevent them. Do extra testing until night lows are no longer a problem.

16.2 How To Prevent Night Lows

Low blood sugars often occur around 2 a.m. because the body is most sensitive to insulin between midnight and 3 a.m. In a person without diabetes, the body reduces the insulin level automatically at this time so that a low blood sugar will not occur. An insulin pump can be set to mimic this action, reducing basal insulin delivery around 2 a.m if the overall basals are set correctly.

If you suspect you are having lows at night, test at 2 a.m. for a few nights or wear a continuous monitor. If your blood sugar is low during the night, reduce your basal rate starting at 10 p.m. or earlier and then test at 2 a.m. until your nighttime blood sugar drops no more than 30 mg/dl (1.6 mmol) at any point during the night.

Triggers To Nighttime Lows

- Prolonged exercise or activity will cause the blood sugar to fall for 24 to 36 hours afterward. After a day of increased exercise or activity, reduce the carb bolus given for dinner and use a temporary basal rate reduction that evening and over night. Extra carbs at bedtime may also be needed to prevent an unexpected low.

- Covering a high bedtime blood sugar with too large a correction bolus is a common trigger for night lows. When you have a high reading near bedtime, allow your smart pump to calculate any BOB and recommend a dose. Then try a dose below this recommended amount. You can also use a larger correction factor or raise your target blood sugar in your pump during bedtime hours.

Prevention

The best approach for all lows is to prevent them in the first place. Important steps for prevention are listed in Table 16.4. Keep in mind that one low blood sugar increases the risk of another. The chance for having a followup low after an initial one is very high: 46 percent in the next 24 hours, 24 percent on the second day, and 12 percent on the third day after the original low.[78] Awareness of the extra risk that follows a first low can prevent a second one. Stress hormone release during the first low blood sugar reduces the body's stores for the next two to three days so symptoms during the second low will be milder and harder to recognize.

> ## 16.3 Good Control Starts By Stopping LOWS!
>
> When low blood sugars become frequent or severe, reduce your TDD by 10 percent. From this new TDD, calculate new basal rates and boluses, and establish a safer pattern.

After a low blood sugar happens, take steps to keep your blood sugar higher for the next 24 to 36 hours, such as setting a temporary basal that is 10% lower for much of this time, to avoid a second low. Alternatively, you may want to lower carb boluses by 20% or allow 10 to 15 grams of free carb into your usual boluses for 24 to 36 hours after a low.

Lows have many causes and this may take time to analyze and correct. Frequent or severe lows mean that too much insulin is being given, especially when lows occur within one to three hours after a bolus, when more than 15 grams of glucose is required to bring the blood sugar back to normal, or when lows occur during sleep or before breakfast. If one of these is happening, call your physician or health care team immediately to discuss an appropriate redistribution of your doses.

Lows are most likely

1. When too much insulin is taken
2. When a meal bolus is taken but the meal is missed, delayed, or interrupted
3. When carbs are counted incorrectly
4. When normal correction boluses are increased to hasten a fall in blood sugar
5. When the duration of insulin action is set too short and hides BOB
6. After drinking alcohol, especially on an empty stomach
7. During and after exercise, especially that night
8. On vacation when stress is reduced, activity is increased, or eating is irregular

Be alert for changes in your daily routine (travel, vacation, weight loss, stress, etc.) that may cause lows. People who exercise strenuously or for prolonged periods will benefit from frequent basal and bolus adjustments to match these changes in activity. More activity, less insulin. Less activity, more insulin. Alternate basal profiles can be set up to easily switch basal profiles for activity, menses, weekends, or vacations.

16.4 How To Prevent Lows

- Test often if you are unsure of your blood sugar. Use a continuous monitor.

- Eat every meal or snack that you have taken a bolus for.

- Count the carbs in each meal and match your carb bolus to the carb count, your carb factor, and your current blood sugar.

- Use your past experience to add a between-meal snack if needed or to adjust your insulin doses and carbohydrates at mealtime. For example, if low blood sugars often occur in the afternoon, either an afternoon snack, a smaller bolus for lunch, or a lower basal rate in the afternoon can help.

- Raise your premeal blood sugar target to 100 – 150 mg/dl (5.6 to 8.3 mmol) if you are having repeated lows. Reach this target by lowering your basal rates and raising your carb and correction factors.

- Test before, during, and after long or unusually strenuous periods of exercise. Activity can lower the blood sugar for as long as 36 hours afterwards.

- Always check blood sugars before driving and during long drives. The most serious consequences of a low blood sugar often occur on the highway. Keep glucose tabs in sight when going on trips and eat some before you start the car. Don't take chances, especially when traveling alone.

- Be careful when drinking alcohol. Excess alcohol shuts off the glucose normally released from the liver and makes a low more likely. Inebriation and hypoglycemia are hard to tell apart, so if you go low, you may be treated as being drunk rather than getting the medical help you need.

Reduce Your TDD

- when reactions are frequent or severe.

- as soon as you start planned or unplanned weight loss.

- when committing to a new and strenuous exercise activity.

- when stress levels drop (such as on vacation).

Reduce Your Carb Bolus By Raising Your Carb Factor

- if lows often occur within one to three hours after boluses.

- before, during and after exercise, especially if it is moderate or strenuous and lasts longer than 40 minutes.

- anytime daily activity, such as shopping or cleaning house, is increased.

Reduce Your Correction Bolus By Raising Your Correction Factor

- if lows often occur after you correct high blood sugars.

When making these changes call your physician/health care team to discuss whether your lowering of basals and boluses is reasonable.

Every time you test your blood sugar, check to see if you have any BOB that may push you low later. For instance, if your blood sugar is 120 mg/dl (6.7 mmol) two hours after a bolus, you may need to eat to avoid a pending low blood sugar. Different pumps show BOB differently, so be sure to learn how your pump displays this information. How to set an appropriate bolus duration time for different pumps is addressed in Figure 5.4, while testing of the duration of insulin action More information can be found at www.diabetesnet.com/diabetes_technology/dia.php on new pumps and DIA testing.

Treatment

Treat lows with products you find tasty and easy to keep on hand. You want carbs that will end the low and relieve symptoms quickly. You will feel better and your brain, muscles and other organs will thank you for rapidly resupplying the glucose they need. Quick treatment minimizes release of stress hormones and makes it less likely a high blood sugar will follow the low. It also preserves internal stores of stress hormones and makes it easier for you to recognize the next low.

16.5 Quick Carbs To Keep On Hand
Each provides 15 grams of quick carbs:
1   Tablespoon of honey
3   BD Glucose Tablets
3   Smartie Rolls (in cellophane)
4   CanAm Dex4® Glucose Tablets
5   Dextrosols Glucose Tablets
5   Wacky Wafers®
6   Sweet Tarts® (3 tabs/packet)
7   Pixy Stix
8   Sweet Tarts® (3/4" diam roll)
14   Smarties® (3/4"diam roll)

Glucose is the best treatment for a low. Referred to as glucose or dextrose on food labels, it can be found in glucose tablets, in certain candies like Sweet Tarts, and in certain drinks like Gatorade, which are all easy to keep on hand. These products act quickly and are excellent choices for raising the blood sugar. Table 16.5 lists a variety of quick carbs that contain 15 grams of fast carbs that will raise the blood sugar 45 to 75 mg/dl (2.5 to 4.2 mmol) in most adults.

Table sugar or sucrose in soft drinks and most candies is different from glucose or "blood sugar". Table sugar contains one glucose molecule and one fructose molecule. After it is broken down in the stomach, only half of its carbs are available as fast-acting glucose. Fruit juices provide a psychological lift, but are a poor choice for quick treatment of serious hypoglycemia, as are regular candy and desserts. The glycemic index in Table 7.14 provides a good guide for the best foods to use to treat lows. Foods with the highest glycemic index numbers will raise the blood sugar the fastest.

Avoid Panic So You Do Not Overtreat

The urge to overtreat lows is natural. Release of stress hormones during a low causes panic that may lead to overdosing on orange juice, chocolates, or the entire contents of your refrigerator. This makes your goal of stable blood sugars hard to achieve. If your blood sugar often goes high after lows, overtreatment is likely or stress hormone release is excessive. One reason to avoid letting panic take over is to avoid gaining excess weight from over-treating lows. If lows are frequent or severe, reduce your TDD and avoid losing this battle.

16.6 How Much 1 Gram Of Carbs May Raise Your BG	
If your weight is:	**1 gram will raise you about:**
50 lbs (23 kg)	8 mg/dl (0.44 mmol)
75 lbs (34 kg)	7 mg/dl (0.39 mmol)
90 lbs (41 kg)	6 mg/dl (0.33 mmol)
120 lbs (55 kg)	5 mg/dl (0.28 mmol)
160 lbs (73 kg)	4 mg/dl (0.22 mmol)
200 lbs (91 kg)	3 mg/dl (0.17 mmol)

© 2006 Diabetes Services, Inc.

Prepare for lows by having a predetermined quantity of quick carbs handy at your bedside, in your pocket or purse, at your desk, in the glove compartment or on the seat beside you, and where you exercise. A low does not mean unlimited treat time! Use your smart pump to determine how many carbs you actually need to counteract a low. Wait until your fast-acting carbs start to reduce your panic-driven appetite to avoid overcorrection.

Have A Treatment Plan

You may not be able to think clearly during a low, so you and your family or friends need to know ahead of time exactly what needs to be done, especially how much glucose is needed and where to find it. One gram of glucose raises the blood sugar about 4 mg/dl (.22 mmol) for most adults (see Table 16.6). A 5-gram glucose tablet should raise the blood sugar 15 to 25 mg/dl, depending on weight. Be sure to factor in recent activity and any BOB.

Know how many grams of carb are in each fast carb you typically use to better judge how many will be needed to counteract a particular low. Retest your blood sugar 15 to 20 minutes after treatment to ensure the low has been corrected.

Have 10 to 15 grams of quick carbs, such as glucose tablets, Sweet Tarts™ or honey. After this is consumed, an additional complex carb and protein snack, like peanut butter and crackers, can help keep the blood sugar from dropping later.

When a low happens four or five hours after the last bolus, only 15 or 20 grams of carbs would typically be needed. But if a low happens only two or three hours after the last bolus, there will be more BOB and more carbs will be required. Always check your current BOB when a test is done to determine how many carbs are needed if you are low or whether additional carbs may be needed to offset any BOB that is still working.

A recent bolus of insulin, extra exercise, or a missed meal may require that more carbs be eaten to treat a low. Both protein and complex carbs may help prevent a drop in blood sugar over time. Special nutrition bars like Extend contain raw cornstarch, a complex carbohydrate that breaks down slowly and provides another choice as a precautionary nighttime snack.

16.7 Treatment Plan For Hypoglycemia

1. Eat 15 to 20 grams of quick carbohydrates immediately. (See Table 16.5)

2. When your mind becomes clear, consider how much BOB is still active and decide how many more carbs you may need (See Table 5.5). Add slow acting carbohydrates and/or protein to keep you stable until your next meal. Cheese and crackers, bread with peanut butter, half an apple with cheese, a cup of milk, or other carb/protein combinations are good choices after eating the quick carbs.

3. Test your blood sugar 30 minutes later to make sure it has risen. Some pumps will remind you to do this. Repeat Step 1 if necessary.

4. After a moderate or severe low blood sugar has returned to target, wait 30 to 45 minutes before driving or operating any machinery. A return to normal coordination and thinking lags behind the return to a normal blood sugar.

When More Than 20 Grams of Quick Carbs Are Needed:

- you took a carb bolus for a meal but forgot to eat.

- you took a bolus too soon since your last bolus so you have BOB.

- you have been more physically active than you prepared for.

After you have a low, normal thinking and coordination will lag behind the return to a normal blood sugar. Wait 30 to 45 minutes after the blood sugar returns to normal before driving a car or operating machinery.

Things To Do To Minimize Hypoglycemia

- Always carry quick carbs like glucose tablets or sugar candy. Know how much to eat. Do not use chocolate – you may feel better but it's too slow for lows.

- Test if you are able. If not, have two glucose tabs and test ASAP but only after washing your hands free of the glucose!

- Wait about 15 to 20 minutes for fast carbs to work, then retest to ensure your blood sugar has risen. Retreat if necessary.

- Assume the primary responsibility for handling your own low blood sugars. This includes always being willing to accept help and advice from others.

- Use your mental radar to notice anything unusual. Does the world around you look normal? Do you feel normal? Test immediately if you have any doubts.

- Let your family, friends, and those you are with know about your diabetes and what they can do to help if you become confused or weak suddenly.

- Tell family and friends when you vary your regimen or lifestyle in ways that make you more vulnerable to lows. Share what is happening with your blood sugar control so that others will be prepared to help you if you need it.

- Be more watchful of lows and test more often any time you change your insulin doses, food choices, activity, or go on vacation.

- Be very careful when lows become frequent or you may be having night lows because these cause hypoglycemia unawareness. Lower your TDD immediately.

- If you ever become unconscious or too incoherent to treat a low, discuss this with your physician as soon as possible. You will likely need to change insulin doses or modify your lifestyle.

- Work with a physician who understands and specializes in insulin delivery to improve your control and reduce your risk for lows.

Treatment Of Severe Hypoglycemia

Severe hypoglycemia occurs when you can no longer handle a low by yourself. This becomes dangerous if it happens while driving, when you are alone, or if it results in loss of consciousness or convulsions. In one Danish study, severe hypoglycemia occurred in 40 percent of people with Type 1 diabetes. Those who had it experienced an episode about once every 9 months and unconsciousness occurred every two and a half years.[79]

For severe hypogly-cemia, glucagon is the best treatment. Glucagon is also made by the pancreas, but unlike insulin, it rapidly raises the blood sugar by releasing glucose stores from the liver.

16.8 Glucagon: How Much Do You Need?

Each 0.15 mg of glucagon or 1/6 of a standard dose raises the blood sugar 30 mg/dl! Avoid taking too much glucagon as this raises the blood sugar too high and may cause nausea.

An injection of glucagon can bring someone out of unconsciousness or a seizure, and can also be helpful if someone is resisting treatment due to hypoglycemia unawareness or if nausea does not allow carbs to be eaten.

Keep glucagon handy at all times. Glucagon kits are available by prescription and should be kept at home by everyone on insulin. A glucagon kit contains a syringe with saline and a small vial of dry glucagon powder that must be freshly mixed prior to injection. To prepare glucagon, inject the saline into the glass vial and shake the vial to suspend the glucagon. Draw the suspended glucagon back into the syringe for injection into the upper arm, leg or buttock.

Glucagon can be stored at room temperature or in the refrigerator. The expiration date should be checked periodically to ensure potency. Using out-of-date glucagon is always better than not using glucagon. Be sure that a family member or a friend has been trained in how and when to inject glucagon. Anyone who is likely to be present during a severe low blood sugar should be instructed by a Certified Diabetes Educator, a trained nurse, or a pharmacist on how to inject glucagon.

The dose in the vial is 1 mg. of glucagon. Half this dose is usually enough for many children or trim adults. A response should begin within 15 minutes.

If someone with diabetes is unconscious, assume this is caused by a low and treat it accordingly. If they do not respond to glucose or glucagon, call 911. This may also be necessary if the person having the low blood sugar is too irate or irrational to accept help and is larger or stronger than those trying to help. In an emergency, stay calm and keep your emotions under control. Tell the emergency operator right away that the person has diabetes, is on insulin, and appears to be having a severe low blood sugar. Give instructions, if needed, on how to get to your location. Let the paramedics who are well trained to do blood glucose tests, give carbohydrates or an injection of glucagon, or start IV glucose, take over.

16.9 Clever Pump Tricks

When You Overeat Carbs To Treat A Low

If you overeat when a low occurs, count the number of carbs you ate as soon as your thinking clears. Enter this total into your pump along with your low glucose reading. Your pump will recommend an appropriate bolus dose to cover the excess carbs that you ate to prevent the high reading that will follow. For safety, reduce this recommended dose slightly to avoid going low again. Check your blood sugar again in 20 minutes to ensure your sugar has risen and in 2 hours to determine whether an additional bolus or carbs are needed..

How Others Can Help

Many problems associated with hypoglycemia are caused by the person's sudden inability to think clearly. The brain uses only glucose as fuel, and as the glucose level falls, the ability to think, reason, and solve problems becomes more impaired. During a low blood sugar, a person's actions may range from anger and hostility to lethargy and incoherence, depending on how fast and how far the blood sugar drops.

Anger during a low blood sugar may be triggered by release of stress hormones. Ordinarily, the release of these hormones will help return the blood sugar levels to normal, but they also have a darker side that makes it difficult to treat the person who desperately needs help. If others can recognize that a low blood sugar is taking place, they may be able to ignore the anger and treat it quickly with fast sugar or glucagon.

If irrational thought, anger, irritability, silliness, running away, or an insistence that "I feel fine" occurs, a low blood sugar is almost certainly the cause. Since the person may be unwilling and unable to acknowledge the problem, insistent but gentle coaxing and encouragement may be needed before fast-acting carbs can be given to treat the low. A confrontational attitude does not help. The best approach is to coax the obstinate person into drinking or eating something sweet. When their thinking becomes more normal, ask them to test their blood sugar.

When a person's defiance makes it difficult to assist them:

- Control your emotions. If the person you are helping is stubborn, acts silly or becomes angry, do not take it personally. Recognize that mental function is impaired and be prepared ahead of time to deal with the variety of hypoglycemia attitudes you may encounter.

- Take charge of the situation. Use a gentle but firm tone. A nonconfrontational stance, such as sitting or standing beside the person may help.

- Say, "Here, have this piece of candy," or try "I'm going to drink a soda, here, have a sip." If the person refuses to be persuaded, be kind but firm and say, "You need to drink (or eat) this."

- Avoid direct questions like "Are you low?", "Do you need to test?", or "Do you need to eat?" The person who is unable to think clearly will likely say "NO" and become defensive. You may need to be more forceful than you want to be, but only in that way can you help.

- Do not let the person drive a car, run machinery, or become involved in other dangerous activities that require coordination and thinking.

- Ask for help from others if you cannot treat the person yourself. Keep embarrassment to a minimum and cooperation to a maximum.

Hypoglycemia And Driving

Always test before getting behind the wheel and have glucose tablets or quick carbohydrate easily accessible in your pocket and vehicle. Some people always eat carbohydrate before driving just to be safe. This is a good accident-prevention technique.

Driving a car can be hypnotic or trancelike. With attention focused on the road, you may not notice that your ability to think, make decisions, and interact with others has changed. If the blood sugar drops slowly during a longer drive, a low becomes hard to recognize, especially if you are alone

---

16.10 Clever Pump Tricks

Treat A Low With The Right Number Of Carbs

If you go low only two or three hours after your last bolus, remember that you still have BOB. If you cannot think clearly, eat 15 grams of fast carbs right away. After your thinking clears, quickly determine how many more carbs you need. Using the meal bolus function, enter your low reading, then enter an increasing number of carbs until your pump says you need a bolus. This is the tipping point.* The tipping point shows how many grams of carb are needed for this low. No bolus is needed for these carbs, of course.

No more "15 grams" for all lows. Assuming your pump settings are correct and excess activity is not involved, your smart pump can give an accurate carb recommendation for each low you have. Bolus Tipping is particularly helpful for bedtime and middle of the night lows.

*On Paradigm 500 or 700 series pumps, the tipping point is where the BOB, or active insulin, equals the sum of the carb bolus plus correction bolus.

195

or your partner is sleeping. On long drives, test at least every two hours, and always test immediately if someone else in your vehicle requests that you do so. If you become involved in an auto accident due to a low blood sugar, an automatic suspension of your license is likely.

Pull over and test your blood sugar if you have any doubts. The risk of injury or death to yourself and others is raised if you drive while low.

Prevent Death In Bed

The most serious complication of hypoglycemia is death. Though uncommon, this happens to otherwise healthy people who are usually having frequent or severe lows (sometimes in an overzealous attempt to stay "normal"). The term death in bed is derived because death typically occurs at night in bed where hypoglycemia goes undetected for a long time and becomes severe. Death appears to result from a prolonged and severe hypoglycemia event that releases enough stress hormones to trigger a cardiac arrhythmia long enough to create a "heart attack". It is believed to cause 3% to 6% of all deaths among people with diabetes under the age of 40.[80,81]

Tips to take to protect yourself against a fatal low:

- Use a continuous monitor to detect unrecognized night lows, or test your blood sugar in the middle of the night once or twice a week to eliminate night lows
- Never let your blood sugar go below 50 mg/dl (2.8 mmol)
- Use the Auto-Off feature of your pump if you live alone
- Use a temporary basal reduction at night following any day with increased activity
- Discuss use of a beta-blocker with your physician. These blood pressure medications reduce the risk of arrhythmias by reducing the release of stress hormones. Even though they have a weak reputation for increasing the risk for hypoglycemia unawareness, their use here may produce major rewards
- Unproven methods: if your health allows, take a 400 mg. tablet of magnesium and eat nuts regularly to reduce the likelihood of an arrhythmia.

What we hope to do with ease, we must do with diligence.

Samuel Johnson

16.11 Clever Pump Tricks

Alarms

If you need an alarm, for example, to wake up a couple of hours after putting in an infusion set or giving a correction bolus at bedtime, set up your pump to alarm 2 hours after boluses. When you give a bolus, this alarm should automatically awaken you 2 hours later. If you change an infusion set at bedtime (not recommended), give a minimal bolus, such as 0.05 u. Your alarm will then awaken you 2 hours later.

If you have trouble hearing alarms and may sleep through them at night, set the pump to vibrate instead of alarm and wear the pump in a pump case, such as a Round About or Waist It, that keeps it close to your body.

Reverse Hypo Unawareness

One of the most distressing problems in diabetes is hypoglycemia unawareness. Normally the person going low recognizes it due to shaking and sweating caused by release of stress hormones. However, stress hormones become depleted after several lows, resulting in a loss of warning symptoms. This causes thinking to become impaired before the person recognizes they are low.

Even if the person does a blood sugar test while low, they may no longer be rational enough to remember how to treat the low number on their meter. Unless the hypoglycemia is recognized and treated by someone else, serious problems, such as bizarre behavior or grand mal seizures, can follow.

This chapter presents

- Causes of hypoglycemia unawareness
- How to reverse hypoglycemia unawareness

What Causes Hypoglycemia Unawareness?

Hypoglycemia unawareness is not rare. It is present in 17 percent of those with Type 1 diabetes. Symptoms for lows become weaker in people who have had diabetes for several years and people who are older because repeated lows impair the body's release of stress hormones. Anyone with Type 1 can have unawareness following a series of frequent lows close together. Nighttime lows, in particular, deplete stress hormones because these episodes typically last longer.

The body has a backup system to bring a person out of a low if they are unaware and unable to treat the low themselves. This is glucagon, a major counterregulatory hormone that leads to the release of glucose from the liver. Unfortunately, this response is reduced in most people with Type 1 diabetes after two to ten years. Loss of the glucagon response makes unawareness more likely. Women, with or without diabetes, have less counterregulatory hormone response than men. They have a pronounced reduction in their hypoglycemia symptoms and are more prone to unawareness.[82]

Drinking alcohol decreases awareness of symptoms and increases the risk of an unrecognized low. After one or two drinks, alcohol blocks the glucagon response and the liver no longer creates and releases the glucose needed to raise the blood sugar.[83] Alcohol makes symptoms hard to recognize and slows recovery.

The lower a person's average blood sugar, the higher the risk for hypoglycemia unawareness. It was three times more common in the intensively controlled group compared to the conventionally controlled group in the Diabetes Control and Complications Trial with 55% of episodes occurring during sleep. People wake up for less than half of the lows that occur at night. Not realizing night lows are occurring makes daytime hypoglycemia unawareness more likely.[84]

Hypoglycemia unawareness is less common in people who have Type 2 diabetes because hypoglycemia is less common. A study elevating tight control in Type 2 diabetes done by the Veterans Administration showed that severe lows were about 20 times more common in Type 1 diabetes than in Type 2.[85]

Hypoglycemia unawareness is caused by

- Excessive doses of insulin that cause frequent lows
- Attempts to control the blood sugar too tightly
- A rapid fall in the blood sugar
- Having diabetes for many years
- Stress or depression
- Situations where self-care is a low priority
- Alcohol intake in the last 12 hours
- A low blood sugar within 24 to 48 hours of a previous low
- And although the class of blood pressure medications called beta blockers do provide cardiovascular protection, they may reduce hypo symptoms

Unrecognized night lows and frequent lows cause hypoglycemia unawareness. Dr. Thiemo Veneman and his research team studied 10 people who did not have diabetes on two occasions.[86] While the participants slept in a hospital, the researchers used insulin to lower their blood sugar below 45 mg/dl (2.5 mmol) for two hours in the middle of the night. As occurs during most nighttime lows, they did not wake up.

Five people were put through a nighttime low on the first visit and the other five on the second visit. On waking in the morning, all were given insulin to lower their blood sugar to see when they would recognize the symptoms of a low blood sugar.

After sleeping through a low at night, Dr. Veneman found that people had more trouble recognizing a low the next day. Warning symptoms became less obvious because counterregulatory hormones, like epinephrine, norepinephrine and glucagon, are released more slowly and in smaller concentrations after a prior severe low blood sugar. A low blood sugar in the previous 24 to 48 hours depletes stored stress hormones and makes it harder to recognize the second low. The reduced awareness in people without diabetes in this study makes it is even more likely that similar lows would cause hypoglycemia unawareness in someone with diabetes and a history of low blood sugars.

How To Reverse Hypoglycemia Unawareness

Avoidance of night and frequent lows allows many people to regain their warning symptoms when they become low.[87] A study in Rome by Dr. Carmine Fanelli and other researchers reduced the frequency of lows in people with hypo unawareness to see whether they could regain awareness if their hormone reserves had time to build up again.

When the researchers raised the subjects' target for premeal blood sugars to 140 mg/dl (7.8 mmol), the frequency of hypoglycemia dropped from once every other day to once every 22 days. After avoiding low blood sugars for 22 days, people regained their low blood sugar symptoms and recognized when they were low. Pre-

> ### 17.2 How To Stop Frequent Lows
>
> 1. Identify the time of day during which the most severe lows occur.
>
> 2. Identify whether the basal rate or a bolus is the primary source of insulin working at this time of day. Check your basal/bolus balance to make sure each makes up about 50% of your TDD.
>
> 3. Reduce the dose of insulin that is most likely responsible, remembering that an excess of either basal or bolus doses can cause lows.
>
> 4. If lows are frequent and severe, your TDD will need to be lowered by 10% or more. If lows are occasional and mild, a 5% reduction may be perfect.

venting all lows for about three months resulted in a return to nearly normal symptoms.

To reverse hypoglycemia unawareness, set blood sugar targets higher, readjust doses to closely match your diet and exercise, and stay more alert to physical warnings for 48 hours following any low blood sugar. Wear a continuous monitor and confirm readings with a finger stick test before treating the result. Frequent testing is critical for making needed basal or bolus reductions and to prevent lows before they happen with tools like bolus tipping (see Textbox 5.5) to predict lows. Consider any blood sugar below 60 mg/dl (3.3 mmol) as serious and reduce your boluses or basal rates so that you do not get another one. Use your records to find when lows are most likely to happen.

Deal quickly with problems that arise from stress, depression, and other sources of poor self-care. Avoid alcohol or limit consumption to less than one or two drinks a day to avoid shutting off the liver's release of glucose. On active days, reduce insulin during

17.3 How To Reverse Hypoglycemia Unawareness

- Try to avoid all low blood sugars below 70 mg/dl(4 mmol) for 3 weeks to 3 months.

- Set your blood sugar targets higher so that you will experience no more than one or two insulin reactions per week. A range of 80 to 150 mg/dl (4.4 to 8.3 mmol) works well if you can ensure that no readings go below 80 mg/dl (40 mmol). Otherwise, aim for 100 to 150 mg/dl (5.6 to 8.3 mmol).

- Be especially careful to avoid lows which may be more likely to occur in the 24 to 36 hours after a low occurs.

- Test blood sugars often to detect a falling blood sugar before it goes low. Use a continuous monitor.

- Prevent night lows by testing in the middle of the night at least once or twice a week.

- Always match your basals and boluses to any current change in your lifestyle.

- Eliminate alcohol consumption or reduce intake to one or two servings a day.

© 2006 Diabetes Services, Inc.

increased activity and for several hours afterward. An occasional 2 a.m. blood test can do wonders in spotting unrecognized nighttime lows and preventing them. Using a continuous monitor can alert you and your health care team to occurrences of unrecognized hypoglycemia. They warn of night lows, awaken the wearer, and enable early treatment.

If you require help from others to get out of a severe low, call your doctor immediately. You want help right away because it is very likely to happen again. You may be told to raise your target range for safety's sake. Discuss how to make immediate dose reductions and how to test at critical times, even if it means doing so at 2 a.m. A little lost sleep is a minor problem compared to an exhausting or dangerous low.

17.4 Do Not Overdo Control

For some people, a strict adherence to tight control creates its own problems. A desire to have near-perfect blood sugar readings as a way to avoid complications can become counterproductive. Achieving a lower A1c does not need to come at the price of unconsciousness or grand mal seizures, impaired coordination or thinking, temper tantrums, a car accident, or death.

Health care providers who recognize these tendencies in overly conscientious individuals often advise them to use less insulin and set goals that are safer. This may mean raising a premeal target to 100 - 150 mg/dl (5.5 to 8.3 mmol) and strict avoidance of any glucose level below 70 mg/dl (3.9 mmol) or even below 90 mg/dl (5.0 mmol), particularly for those people who live alone. More reasonable goals often result in more consistent readings and can often be done with little or no rise in the A1c. Anyone who is overly conscientious about control may want to discuss use of an antidepressant medication with their doctor. An antidepressant can sometimes change an obsession into more reasonable and sometimes more effective goal achievement.

Spot Patterns And Stop Lows

18

Low blood sugars that occur in particular pat-terns can be analyzed to find their cause. Appropriate basal and bolus or other adjustments can then be made. Frequent lows are a sure sign that too much insulin is be-ing given. Low blood sugars are addressed first because this stops unwanted lows and often reduces the number of highs caused by overtreatment or excess stress hormone release. This chapter shows how to recognize trends and patterns as-sociated with lows and suggests adjustments to be made.

This chapter presents

- How to look for patterns
- How to correct unwanted low patterns to help you stop lows
    - Frequent lows
    - Lows after eating
    - Afternoon lows
    - Low to high
    - Overtreating nighttime lows
    - Lows that follow highs
    - Lows after exercise

A patterns is any consistent repetition in your blood sugar over several days' time. At least a week's worth of records are needed to spot a pattern. Recognition of unwanted patterns allows basal rates and boluses to be adjusted so they fit your lifestyle and improve control.

How To Look For Patterns

Some people avoid looking at their blood sugar readings because they want no reminder of how bad things are or they have little hope of understanding and changing it. Unfortunately, this may hasten the path to complications or increase the frequency and severity of hypoglycemia. A person's readings reflect what is going on with lifestyle and health and this is not changed if they are ignored.

It may help to pretend your own readings belong to someone else if that makes it easier to study them and make changes. Consider your blood sugars as a game to play or a challenge to solve. Readings outside your target range are simply a learning device. Believe in your ability to tackle any blood sugar problem you may be having. For help, show your records to a friend, your spouse, or a family member and ask them to help you spot your patterns.

When your blood sugar is not as controlled as you want, review your readings once a week to identify any changes you may need to make in doses, carb intake, or activity. Unless the control problem is severe, wait for a week's worth of readings to find a pattern. Identify problem patterns and make one correction at a time until you have a better pattern.

Patterns may occur several days in a row or may be random and occur only occasionally. If patterns are random, try to connect them to certain events. Listing likely causes helps. For instance, if you often have a low or high reading after a particular food or exercise, you have a much better idea of how to correct it.

Steps To Find Your Patterns

- Collect or download a week's records to carefully review
- Identify readings above and below your target range and when they occur
- Find a sample pattern in the pages that follow that matches your pattern
- Try one of the changes recommended to improve that pattern

To make it easier to spot patterns, test often and write down your results. Use a detailed record system like *Smart Charts* or an *Enhanced Logbook*, (See Figures 8.3 and 8.9 for examples.). If possible, regularly download the data from your pump and meter and use software to analyze these readings. Good records help you identify and solve blood sugar problems. When you record your blood sugars, food, exercise, stress, and insulin, you also give your physician or diabetes educator the data they need to help you correct unwanted patterns. Give them a call if you can't understand your readings on your own.

Some control problems may be caused by unusual circumstances, such as an infection, or starting a new herbal weight-loss medication that contains ma huang or ephedra, or insulin that has lost its potency. Highlighted records allow occasional problems like these to be remembered and corrected more easily. Patterns are considered occasional when they occur only in specific circumstances, such as eating bean burritos for dinner.

People who visually process information will see patterns quickly in a graphic record system like *Smart Charts* or the graphic display from a software program, whereas others who think in a more numeric or analytic way may see patterns best in a standard or enhanced logbook that lists numbers in columns. Any approach can work and both graphical and numeric are presented, though space allows only one graph and a simple rather than enhanced logbook to be illustrated. Use the method that fits your thinking process best.

A normal pattern, followed by common low blood sugar patterns throughout one day on a chart and several days on a logbook are shown in this chapter. Your own patterns may not stand out as clearly as the ones in these examples, but each example can assist you in recognizing patterns in general. Patterns for highs are shown in the next chapter. These patterns are ones you may encounter in your charts or logbooks. To spot a pattern on a chart or logbook, see if similar readings repeat several times over a few days in a row on your charts. Make lows and highs easier to spot on your charts or logbook by highlighting them in different colors or shapes.

The logbook that is used in the examples displays a simple logbook with only blood sugar readings and is not the most effective way to analyze patterns. However, they can be identified even with this simple tool. An enhanced logbook includes blood sugars, insulin doses, carb intake, exercise, and the time for each to help you find solutions more easily. For instance, if your breakfast carbs vary from 30 grams to 90 grams but you always take a 5 unit bolus to cover them, it is easy to see why your lunch readings are erratic. Simple logbooks do not allow you to record this detail, but an enhanced logbook does.

The blood sugar ranges on the left of the charts are given in both mg/dl for the U.S. and in mmol for Canada, Europe, and other countries. Suggestions to correct each pattern are given below them. For patterns that repeat regularly (i.e., high all the time or often low in the afternoon), insulin dose adjustments are usually needed. For occasional patterns, find a fix that can be reused whenever the circumstance that causes it arises.

Normal Blood Sugars

A normal blood sugar pattern is like the one shown here. It shows the normal rise and fall in the blood sugar before and after someone

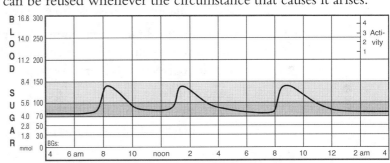

without diabetes eats. The blood sugar rises after eating, but the readings remain in a normal range. This is difficult with diabetes. If your readings come close to this graph, keep up the great work! Recording great readings becomes a reward of its own. A logbook of normal readings would show values in the shaded 70 to 150 mg/dl (4 to 8.4 mmol) range before and after meals, at bedtime and at 2 a.m.

How To Correct Low Patterns

Some low patterns occur often, while others tend to be random. Patterns of frequent lows, such as lows after eating, afternoon lows, or night lows, are usually easy to spot when highlighted with a colored marker. Other patterns, such as low-to-high, high-to-low, or exercise-related lows, occur less often. Some random low patterns are easy to spot, while others require careful logging of associated events, such as changes in the time you exercise or eating unusual foods.

Frequent Lows

A pattern of frequent or severe lows requires a decrease in one or more insulin doses to prevent problems. When the insulin reduction is done carefully, the

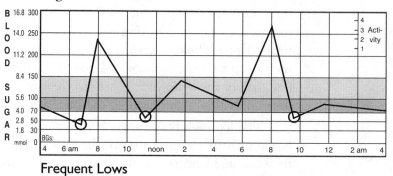

Frequent Lows

A1c will remain close to normal with less glucose variability. Try to prevent lows rather than having to treat them. A consistent blood sugar is what the body needs.

Frequent lows, such as the ones shown in the *Smart Chart* here, often cause high or erratic blood sugar readings. The chart and the accompanying logbook below show a pattern of lows that occurs when too much insulin is being given. The low blood sugar readings in this chart are circled.

What To Do

- Frequent lows are a sure sign of excess insulin. Lower your TDD by 5 to 10% as described in Chapter 10. Discuss how to reduce specific doses with your physician.

- Review your basal rates, bolus doses, and basal/bolus balance to determine where the excess insulin might be coming from. With your doctor's help, calculate new carb and correction factors after reducing your TDD.

- Use glucose tabs or fast carbs to treat all low blood sugars. Glucose tablets relieve symptoms fast and can be measured precisely to prevent overtreatment. Follow them with a cracker if you will not be eating right away.

Case Study

Frequent lows began to appear in Jeanine's logbook after she started a diet to lose an extra 15 pounds. Because she was eating fewer carbs, her doses at mealtime were lower but she had not lowered her basal rates.

When lows become frequent, the first thing to check is the basal/bolus balance to see which dose is greater. If either basals or boluses are considerably larger than the other, the larger one is likely the source for the lows. If they are close to each other, both may be contributing some of the excess insulin. Jeanine looked at a 7-day average of her doses and found that her TDD was 41.1 units, with 9.9 units a day (24.1%) used for carb boluses, 2.5 units (6.1%) for correction boluses, and 28.7 units (69.8%) a day for basal delivery. Her current basal rates make up 69.8% of her TDD, so this is most likely the source for the low readings she is experiencing.

In Jeanine's log-book, notice her blood sugar at bedtime on Wednesday night. This test was taken five hours after her dinner bolus so very little of her dinner bolus

Sugar	Breakfast Before	Breakfast After	Lunch Before	Lunch After	Dinner Before	Dinner After	Night Bed	Night 2 a.m.
Sun	(41)	163	(51)	147	90	196	(56)	92
Mon	(37)	186	89	121	(53)	203	128	132
Tues	63	119	(47)	174	66	163	(59)	177
Wed	94	131	63	110	(41)	237	184	139
Thurs	73	162	(38)	394	207	110	(48)	211
							65	70

Jeanine's logbook showing frequent lows

was still active. She took no correction bolus for this but her bedtime blood sugar fell anyway from 184 mg/dl (10.3 mmol) to 139 mg/dl (7.7 mmol) at 2 a.m. on Thursday and then to 73 mg/dl (4.1 mmol) at breakfast the following morning. This drop of 111 mg/dl (6.2 mmol) overnight is well beyond the 30 mg/dl (+0.8 to -1.7 mmol) rise or fall that is preferred during the overnight period. Other nights show a similar pattern and clearly indicate that Jeanine's overnight basal rates are too high.

Her daytime basals are probably too high as well, given the high percentage of the TDD being used for basal delivery. It would be reasonable to lower the basal rates around the clock as a first step until further basal and bolus testing can be done. From Table 11.3, a basal reduction of about 1.3 total units overnight (a TDD close to 40 units with a drop of 111 mg/dl or 6.2 mmol overnight) and a reductions of about twice this amount for the 16 hours of her daytime basal will be needed.

When carb and calorie consumption is reduced at the start of a diet, there is an immediate need to lower carb boluses. Although the exact timing cannot be predicted, the basal rate usually needs to be reduced after a few days of successful dieting.

Jeanine had not told her doctor she was starting a diet, but when she finally called because of the lows, he recommended she lower her basal rates by 0.15 unit per hour around the clock right away. This equals 3.6 units over a 24 hour period. During the 8-hour overnight period, one third of this 3.6 units equals 1.2 units which multiplied by Jeanine's correction factor of 60 equals 72 mg/dl (4 mmol) less fall in her overnight blood sugar. This should bring her much closer to her target of falling no more than 30 mg/dl (1.7 mmol) overnight. Her doctor recommended that she test her new basals to validate them.

Lows After Eating

The pattern on the chart to the right looks similar to the previous pattern of frequent lows, but here the overnight basal appears to be fine because the blood sugar stays level overnight. The

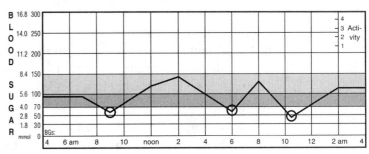

Lows After Eating

fall in the blood sugar is more likely caused by the excess carb boluses, especially if the daytime basal rate is no higher than the overnight basal, or if daytime basal testing shows daytime rates to be appropriate.

What To Do

When lows occur after carb boluses, the solution is to increase the carb factor number to make carb boluses smaller. A check of the daytime basal rates would be needed to confirm that they are not the source of the excess insulin. Also check the basal/bolus balance. If carb boluses make up more than half of the TDD, raise your carb factor number to reduce carb boluses. For instance, if you use 1 unit for every 16 grams, try 1 unit for every 17 or 18 grams. If you are not certain about the accuracy of your carb counting, visit your dietitian and bring with you a detailed three-day diet diary to verify your carb counting.

Case Study

In Jeff's logbook to the right, his blood sugar goes low either right after a meal or before the next meal. He checked the history on his pump and

Sugar	Breakfast		Lunch		Dinner		Night	
	Before	After	Before	After	Before	After	Bed	2 a.m.
Sun	97	(60)	123	146	(53)	129	(42)	110
Mon	89	71	95	123	(37)	121	103	99
Tues	89	152	(45)	207	111	(56)	106	101
Wed	78	144	84	(41)	214	98	65	122
Thurs	100	137	92	151	83	141	107	154
					78		95	110

Jeff's logbook showing lows after eating

found that his TDD averaged 40 units a day with 25.5 units (63.8%) for carb boluses, 0.8 units (2%) for correction boluses, and 13.7 units (34.2%) for his basal rates. He averaged 255 carbs a day in his diet and his basal/bolus balance was 34% for basal and 64% for boluses, suggesting his carb boluses were too high.

When his blood sugars go low only a couple of hours after eating, his carb boluses are obviously too large, especially since he uses such a low percentage of his TDD for his basal rates. His lows could also be caused by overcounting his carbs at meals, but this is unlikely because most pumpers undercount their carbs by about 30%.

On Wednesday morning, Jeff's blood sugar was a bit low at 78 mg/dl (4.3 mmol), so he reduced his carb bolus from 7 units for 70 grams (1 unit for every 10 grams is his current carb factor) down to 5.8 units (or 1 unit for every 12 grams). That morning he did not have a low after breakfast. At lunch, he returned to using his normal carb factor of 1 to 10 but went low that afternoon and again at bedtime. On Thursday morning, Jeff decided it would be better to use the larger carb factor of one unit for every 12 grams for all his meals. He set aside time to recheck his daytime basal dose on the coming weekend.

However, he decided to call his doctor to discuss the situation. Jeff's doctor pointed out that even though he might have reduced the number of lows, he would continue to be getting a relatively high percentage of his TDD from carb boluses compared to his basal insulin. About six weeks earlier, Jeff had lowered his daytime basal rate from 0.8 u/hr to 0.5 u/hr because he was having so many lows. His doctor suggested he lower his carb boluses even further by raising his carb factor number to 14 but then raise his daytime basal rates from 0.5 u/hr to 0.7 u/hr.

One way to determine whether the problem originates from basal or bolus insulin is to compare the contribution of each during a six hour period prior to the low blood sugar. For instance, when Jeff compared his basal rates and carb boluses prior to the low blood sugar of 45 mg/dl (2.5 mmol) at lunch on Tuesday, he found that he had gotten only 3.0 units of basal insulin over the previous 6 hours (0.5 u/hr times 6 hours) compared to the 6.5 units he had taken for 65 grams of carb for breakfast that morning. This suggests but does not prove that his carb boluses are causing the lows.

Afternoon Lows

Low in the afternoon, shown on this chart, occurred 4 out of 7 days this week for Jody who works days as a parts picker in an automobile parts distributor plant.

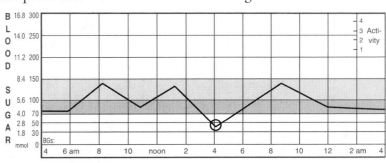

Afternoon Lows

The late afternoon is a common time for many people to have lows, especially those who are physically active at work or school. An excess of insulin may accumulate at this time from the combination of the bolus dose given for lunch plus a basal rate that is too high in the morning and afternoon hours.

What To Do

To stop lows in the afternoon, lower the noon bolus or the late morning and afternoon basal.

Case Study

Jody's readings on Sunday and Monday are typical of her problem with afternoon lows. On Wednesday morning, however,

Sugar	Breakfast		Lunch		Dinner		Night	
	Before	After	Before	After	Before	After	Bed	2 a.m.
Sun	101	167	89	(43)	96	117	144	105
Mon	124	138	92	(51)	163	176	103	99
Tues	83	149	84	67	94	143	92	
Wed	88	241	143	103	(41)	139	107	93
Thurs	83	133	76	184	(52)	158	129	121
							115	100

Jody's logbook showing afternoon lows

Jody stopped to eat breakfast at a local restaurant and apparently underestimated how many carbs were in her pancakes. Her blood sugar rose from 88 mg/dl (4.9 mmol) before breakfast to 241 mg/dl (13.4 mmol) afterward. She did not take a correction bolus for this high reading, so she was still high at 143 mg/dl (7.9 mmol) before lunch.

Because of her afternoon lows, she decided not to add any correction bolus for Wednesday's high lunch reading. Even though she took no correction bolus for lunch

207

that day, her blood sugar again went low before dinner. The low occurred just before dinner rather than in the middle of the afternoon because she started higher at lunch.

Jody checked her basal/bolus balance in her pump's history and found she had averaged 15.5 units (51%) for basal and 14.7 units (49%) for boluses in the previous week. Because her basals and boluses are fairly even, she lowered her basal rates through the morning and afternoon hours from 8 a.m. to 4 p.m. by 0.05 u/hr and raised her carb factor for lunch from 1u/17 grams to 1u/19 grams. The combined dose reduction was enough to prevent all but one mild low over the next week. Jody felt better at work and safer on her drive home afterward.

Low To High

Eating too many carbs to compensate for lows will cause high readings an hour or two later. If your blood sugar often goes higher than 150 mg/dl (8.3 mmol) after lows, it is likely you are eating more than you need to treat these lows. Stress hormones released at the time of the low cause sweating and shaking and can raise the blood sugar, but will

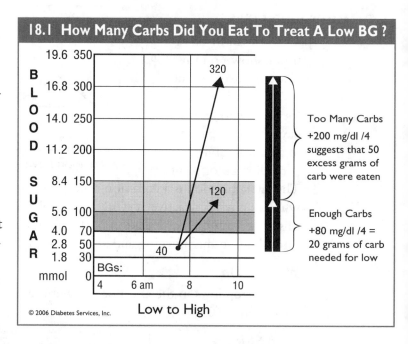

not cause a rapid rise over a short period of time as seen in the jump from 40 to 320 mg/dl (2.2 to 17.7 mmol) in Fig. 18.1 which is likely the result of overeating.

Look over your records or back through a download of your meter to see whether readings below 60 mg/dl (3.3 mmol) are followed by readings of 150 mg/dl (8.5 mmol) or higher. If highs often follow lows in your charts, you have a low-to-high pattern that is likely caused by overtreatment. One gram of carbohydrate raises the blood sugar between three and five points for most adults, so only 15 to 20 grams of quick carbohydrate is typically needed to stop most lows.

If a blood sugar is done when you are low, your pump can tell you how many carbs you need to treat that particular low (see Textbox 5.5). If you are too confused to do bolus tipping right away, eat 20 grams of carbs and check your pump for its suggestion once you can think clearly.

What To Do

Be patient when treating lows. Fast carbs require 15 or 20 minutes to raise the blood sugar. Once stress hormones have been released, they can make you feel hungry for much longer than this. Get in the habit of using only glucose tablets or fast-acting carbs for lows if you have been overtreating them. Do not eat more than 20 grams of fast carbs unless there is a clear reason to do so. More than 20 grams may be needed if you have BOB from a recent carb or correction bolus or if extra activity is the reason for the low.

| 18.2 How Much 1 Gram of Carbs May Raise Your BG ||
If your weight is:	1 gram will raise you about:
50 lbs (23 kg)	8 mg/dl (0.44 mmol)
75 lbs (34 kg)	7 mg/dl (0.39 mmol)
90 lbs (41 kg)	6 mg/dl (0.33 mmol)
120 lbs (55 kg)	5 mg/dl (0.28 mmol)
160 lbs (73 kg)	4 mg/dl (0.22 mmol)
200 lbs (91 kg)	3 mg/dl (0.17 mmol)

© 2006 Diabetes Services, Inc.

If you do overeat, calculate how many grams of carb you actually consumed, and enter this amount as carbs to be eaten into your pump, along with your blood sugar reading, and let your pump calculate the bolus you need to cover these carbs. (Use this method only if your pump automatically discounts your BOB from your carb boluses, as discussed on page 48.) A slightly smaller bolus than the one recommended can be taken for safety if you wish. Taking a bolus may seem strange when you are low, but it's exactly what is needed to cover the excess carbs and prevent a high reading later. A test of your blood a couple of hours later will ensure you did not bolus too much.

Take time to think through what caused the low and whether any changes are needed in your basal doses, carb factor, or correction factor so that you will not encounter another one.

Case Study

Several times in the last couple of weeks Joe has had low to high readings. On Monday, Joe was low before lunch, ate two

Sugar	Breakfast		Lunch		Dinner		Night	
	Before	After	Before	After	Before	After	Bed	2 a.m.
Sun	193	287	212	127	(40)	320	273	142
Mon	132	125	(48)	219	171	152	107	91
Tues	84	73	216	(58)	248	(39)	211	71
Wed	(53)	347	227	184	132	63	188	142
Thurs	134	167	118	169	126	141	(53)	277
							95	110

Joe's logbook showing low to high

candy bars, and went high afterward even though he took his usual bolus for lunch. It took over six hours to bring his reading back down. The physical or emotional discomfort of being low can cause a person to overtreat it to try to feel better right away. Focus first on preventing lows, but remember it is important to not overtreat them and cause rebound highs.

Joe called his physician to review what to do about having so many lows. His doctor scanned the readings he had faxed and told him he needed an immediate reduction in his TDD from 38 units to 35 units a day. To do this, Joe raised his carb factor from 1/13 to 1/14 and lowered his basal rate by 0.05 u/hr from 5 a.m. through 9 p.m. On the way home from work that day, he stopped at his pharmacy and bought a large bottle of glucose tablets to have available whenever he goes low so he would not overtreat it. These steps helped smooth out his blood sugars and he felt a lot better. His A1c dropped from 7.4% to 6.6% four months later, and he felt much more capable of controlling his readings.

Overtreating Nighttime Lows

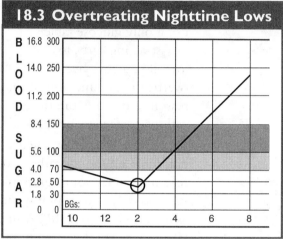

When the blood sugar goes low during the night and you awaken sweating and shaking, it is especially hard to be rational. You may not be thinking clearly and the fear and confusion plus extreme hunger that accompany a low makes emptying the refrigerator seem quite sane. Overeating, however, only makes your blood sugar sky-high the following morning and for several hours through the day. The graph shows a low during the night and the blood sugar as it climbs high before breakfast after excess carbs were eaten during the night to treat the low.

What To Do

When you have recovered, determine why your nighttime lows happen. If night lows occur often, reduce the evening basal rate or the dinner carb bolus as needed to stop them. If the low happens only after increased daytime activity, eating extra carbs at bedtime on active days may be the perfect solution. If nighttime hypoglycemia occurs only after a correction bolus is taken for a high blood sugar at bedtime, use a larger correction factor for the after dinner hours to make the correction boluses taken near bedtime smaller.

Keep glucose tablets or other fast-acting carbs at the bedside and use them routinely for all night lows. Even in the panic of a serious nighttime low, it is harder to overdose on glucose tablets than it is with cookies and candy. Once sufficient fast carbs are eaten, wait five or ten minutes for your appetite to ease. Then have a small amount of slow-acting carbs to ensure against another low.

Case Study

As can be seen in his logbook, Jared has been overtreating his night lows. He found he could stop the high breakfast readings by keeping glucose tablets

Sugar	Breakfast		Lunch		Dinner		Night	
	Before	After	Before	After	Before	After	Bed	2 a.m.
Sun	185	341	188	162	76	142	96	(37)
Mon	284	289	204	187	123	163	132	(53)
Tues	259	323	225	156	98	138	105	89
Wed	102	291	198	182	143	189	116	(46)
Thurs	287	284	233	142	107	154	93	(48)
					73		122	72

Jared's logbook showing overtreating lows

on his night stand and using only three tablets. To stop the night lows, he reduced his basal rate between 6 p.m. and 2 a.m. by 0.1 u/hr. This stopped his night lows

Lows That Follow Highs

Plummeting from a high to a low blood sugar over a two- to-four hour period may be caused by a correction bolus that is too large, by two or more boluses that overlap, or by a duration of insulin action that is set too short in your pump. A high to low pattern is shown in the graph to the right. If this pattern is seen several times on your charts, you will need to discuss it with your doctor.

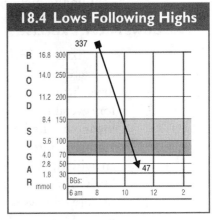

18.4 Lows Following Highs

What To Do

If you frequently go from highs to lows, the size of your correction boluses needs to be reduced. Even if it happens only occasionally, you want to be able to lower high readings safely. When lows follow highs, the most likely cause is a correction factor that is too small, which makes your correction boluses too large. Calculate and retest your correction factor. Raising your correction factor gives you less insulin in your boluses. For instance, if your correction factor is 50, use 55 or 60 instead. Recalculate by using your current TDD and the 2000 Rule in Table 13.1 to determine how many points you are likely to drop per unit. Stop these lows first, then work on any highs if this is still a problem.

Be sure that your duration of insulin action is set for a long enough time, usually 4.5 to 6.5 hours. A short duration of insulin action (DIA) makes residual insulin from previous boluses appear to be less than it actually is, causing high readings to be overtreated and excess insulin to be taken for any carbs eaten during this time. Once the DIA is correctly set, your pump will not give a correction bolus that is too large.

On a smart pump, only a single premeal target and a correct DIA are needed for the pump to accurately calculate boluses. However, if you ever need to calculate your own correction doses on a syringe, keep in mind that your postmeal target will be a higher one than what is used before meals. For example, if 100 mg/dl (5.6 mmol) is the premeal target, a realistic postmeal target would be 150 mg/dl or 180 mg/dl (8.3 or 10 mmol). Be sure to consider how long after a meal a blood test is taken when considering whether a reading represents an actual high.

If you feel frustrated or uncomfortable when you are high and use boluses that are too large to

Sugar	Breakfast Before	Breakfast After	Lunch Before	Lunch After	Dinner Before	Dinner After	Night Bed	Night 2 a.m.
Sun	96	127	82	337	(41)	168	129	128
Mon	137	179	138	162	107	171	141	125
Tues	119	284	(51)	117	84	136	91	84
Wed	73	121	87	148	121	345	(38)	167
Thurs	155	173	96	71	276	(53)	164	114

Lows that follow highs

lower highs quickly, start practicing some self-restraint. Letting it take a little longer for your blood sugar to come down can prevent many unnecessary lows. Focus on preventing the highs in the first place rather than overdosing to lower them too quickly.

Lows After Exercise

Extra activity or exercise can cause lows during, after, and for several hours following it. The longer and more intense an activity, the more likely that immediate or delayed lows will

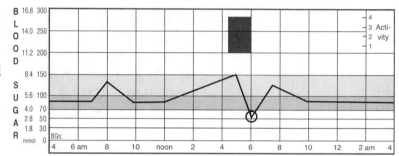

Lows After Exercise

occur. Use your *Smart Charts* or notes to record exercise and match it to your food or premeal bolus so that appropriate blood sugars will follow.

What To Do

As discussed in Chapter 23, the effect that extra activity has on your blood sugar depends on how strenuous it is, how long it lasts, and how much insulin you have in your blood at the time. Mild to moderate activity that lasts less than 30 to 45 minutes will not require as much extra carb intake or as much reduction in insulin doses as longer and more intense forms of exercise. Table 23.5 provides guidance for carb and insulin adjustments for the amount of activity.

First check that your basal and bolus insulin doses are balanced well during the time you exercise. If they are, Excarbs can be estimated using Table 23.6. Use this table to judge how many replacement carbs are needed for your particular activity.

Summary

It is very important to adjust basals and boluses to stop lows. When you encounter low readings, look for any patterns in your blood sugar readings and decide on a plan to stop them. Match your pattern of lows to one of these for suggestions on how to adjust insulin doses to solve the problem.

Solutions For Severe Highs And Ketoacidosis

High blood sugars can turn into serious medical problems, including ketosis in early stages and ketoacidosis (DKA) later. The life-threatening condition of ketoacidosis occurs when little or no insulin is present in the body or when a marginal level of insulin is overwhelmed by infection, stress, or certain medications.

This chapter covers severe highs, ketosis, and DKA

- Causes
- Symptoms and detection
- Treatment and prevention

When the blood sugar is high and the insulin level low, the body will use more fat for fuel because it cannot move the large amounts of glucose in the blood into cells. Glucose needs insulin to enter the cells and provide energy. Burning fat sounds good if you are trying to lose weight, but done excessively, it produces ketones that cause the blood to become acidic. This leads to nausea and vomiting. Vomiting combined with a high blood sugar leads to rapid dehydration. In this situation, immediate hospitalization is necessary. Death is the likely outcome without treatment.

Causes

Ketosis is a severely high blood sugar (usually) with excess ketones in the blood. If left untreated ketosis can turn into ketoacidosis, which is ketosis plus a dangerous acidification of the blood. Ketoacidosis often occurs when Type 1 diabetes is first diagnosed. Later, people with Type 1 may have ketoacidosis when they have a severe infection or other serious illness, when they take certain medications like prednisone, when insulin doses are forgotten or deliberately not taken, or when their insulin has lost potency. Episodes of ketoacidosis are more common in pump wearers due to a displacement or failure of an infusion set, or an empty reservoir after an alarm was not noticed.

In children and adolescents, ketoacidosis can also be triggered by normal growth spurts if basal rates and boluses have not been raised to meet their increased need for insulin. As children grow, they require more insulin, and at puberty, even more insulin is needed. Avoiding DKA in children is especially important as it is believed to lower a child's IQ.[88]

In Type 1 diabetes, hospitalization for ketoacidosis occurs about once for every 30 years of insulin use and is more common in children. Although the likelihood of any individual with Type 2 diabetes developing ketoacidosis is lower, there are many more people who have Type 2 so the actual number of cases of ketoacidosis is greater among those with Type 2 than Type 1. The death rate from ketoacidosis is higher in people with Type 2 diabetes because of older age and because it is more likely to be triggered by a severe illness like pneumonia or a heart attack.

19.1 Causes Of Severe Highs And Ketoacidosis
• Onset of Type 1 diabetes
• Severe infection
• A serious illness, heart attack, or serious infection
• Insulin doses that are skipped or too low
• Nondelivery from a pump caused by a displaced infusion set or pump problems
• Leaving infusion sets in longer than 2 - 3 days
• Growth spurts in kids and adolescents
• Certain medications, such as prednisone
• Stress

Symptoms And Detection

Early symptoms of ketoacidosis include tiredness, excessive thirst, frequent urination, dry skin, a fruity odor to the breath, abdominal pain, and nausea. Advanced symptoms include vomiting, shortness of breath, rapid breathing, and unconsciousness. Early symptoms may be confused with the flu or food poisoning, but because they may be due to ketone poisoning, they should never be ignored. As soon as a person begins to vomit or has difficulty breathing, immediate treatment in an emergency room is required to prevent coma or death.

Know how to recognize and treat ketoacidosis. Ketones can be detected in the urine with Bayer Ketostix® or Ketodiastix® urine test strips available at any pharmacy. Keep ketone strips on hand, but store them in a dry area and replace them as soon as they are outdated. Most people will only occasionally use ketone test strips, so individually wrapped ones are better. Have them available and know how to use them.

The Precision Xtra™ meter is able to measure not only blood sugar but also ketone levels in the blood. It uses a special type of strip, individually wrapped in foil for freshness, to measure blood ketones. These strips as well as blood sugar strips must be kept on hand. Ketone measurement in the blood offers a tremendous advantage for anyone who is prone to ketoacidosis because this detects ketosis two to four hours earlier than waiting for ketone levels to rise or fall in the urine. Blood testing enables a faster evaluation of insulin need than urine testing with urine test strips.

If a test shows an unexpectedly high blood sugar, the blood ketone level can be measured immediately with a Precision Xtra™ meter or later the urine ketone level with urine testing with ketone strips. If ketones are normal, this provides some assurance that there is not a serious pump problem and that a correction bolus will correct a high reading. If ketones are present, however, a problem with insulin delivery from the pump should be suspected. Inspect the infusion site, line, hub, and pump for any problems, then inject a larger than normal correction bolus and give special attention to increasing fluid intake. Call your physician immediately if blood ketones are over 0.6 mmol/L or there are moderate or large levels of ketones in a urine test.

If you have had one episode of ketoacidosis, review what is causing this and discuss with your physician whether you should have a Precision

19.2 Ketoacidosis

Early Symptoms

- any unexplained high blood sugar
- nausea
- increased thirst and dry mouth
- excessive urination
- increased hunger
- excess tiredness or weakness
- confusion
- an acetone or fruity odor of the breath
- abdominal pain
- vague flu-like symptoms

Late Signs

- vomiting
- severe abdominal pain
- rapid breathing
- shortness of breath
- unconsciousness

Immediate medical treatment is required if late signs are present, or moderate or large amounts of ketones are found on a urine or blood test.

Xtra™ meter on hand for ketone testing. Ketoacidosis can be debilitating, painful, expensive, dangerous, and deadly. Take care to avoid it and if it occurs treat it quickly with extra insulin and fluid intake.

Using a continuous monitor should alert you with an alarm to a high blood sugar over a preset threshold. This may be 200 mg/dl (11 mmol) or higher. Always confirm with a finger stick test before treating a high blood sugar.

Treatment and Prevention

When someone with diabetes falls ill, they may stop testing blood sugars and fail to recognize the seriousness of their situation. Extreme tiredness may tempt them to go to bed without testing. When extremely tired, never go to bed without first testing for a high or low blood sugar. Frequent monitoring of blood sugar and ketone levels is critical

19.3 Steps To Prevent And Treat Ketoacidosis On A Pump

Ketones suggest you have a problem with insulin delivery from your pump or a serious illness. If you have any reason to suspect an illness, **call your physician.** Suspect an insulin delivery problem from your pump anytime you have an unexplained high blood sugar or a reading above 300 mg/dl (16.7 mmol). If you have a clear reason for the high reading, take a bolus by pen or syringe and recheck your blood sugar in one hour to ensure it is being corrected. Meanwhile:

1. Test your blood or urine for ketones.

2. Check for pump or site-related problems (Chapter 21). Call your pump company's customer service if you are uncertain what to check. (Their phone number is on the back of the pump)

If Ketones Are OK*:	If Ketones Are Moderate Or High**:
1. Give a normal bolus with the pump. 2. Then drink 8 to 12 ounces of fluid every hour until control is regained. 3. Test your blood sugar again in one hour. If your sugar is not lower in one hour, follow the procedure to the right. 4. If lower at one hour, recheck in another one to two hours and enter this reading into your pump to determine if an additional correction bolus is needed. 5. If your blood sugar remains high or ketones appear, call your physician and follow the second procedure to the right.	1. Start by drinking water or water with a pinch of Nu-Salt™ until **well-hydrated**. Continue to drink 8 to 12 ounces of fluid every hour until control is regained. 2. Correct the high sugar with **injected insulin** from a syringe or pen. You may need more insulin than normal, especially if ketones have been present for several hours or if an illness is causing the problem. 3. Replace the insulin cartridge and entire infusion set, using a new site. 4. Test your blood sugar in two hours. If it is not lower, call your physician immediately. 5. If your blood sugar is lower at two hours, enter the reading into your pump to determine if an additional correction bolus is needed. 6. If your blood sugar remains high or nausea worsens, call your physician. 7. If vomiting begins, **immediately call your physician and go to the nearest ER** for IV hydration and further testing. Call 911 if no one is available to drive you.

* OK = urine ketones are negative or small, or blood ketones are less than 0.6 mmol/L
** HIGH = urine ketones are moderate or high, or blood ketones are above 0.6 mmol/L

Thanks to Geri Wood, RN, BSN, CDE and John Stanchfield, MD, of Salt Lake City for their helpful suggestions.

Laughter is the tranquilizer with no side effects.

Anon.

when ill to prevent unrecognized ketoacidosis from complicating an already serious situation.

A sudden, extreme rise in blood sugar can be caused by nondelivery from a pump. Pump failure can put an unsuspecting person into ketoacidosis within a few hours. Never go to sleep with a high blood sugar on a pump. If you suspect an infusion delivery problem, use injections to bring the blood sugar down and change the entire pump setup. Check your insulin's expiration date and do not use vials that were opened for more than a month.

Some episodes of ketoacidosis occur after several weeks or months of inattention to testing or to its results. Basal and bolus doses may have gradually become inadequate due to growth, weight gain, or stress. When monitoring is not done or high blood sugar readings are ignored for weeks, your body is at risk. Under these circumstances, a missed insulin dose or the start of an infection can cascade quickly into ketoacidosis.

To Treat Ketosis And Prevent Ketoacidosis

• Treat high blood sugars and moderate or high ketone levels immediately with an insulin injection because insulin delivery from your pump may have stopped.

• Correction doses will be much larger than normal when ketones are present. Injected or basal and bolus doses two or three times greater than normal may be needed until the situation is stabilized.

• Drink as much water and noncaloric or low caloric beverages as possible to correct dehydration. Dehydration comes from the excess urination caused by high blood sugars and worsens rapidly when vomiting begins. Drink 8 to 12 oz. every 30 minutes even if you do not feel thirsty. Diluted Gatorade, water with Nu-Salt™, and similar fluids are good because they help restore potassium levels.

• Monitor the blood sugar at least 4 times a day at all times when on a pump. Wear a continuous monitor and check its reading and trend line often.

• Monitor at least every 2 hours when readings are above 250 mg/dl (13.9 mmol).

• Check for ketones for all single readings above 300 mg/dl (16.7 mmol) and for any two unexplained blood sugar readings above 250 mg/dl (13.9 mmol).

• For one unexplained reading of 250 mg/dl (13.9 mmol) or higher, take a correction bolus. If the blood sugar is still that high or higher two hours later, use an injection to give a correction dose, test for ketones, and change the infusion site and reservoir using a new bottle of insulin.

19.5 What To Do When You Are Ill

Illness, such as a cold or flu, or infection may lead to ketoacidosis. These tips for treatment during illness can help you prevent ketoacidosis.

- Test your blood sugar every 2 hours during the day and at least once in the middle of the night.

- DKA and the flu are very similar. NEVER assume your symptoms are just caused by the flu. Always test your blood sugar before going to bed when you are unusually tired.

- Raise your basal rates if an infection or pain are keeping your numbers high all the time. Call your doctor for treatment advice.

- Never completely stop your basal delivery even if you are not eating. Your bodily functions, as well as this illness still require basal insulin.

- Respond to any high blood sugar promptly. Realize you may need to use more than your normal correction bolus amounts.

- Drink extra water or noncaloric fluids when your blood sugar is above 200 mg/dl (11.1 mmol).

- Check for ketones every 2 to 4 hours if your blood sugar goes above 300 mg/dl (16.7 mmol) or use the Precision Xtra™ meter for blood ketone testing or ketone strips for urine testing.

- If you have any doubt about your insulin delivery, take insulin by injection from a fresh insulin bottle to correct the high readings, remembering that this dose needs to be higher than a normal correction dose if your basal insulin was also not effective. Then replace your reservoir and infusion set, using a new infusion set and the fresh insulin.

- If your blood sugar falls below 90 mg/dl (5 mmol), drink regular soda, fruit juice, milk shake, or a sport drink in 4 to 6 ounce servings, or eat soup, ice cream, pudding, or crackers.

- Call your doctor immediately if vomiting begins.

- Call a health care provider if your blood sugar is over 250 mg/dl (14 mmol), ketones are present, and you feel ill.

- Never go to sleep on a pump with a high blood sugar without checking your insulin delivery. If there is any question about insulin delivery from the pump, give insulin by injection and replace the reservoir and infusion set and site.

- If vomiting begins and you cannot drink fluids, call your physician right away and go to an emergency room. Vomiting means you can no longer hydrate yourself. Dehydration is very serious and medical treatment is required.

When an infection or illness causes blood sugars to go high, the underlying problem must be dealt with first to lower the blood sugar. Medications, like prednisone and cortisone, can cause very high blood sugars. Very large increases in basal and bolus doses may be needed to deal with infection, a serious illness, or some medications. Call your doctor right away to discuss how to treat any underlying problem and how much to increase your doses.

Any very high blood sugar or the presence of ketones while on a pump should raise a red flag. If there is not a clear reason, such as illness or infection, the cause may come from the pump itself, from bad insulin, an infusion set that has come loose, or a leak from a hub or an infusion line. Other causes include incorrect basal or bolus settings, forgetting or neglecting to take boluses, and pain or depression that causes personal care to be neglected. Discuss any problems you have regarding high readings, the presence of ketones, or personal issues regarding diabetes with your physician so you can resolve them quickly and avoid them in the future. Trying to solve them without help is not effective enough in these cases.

19.6 Clever Pump Tricks

Use Injections To Replace Some Basal

Anyone who has had more than one episode of ketoacidosis or who needs to ensure that DKA does not occur, such as someone during pregnancy or in someone with heart disease, may want to replace some basal insulin delivery with an injection of Lantus or NPH, especially overnight. About 50% of basal delivery can be replaced with long-acting insulin to ensure that enough insulin always remains on board if an infusion set becomes dislodged or some other disruption of pump delivery occurs. This greatly reduces risk of DKA in those at high risk and in those who must absolutely avoid this possibility. Discuss how to do this with your physician.

19.7 Is Your Meter Accurate When High?

Many meters lose accuracy as the blood sugar goes above 360 mg/dl (20 mmol). When your meter shows a reading higher than 360 mg/dl, your true blood sugar may be much higher or lower than the actual reading.

Consider whether there is a clear reason for the high reading. If a reading is high for no apparent reason, wash your hands and retest. If the reading remains high for no clear reason, change your site, infusion set, and cartridge.

**During even mild episodes of ketosis, staying hydrated is VITAL.
Drink lots of fluids first, then take insulin to start bringing the blood sugar down.**

**If a reading is high for no apparent reason, wash your hands and retest.
You may have touched something with sugar in it before you tested.
Along with all our diabetes knowledge, we want to remember common sense.**

Learn From Crisis Situations

People often ignore serious control problems until a crisis brings it to their attention. A crisis may be a severe low that causes embarrassment or injury, or readings so high they result in ketoacidosis or a hospital visit.

You may survive a crisis or two without consequences, but it is not wise to count on luck. Get the help you need before someone suffers. Review immediate treatments, such as quick carbs, glucagon, or calling 911, for severe lows. For highs, drink water, inject insulin to ensure delivery, exercise if you're not already in ketosis, or call 911 if vomiting begins.

A pattern of frequent mild lows demands immediate attention because this is the most common warning that a severe low is on its way. Frequent lows reduce your usual warning symptoms and set you up to have a severe low.

Unless caused by an obvious error such as bolusing and neglecting to eat, emergencies usually require an immediate change in TDD, basal rates, or boluses, as well as a review of the lifestyle factors that contributed to the crisis. After an emergency occurs, do not fall back into the old routine that created the problem. Determine what you need to change to avoid repeating it in the future.

Let your doctor help you find new ways to maintain better control. It is rare for someone who has erratic readings to leave the office of an experienced pump specialist on the same basal rates and boluses they came in with. An open mind combined with open discussion with others will speed your progress.

19.8 Emergencies

Problem	Can Be Caused By	Can Be Prevented By
Frequent Lows	weight loss, extra activity, insulin doses being too high or dieting	lowering your basals or boluses or eating more, particularly snacks before exercise
Severe Lows	excess bolus or basal insulin, a missed or delayed meal, increased activity or poorly understood management	reducing insulin doses, correcting the situation that causes the low, adjusting targets upward, plus a willingness to learn more about diabetes control
Severe Highs and Ketoacidosis	bad insulin, faulty set, forgetting or skipping boluses, an infection, severe illness or trauma, steroids, or other medical causes	exercising more, raising your basals or boluses, changing your insulin and set, remembering boluses, or getting help for care of serious medical problems

Spot Patterns And Stop Highs

When you have control problems, always work to stop lows first. If readings are often high, determine the time of day when this occurs or find the circumstance that may cause these highs. The best solution to regain control usually is to raise both your basal rates and carb boluses at the time when highs occur. To be safe, make a small increase in one insulin dose at a time and test often to determine the result before trying another.

This chapter presents how to prevent

- Frequent highs
- Highs before breakfast
- Highs after meals
- After-breakfast highs
- Plus fine-tuning

Frequent Highs

The chart below shows the consistently high blood sugar readings that James has encountered over the past few weeks. This pattern strongly suggests his TDD is too low and needs to be raised. Someone with this pattern will have an A1c level that is well above 7%.

What To Do

Check your basal/bolus balance and raise your TDD through a series of increases in either the total daily basal or carb bolus doses. Choose

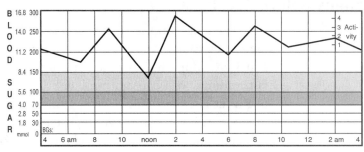

Frequent Highs

the one that is currently lower. Basal and bolus doses are balanced, usually with 50 to 60% of the TDD in basal doses. If your readings are usually between 120 mg/dl and 200 mg/dl range (6.7 to 11.1 mmol), a 3 to 5% increase in your TDD may solve this problem of mild highs. If you frequently go above your target range, review your diet and whether you are covering all the carbs you eat with adequate boluses. Identify whether it is your lifestyle or insulin doses or both that need to be changed. If your readings are not normally as high as recently, consider whether infection, pain, stress, non-potent insulin, a steroid medication, or other new medication might be causing the high readings. In some of these unusual situations, you might need to raise your TDD by much more than 10%, but once the cause is eliminated, your TDD and any specific insulin doses you raised can go back to normal.

Case Study

James' blood sugar is consistently high as shown in the log book. In James' case, a 5% to 10% increase should be considered because his readings

Sugar	Breakfast		Lunch		Dinner		Night	
	Before	After	Before	After	Before	After	Bed	2 a.m.
Sun	163	256	144	292	189	267	212	238
Mon	241	346	212	248	171	283	164	187
Tues	208	219	132	176	143	258	181	206
Wed	233	341	264	217	168	211	145	178
Thurs	204	243	197	236	156	184	173	184
							260	167

James' logbook showing frequent highs

are above 200 mg/dl (11.1 mmol) most of the time. Although he needs to lose weight, he knows his busy schedule as a department store manager during the holiday season will not allow this. After discussing the situation with his doctor, he decided to raise his TDD. Refer to Table 15.3 for suggested increases.

James' current average TDD is 67 units and he uses a single basal rate of 1.5 units per hour for the day. This 36 units of basal insulin (24 hours times 1.5 u/hr) makes up 54% of his TDD. His carb factor is one unit for every 8 grams.

Jeff decided to raise his TDD by about 4.0 units or 6% of his TDD from 67 units to 71 units a day. He raised his basal rate to 1.6 units per hour and his carb factor to one unit for every 7 grams of carb. This increase brought his readings down until he can focus on losing weight after the holidays.

Highs Before Breakfast

The graph on the next page shows different ways in which a high morning reading can be caused by what happens during the night. Readings between 10 p.m. and 8 a.m. show four common patterns that cause a high breakfast blood sugar. If high breakfast readings are a constant problem for you, first determine when your blood sugar begins its rise. You will need more insulin before the rise begins except if it is caused by overtreating a low during the night (line D on the graph). Compare the trend lines in a continuous monitor with Figure 20.1 for help in identifying these patterns.

Four common causes for high blood sugars before breakfast are discussed below.

Already High At Bedtime

Pattern A in Fig. 20.1 is easy to identify because the blood sugar is already high at bedtime and stays high through the night.

What To Do

If your blood sugar is okay during the day but rises after dinner and is still high at bedtime, either a larger carb bolus was needed for dinner or the daytime basal rate may need to be raised. It is also possible that an after-dinner snack has caused this rise. If snacking is a problem, reduce the snack size or fully cover the extra carbs eaten in the evening hours with carb boluses. When you find your blood sugar is high at bedtime, take enough correction bolus to bring the high reading down without causing a nighttime low. This is tricky so be careful. If taking a correction bolus at bedtime corrects the high morning blood sugar

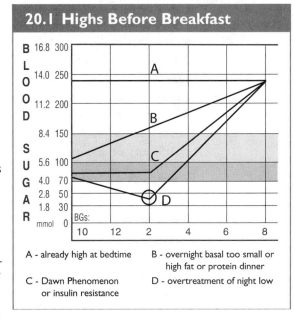

20.1 Highs Before Breakfast

A - already high at bedtime

B - overnight basal too small or high fat or protein dinner

C - Dawn Phenomenon or insulin resistance

D - overtreatment of night low

without causing a low around 2 a.m., your overnight basal dose is fine. Use a continuous monitor to check your overnight basal and to give you a warning if you go low.

If you keep your bedtime reading high because you are afraid you may have a low during the night, discuss this with your physician. You want to recheck your night basal dose to ensure that it keeps your blood sugar flat overnight. Today's pumps allow you to check BOB at bedtime. Any BOB that is still present can be offset with a bedtime snack or with an appropriate temporary basal reduction. Once the basal rate is correctly set and BOB is accounted for, you should be able to go to sleep with a relatively normal bedtime reading and sleep soundly and safely.

Case Study

In Jasmine's situation, her blood sugar rises after dinner as shown in her logbook. She decided to increase her carb bolus for dinner to lower

Sugar	Breakfast		Lunch		Dinner		Night	
	Before	After	Before	After	Before	After	Bed	2 a.m.
Sun	185	212	127	153	76	289	212	207
Mon	204	249	174	156	123	341	238	243
Tues	219	231	84	136	98	207	179	163
Wed	172	187	104	171	143	342	256	268
Thurs	247	233	138	149	107	261	182	196
							260	167

Jasmine's logbook showing highs at bedtime

her bedtime reading into a desirable range. Using a larger carb bolus at dinner is also safer because a dinner bolus will be active while she is awake, rather than having to take an extra correction bolus just before going to sleep.

Low Overnight Basal Rate

Pattern B in Fig. 20.1 and Julie's logbook below shows the blood sugar rising steadily during the night. In her logbook, her Sunday night bedtime blood sugar of 96 mg/dl (5.3 mmol) rises to 151 mg/dl (8.4 mmol) at 2 a.m. and goes higher to 204 mg/dl (11.3 mmol) by breakfast. The rise in the blood sugar through the night hours indicates that the night basal rate is set too low. Remember that a blood sugar test at 1 or 2 a.m. or in the middle of sleep is needed to verify this pattern since the number at 1 a.m. must be significantly higher than the bedtime reading. The graph that covers the last 9 hours on a continuous monitor can help you identify this.

What To Do

Raise the basal dose near bedtime to provide more overnight coverage. Review Chapter 11 on how to test and reset your basal rates.

Sugar	Breakfast		Lunch		Dinner		Night	
	Before	After	Before	After	Before	After	Bed	2 a.m.
Sun	185	341	188	162	76	142	96	151
Mon	204	289	204	187	123	163	132	187
Tues	219	323	225	156	98	138	105	146
Wed	172	291	198	182	143	189	116	163
Thurs	247	284	233	142	107	154	93	127
							122	167

Julie's logbook showing basal too low

When you first raise your evening basal dose, test your blood sugar more often and test at 2 a.m. for a few nights to ensure that no drop in your blood sugar occurs in the middle of the night.

Case Study

Julie was frustrated because her blood sugar always rose during the night, though she ate no bedtime snack. For instance, on Tuesday night her bedtime reading of 105 mg/dl (5.8 mmol) rose to 146 mg/dl (8.1 mmol) at 2 a.m. and then to 172 mg/dl (9.5 mmol) on Wednesday morning. Her physician suggested she raise her basal rate through the night from 1.05 u/hr to 1.15 u/hr, but told her that a readjustment would be needed if she started to have lows during the night or if her morning reading was still high.

High Protein Or High Fat Dinners

Although this pattern is identical to a low overnight basal rate (Both are shown as pattern B), the cause is different. The high breakfast reading only occurs after a large amount of protein or fat is eaten for dinner or as a snack in the evening. The glucose rise from protein eaten at dinner will appear the next morning.

When an 8 to 12-ounce steak, a Mexican dinner with refried beans, or several ounces of nuts are eaten, 40 to 50 percent of the protein in these foods will slowly convert to glucose over several hours. Most meals contain too little protein to affect the blood sugar, but when large amounts are consumed, the blood sugar is sure to rise overnight and stay high.

20.2 The Breakfast Blood Sugar

For most people, the breakfast blood sugar is the most important reading to control because it affects blood sugars for the whole day. When you wake up with a normal reading, it means your basal rates are set correctly during the night. If you have insulin resistance, it means you have increased your basal rate slightly at 1 or 2 am so that your liver is not triggered to make the excess glucose that necessitates larger than normal insulin doses through the morning hours. Alternately, if you have a Dawn Phenomenon it means you have raised your basal rate at 1 or 2 am to match increased insulin need. The rest of the day can go well in either case.

In someone who does not have diabetes, a low insulin level means the blood sugar is also low. The liver responds to the low insulin level by releasing glucose into the blood. The liver responds in the same way to a low insulin level when someone has diabetes, but the blood sugar is high rather than low. Unfortunately the liver does not know this.

Once the liver starts producing extra glucose, whether due to a Dawn Phenomenon in Type 1 diabetes or a rise in insulin resistance during the early hours in Type 2 diabetes, it is difficult to stop. Large correction boluses may be needed before breakfast to lower breakfast readings after eating. Extra care has to be taken to avoid so much morning insulin that an afternoon low can follow.

The inappropriate outpouring of glucose from the liver during the night can best be prevented by having the basal rates correctly set during the night.

High fat meals can also cause the blood sugar to rise over several hours and be high the following morning. Certain varieties of fat found in high fat foods cause insulin resistance to increase. A dual fat/protein effect at work in some food increases the likelihood of a blood sugar rise.

What To Do

• The wise approach is to eat less of the high protein or high fat food.

• If you have eaten more protein than usual in the evening, be sure to correct any high bedtime reading with a full correction bolus.

• If you know from past experience that unusually high morning readings follow eating large portions of protein or fat the evening before, try using a temporary basal rate increase overnight when you eat these foods. Start with 110 or 115% of your normal basal for 6 to 8 hours, and test at 2 a.m. to ensure you are not going low.

• If you are unsure of a meal's effect, wake up halfway through the night and check your blood sugar. Use a correction bolus at that time if needed so that you will be within a reasonable range when you awaken in the morning.

• Use a continuous monitor to see the full effect of protein or fat overnight.

Dawn Phenomenon Or Insulin Resistance

For those with Type 1 diabetes, 50 percent to 70 percent need a higher basal rate starting between 1 a.m. and 3 a.m. to control the Dawn Phenomenon. Of these, 20 to 30 percent need a large basal increase to keep the breakfast reading controlled.[2,53,65] More basal insulin is needed to offset the increased release of growth hormone and cortisol increases in the early morning hours which cause more glucose to be released into the blood. Check with your physician or health care team to make sure you actually have a Dawn Phenomenon before increasing your nighttime basal rate. If you are inconsistently high before breakfast, the problem may have another cause.

In Type 2 diabetes, high morning readings are seen, but for a different reason. In Type 2, excess fat is released from the abdomen into the blood during the night and adds to existing insulin resistance. This causes the liver to increase glucose production unnecessarily and the person to wake up with a high reading. Pumps are ideal for increasing basal delivery at the precise time to prevent this early morning rise. Textbox 20.2 provides an explanation for causes and solutions.

Shown in Jethro's logbook and as pattern C in Figure 20.1, the blood sugar stays level until about 2 a.m. and then begins to rise. When a Dawn Phenomenon causes the

Sugar	Breakfast		Lunch		Dinner		Night	
	Before	After	Before	After	Before	After	Bed	2 a.m.
Sun	185	341	188	162	76	142	96	112
Mon	204	289	204	187	123	163	132	127
Tues	219	323	225	156	98	138	105	121
Wed	172	291	198	182	143	189	116	132
Thurs	247	284	233	142	107	154	93	111
							122	117

Jethro's logbook showing a Dawn Phenomenon

blood sugar to be high before breakfast, it will often remain high after breakfast and require larger than normal correction boluses to overcome the excess glucose production by the liver. To correct a Dawn Phenomenon, more basal insulin is needed during the predawn hours. For those who sleep typical nighttime hours, the basal rate is typically raised between 1 a.m. and 3 a.m. and stays at a higher level until 9 a.m. or 11 a.m.

What To Do

Raise the basal rate early to get the best effect, usually at least two hours before the blood sugar begins its rise. Children may need to raise the basal rate earlier at 11 p.m. or midnight because they may go to sleep earlier and the Dawn Phenomenon may be stronger.

Overtreated Nighttime Lows

Pattern D in Figure 20.1 shows a blood sugar high in the morning caused by an overtreatment of a low blood sugar during the night. See Chapter 16 for how to stop lows at night and how to balance the excess carbs if overeating does occur.

Frequent Highs After Meals

One common and annoying pattern is to have a normal blood sugar before a meal but then go too high after eating. How high the blood sugar rises after a meal depends on the size of the bolus, how early the bolus is given before eating, how many carbs are eaten, activity level after the meal, and the food's glycemic index. Compare the trend lines in a continuous monitor to Figure 20.3 for help in identifying these. Common reasons for postmeal highs are discussed below.

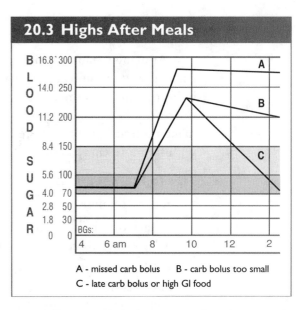

20.3 Highs After Meals

A - missed carb bolus   B - carb bolus too small
C - late carb bolus or high GI food

Missed Carb Bolus

Line A in Fig. 20.3 shows a typical pattern when a carb bolus is not taken for a meal. Forgetting to take a bolus is hopefully rare, but it can be a real problem when it happens.

If you often forget boluses, use the helpful reminders available in today's smart pumps. Change your pattern so that you always take your bolus while the food is being prepared rather than in the bustle of recording numbers or of sitting down to eat. Your smart pump alarm can remind you, or you can wear a wristwatch with up to 12 alarms per day that you can preset to remind you to bolus for meals. If you are unsure whether a bolus was actually given for a recent meal or snack, check the history in your pump to confirm this.

Carb Bolus Too Small

Line B shows a typical pattern when the carb bolus for a meal is too small for the number of carbs eaten. Carb boluses can be too small if carbs are not counted or counted inaccurately, when portions are not measured, when snacks are not fully covered, or if there is hesitation to cover carbs due to a fear of hypoglycemia. Even if you usually count carbs accurately at home, you may misjudge carb boluses for meals that are eaten out or when a casserole or other combination food is eaten.

What To Do

Learn how to do carb counting thoroughly and accurately. The time spent on this will benefit you day after day. If you already practice carb counting, you may want to review the numbers again. Learning how to quantify the effect foods have on your blood sugar becomes invaluable to your control over time. Review Chapter 7 on carb counting to be sure you have a good understanding of this excellent tool.

You may want to retest your carb factor to ensure that the size of your carb bolus is correctly matched to your meals. If a carb factor number is too high, it will result in a high blood sugar when a large amount of carbs is eaten even if it works for meals that have fewer carbs. Larger quantities of carb may uncover an inadequacy in the carb factor that smaller quantities do not reveal.

At many restaurants, nutritional information is available to guide your doses. Pay particular attention to meals that consistently cause high readings so that you choose a bolus that matches the carbs when you return and order the same meal. You may want to create a personal list of restaurant meals with their accompanying insulin doses to make postmeal readings more reliable. With this list in your pocket you can eat out with far more enjoyment.

Tips To Prevent Highs After Meals

• Set a reminder in your pump or a watch so you won't forget to take boluses.

• Take carb boluses 15 to 20 minutes before eating when possible. Be careful not to delay eating. Keep quick carbs available in case the meal is not ready on time.

• Check the glycemic index of any suspect foods. Replace problem foods with ones that have a lower glycemic index. For breakfast, try old-fashioned oatmeal, a high-fiber cereal topped with strawberries, or plain yogurt with fresh fruit sliced into it. More fiber also lessens constipation.

• If you plan to eat a high glycemic index food (white bread, white rice, etc.), be sure to take the carb bolus at least 20 minutes before the meal.

• Review carb counting so that you can avoid a mismatch between carbs you eat and the bolus you take to cover them.

• Add extra fiber like psyllium (sugar-free Metamucil) or guar gum to a meal to reduce its glycemic index. A tablespoon or two of psyllium added to cold cereals can dramatically lower postmeal readings, and lessen both constipation or diarrhea.

• Get 30 to 45 minutes of exercise shortly after the meal. If you have heart disease, get your doctor's approval ahead of time.

• Discuss with your doctor use of a prescription medication like Symlin (pramlintide), Byetta, Precose (acarbose) or Glyset (miglitol) to slow the digestion of carbohydrates and to avoid a postmeal spike.

If you continue to have postmeal spikes, check the balance between your basal and bolus insulins. If the basal insulin is less than 50% of your TDD, raise your basal insulin during the day. Having a higher basal insulin level in the blood prior to eating while using the same or even lower carb boluses can often reduce postmeal spikes. Lower your carb boluses if necessary.

Late Carb Bolus Or A High GI Food

Line C in Fig. 20.3 shows a spiking blood sugar that returns to normal as the insulin finally catches up 4 or 5 hours later. After meal spikes that rise above 150 mg/dl (8.3 mmol) should be avoided whenever possible to lessen glucose exposure and variability.

Carb breakdown starts very quickly after eating begins. Many foods will largely break down and enter the bloodstream within 45 to 60 minutes, unless gastroparesis (see page 170) is present. To offset this, a carb bolus should be taken 15 to 20 minutes before eating.

When boluses are taken just before eating, the blood sugar spikes because even rapid insulins cannot start to work quickly enough. Learn the glycemic index of the foods you eat, and take your carb bolus earlier than usual, such as 30 minutes for foods that have a high glycemic index or eat those foods late in the meal. This may not completely solve the problem but will help lower the spiking.

If you eat a breakfast of old-fashioned oatmeal, your blood sugar will not rise as fast or as high as it will after eating most cold cereals. These cereals, like many other breakfast foods, such as instant oatmeal, yogurt with fruit syrup, or a toasted cheese sandwich, are high glycemic index foods that cause postmeal readings to spike even if the size of the carb bolus is correct.

After-Breakfast Highs Caused By Unrecognized Night Lows

The pattern to the right shows a typical response during the morning hours following unrecognized nighttime hypoglycemia. Note that the blood sugar is normal before breakfast but rises steadily after breakfast because of the stress hormones that were released earlier in the night. Stress hormones often raise the blood sugar for 8 to 10 hours following a major low blood sugar. This can cause a spike after breakfast even though the breakfast carbohydrate has been correctly covered with a carb bolus. The blood sugar may remain higher than usual at lunch and into the afternoon hours.

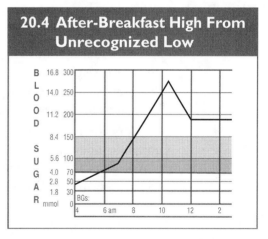

If you have unusual spikes in your reading after breakfast, consider whether you may be experiencing unrecognized nighttime lows. For information on setting and testing overnight basal doses, see Chapter 11.

What To Do

This pattern appears similar to taking a carb bolus that is too small for the breakfast carbs, but it is created by an entirely different problem. Learn to recognize the symptoms that may occur the morning after nighttime hypoglycemia on page 186-187. Set an alarm for 2 a.m. to check whether your blood sugar drops in the middle of the night. If it does, reduce the evening basal dose or eat a small bedtime snack. It is wise to test the blood sugar at 2 a.m. every week or so, even when you don't seem to be having any problems. New ones won't creep up on you that way.

Use of a continuous monitor provides an easy way to identify nighttime lows. Set the alarm feature, and it will warn you every time your blood sugar drops below the limit you set. Review your overnight trend line regularly or download the data into a PC to see several night's readings. Use of a continuous monitor can open your eyes to a problem you never knew existed.

Fine Tuning

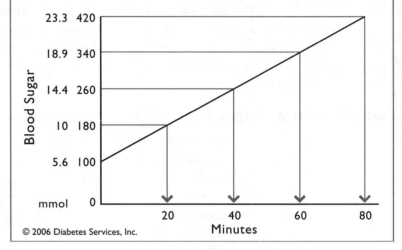

20.5 Fastest Time To Reach 100 mg/dl

How fast can the blood sugar fall? Continuous monitoring studies show that 99 times out of 100 the blood sugar falls less than 4 mg/dl (0.22 mmol) per minute. This chart shows the fastest time you can expect to reach 100 mg/dl (5.5 mmol) when your reading is high. For example, if your blood sugar is 260 mg/dl (14.4 mmol), it will take at least 40 min. to reach 100 mg/dl (5.5 mmol) after a combined carb and correction bolus.

© 2006 Diabetes Services, Inc.

Eventually, you will have adjusted your doses or have changed the timing or type of your insulins so that lows and highs are no longer a major concern. Keeping your readings within your target range then becomes your main priority.

Pay attention to matching your meal doses precisely to grams of carbs and their glycemic index, and make the needed adjustments for changes in activity. Although the results of fine tuning may not be dramatic, making these subtle adjustments every day keeps you actively involved in your control and lets you see even better readings and A1c results.

Celebrate small victories. Never feel guilty or blame yourself for a blood sugar reading that is out of your target range. Use it to learn from. Recognize that if you don't test because you dread seeing the result, any out-of-control blood sugar still affects your body. Only testing allows you to attain really optimal control. When you encounter an unwanted reading or series of readings, focus calmly on figuring out what happened and how you can adapt for better control. Aim to get your next readings back into your target range as soon as possible. With this attitude, your mastery over your blood sugar will continue to evolve and improve.

A few people get up bright and early, but most of us get up early.

Anon.

Unexplained Highs

First Sign Of A Pump Problem

When an unexplained high blood sugar occurs, most pumpers blame excess carbs as the cause. Although this may be the case, the person on a pump must always keep in mind that the cause may originate from the infusion site, the infusion line, the hub, the O-rings in the reservoir, their pump programming, or with the insulin they are using. Although the pump itself rarely fails, any of the parts involved can affect insulin delivery and result in a high blood sugar. When this happens, immediate attention must be directed at finding and solving the cause of the problem.

In this chapter, we cover

- Troubleshooting pump problems
- Clogs
- Leaks
- Tunneling of insulin

A mismatch between a carb bolus and the number of carbs eaten is the most likely cause of a high reading. The next most likely cause is a problem with insulin delivery at the infusion site. When non-delivery is causing a high reading, attempting to give an additional bolus with the pump will not bring the high down. The pump user must keep in mind that the source of their problem could be the pump, infusion set, reservoir, or insulin. If any of these could be the source of an unexplained high, always give an injection with a syringe or pen to get the blood sugar under control until the problem has been sorted out.

An insulin pump enhances control when it is working properly, but it is a mechanical system that can also fail to function. Common pump problems are usually encountered in the first six months of use. It is important to know how to troubleshoot them to speed correcting the problem and minimizing its severity. Fortunately, pump and infusion set problems decrease in frequency as the pumper's experience grows.

Determining The Pump Problem Causing A High

The first sign of a pump problem is usually an unexplained high blood sugar. A high blood sugar will usually begin within 2 to 4 hours after insulin delivery is interrupted. Any complete interruption of delivery can trigger early ketoacidosis as soon as 4 to 5 hours after it occurs. If your blood sugar is unexpectedly high, such as above 250 mg/dl (13.9 mmol) on two consecutive tests, always take an injection to lower it before starting to troubleshoot the pump. Always test for ketones. If moderate or large ketones are present, it is likely that insulin delivery is not occurring or there is a serious medical problem underway.

When an unexpected high blood sugar occurs, keep site problems, mechanical problems, and bad insulin in mind as possible causes. Pumps have audible alarms for some problems. They are designed to sound an alarm if there is a clog or other mechanical problem. As soon as you hear an alarm, check for its source and make any needed corrections.

Other problems like bad insulin or a displaced infusion set will not trigger an alarm. If bad insulin may be causing high readings, change to a new bottle when filling the reservoir. Textbox 21.1 describes what bad insulin looks like. Opening a new vial and filling the reservoir with insulin from it could be your answer.

Steps To Take For Unexplained Highs

When an unexplained high blood sugar occurs without an alarm, start at the infusion site and work back to the pump.

1. Feel around the site for a lump caused by bleeding under the skin or an infection

2. Check whether the infusion set is displaced or loose

3. Look for blood in the line (a good sign of bleeding under the skin)

4. Check for air in the infusion line

5. Look for any damage to the infusion line (smell for an insulin leak)

6. Check that the hub is firmly attached to the reservoir (smell for an insulin leak)

7. Look for any leak between the O-rings on the reservoir

8. Consider bad insulin

Be sure to check when you took your last bolus and consider whether the number of carbs you consumed matched that bolus. If the bolus seems to be accurate, take an injection to cover the high blood sugar, and then replace the reservoir and infusion set using a new infusion site and a new bottle of insulin.

Troubleshooting Pump Problems

Pump problems need to be corrected quickly. To do this, you want to clearly understand how to troubleshoot them and how to deal with them. Become familiar with your insulin delivery system so you can check and correct problems efficiently.

Anytime you have unexplained high blood sugars, check the expiration date and visually check your insulin. Grasp the insulin bottle by the neck, turn it upside down, and swirl it a few times against a light background. Bubbles always rise, but the tiny clumps found in bad insulin, which are very small and hard to see, will fall or attach themselves to the inside wall of the bottle. If you see any particles, your insulin is likely bad. Tiny particles usually appear first, but after a few weeks bad insulin eventually develops a slightly yellow or brown color. The insulin used in a pump always appears as clear as water if it is good.

Insulin is likely to go bad more quickly in a pump reservoir than in the insulin bottle. Insulin in the bottle may still be ok even when it has gone bad in the reservoir. Look for particles through the reservoir wall. If there is any question of potency, usually noticed as an unexplained high blood sugar, replace your reservoir and infusion set immediately. To quickly correct the high blood sugar, take an injection using a new bottle of insulin. It's best to use a fresh bottle with a different lot number, even if you need to make an extra trip to your pharmacy.

Insulin goes bad when exposed to sunlight, heat, or cold. When insulin is in your pump against your body, your body temperature is not high enough to damage your insulin. Exposure to temperature extremes may occur during transit to a distributor, to your pharmacy, or to your home. Freezing insulin or storage in a refrigerator close to 32°F (0°C) may cause problems that become apparent only after unexpected highs. A vial of insulin may be stored at room temperature for 30 days without a problem. An opened vial should not be used more than a month.

Clogs

Fortunately, today's insulins and infusion sets make clogs in the infusion line rare. Clogs can occur, however, with low basal rates (0.4 or lower), after a pump is left in suspend mode for several hours, or if bad insulin is used. If you can see specks or particles in your insulin vial, you can be sure the insulin won't work well in your pump.

Any foreign material, such as betadine or alcohol, that comes in contact with the reservoir or infusion line may cause clogging. Hand lotions, hair sprays, or solvents on your hands, skin, clothing, or in the air may penetrate the infusion tubing and cause clogging. Avoid reuse of reservoirs and infusion lines because it increases the risk of delivery problems as well as the risk of infection.

Insulin is a protein just like an egg white that needs to be kept away from heat and sunlight. If your tubing comes in contact with very hot water, such as in a steaming shower or hot tub, heat may coagulate the insulin. It is wise to disconnect before coming in contact with hot water to avoid this problem.

Pumps have sensors that detect clogs so an alarm should sound once a unit or two is not delivered. If only basal insulin is being delivered, it will take longer for pressure

21.2 Clogs

Problem	Causes	Solutions
Insulin and the plastics in reservoirs and infusion sets are not totally compatible. A clog may occur if insulin comes out of solution and crystallizes, usually near the end of the infusion line or out of sight inside the teflon tubing at the end.	May be a sign that insulin is contaminated. More likely to occur when infusion sets are used beyond 3 or 4 days, when basal rates are low, and when hair spray, hand lotion, or any other solvent is close to the infusion line.	Check that a clog is the problem by removing the entire infusion set including the insertion part. After removal, give a 5 unit bolus. If you see insulin coming out easily, a clog is not the cause. If no insulin comes out, a clog is likely. Change the reservoir, infusion set and insertion set before starting back on the pump. Filling the reservoir with insulin from a new bottle will let you cover both possible causes of the high at one time.

Will Pump Alarm? Maybe

to build in the line and trigger an alarm. With a low basal rate, this delay could be several hours, and a blood sugar may already be high by the time the alarm sounds.

Most common sign of clogging: an alarm or a high blood sugar.

Leaks

If insulin leaks from your reservoir or infusion set, it will evaporate and be difficult to see or feel. Unfortunately, your pump cannot warn you that you have a leak.

Insulin does have a distinctive smell, often described as smelling like creosote, railroad ties, or Band Aids. Smelling the hub is a good way to detect a leak in that location caused by a loose or cracked hub. Smelling the infusion line may help find a leak. A leak between the O-rings at the back of the reservoir cannot be smelled but can often be seen when looked for (see Fig. 9.4). Fortunately, leaks tend to be rare when the setup technique is good.

Most common sign of a leak: a high blood sugar.

How To Check For Leaks And Clogs

After two unexplained high blood sugars in a row, remove the whole infusion set from your body, including the insertion set and metal needle or Teflon tubing. Then follow these steps:

• Send a 10-unit bolus through the tubing to check for clogs. If insulin appears immediately at the tip, there is no clog. If no insulin appears at the tip, the infusion set is clogged and the 10-unit bolus should trigger a high pressure alarm.

21.3 Leaks

Problem	Causes	Solutions
O-Rings		
The seal between the O-rings and the reservoir wall is bad. The leak will be at the back of the reservoir.	When reservoirs sit too long in a warehouse or pharmacy, the lubricant needed for a tight seal between the O-rings will pool at the bottom of the reservoir.	Relubricate the O-rings (see Figure 9.4) before filling a new reservoir with insulin. Use care in handling, especially while inserting the reservoir into the pump. Replace the entire infusion set and use a new site.
Hub		
The fit between the infusion line and the reservoir is not snug enough to prevent insulin loss.	Occurs if your hand grip is weak or inattention leads to twisting the hub too much or too little.	Look for fluid around the hub. Check for the smell of insulin. If the hub feels loose, retighten it gently, using small pliers if necessary
Line		
A break in the line has occurred.	Catching the line in door or drawer, or damage from curious child or pet. Rarely caused by manufacturing defect.	Feel and look for any damage along the infusion line. After giving a bolus, check for any drops of insulin along the line. If any appear, replace the infusion set and prime the line as well as the set itself.
Will Pump Alarm? No		

• Now check the infusion line, hub, or O-rings for leaks. If insulin can be seen or smelled at the hub or is visible along the infusion line or between the O-rings, a leak is responsible for the high blood sugars.

• If neither a clog nor leak is present, replace the infusion set and consider other causes for high blood sugars. Are you having any other health problems or excess stress?

Tunneling Of Insulin

Another cause for unexplained highs occurs if the insulin that is infused beneath the skin leaks back to the skin surface along the infusion line. The skin may reject a foreign object like metal or the surfactants on the outside of a Teflon set. When you slide the needle of an infusion set through the skin, the surrounding tissue becomes mildly inflamed and swollen, which you may not notice. As time passes, however, the tissues around the Teflon or metal needle begin to heal, and this process can lead to what is called tunneling.

This healing process sometimes allows a small path to form along the length of the Teflon tubing under the skin. Any movement of the set, such as that created by an active game of golf or tennis, can then allow insulin delivered at the infusion tip to leak back to the surface of the skin. Once this begins, control will be impossible with this infusion set, and it must be changed.

Tunneling is more common with use of Teflon infusion sets that go straight in and have a shorter length of Teflon than slanted sets. Unfortunately, straight-in sets also cover their entry point, so any leakage of insulin back to the skin surface cannot be seen. When tunneling occurs with slanted Teflon sets, a drop of insulin will occasionally be visible around the set's entry point after a large bolus. Tunneling also can happen with metal needles, but it seems to be less common.

21.4 Tunneling		
Information	**Causes**	**Solutions**
Blood sugars rise unexpectedly due to leakage of insulin along the teflon infusion set or metal needle back to the surface of the skin. More common with Teflon insertion sets, especially those inserted at 90 degrees, or after prolonged use of sets in one spot. Very common after 6 or 7 days. Often seen following activities like golf or tennis.	Because Teflon is inert, it may encourage tissues touching it to "heal" and harden. Bumping or movement of the infusion set then can loosen contact between the teflon and tissue, and open a path for insulin to escape to the outside surface of the skin.	Use any one insertion set no longer than 3 to 4 days. If tunneling happens frequently, try angling the teflon cannula or metal needle as you insert it. Replace the reservoir, infusion set and insertion set when tunneling causes a problem.
Will Pump Alarm? No		

Most common sign of tunneling: a high blood sugar.

Do Not Leave Infusion Sets In Too Long

Another cause of high blood sugars is leaving your infusion set in too long. When an infusion set is left in longer than three days, it may loosen and allow tunneling to occur around it, or it may cause irritation or infection that will drive up the blood sugar. Check for redness of the skin at the site. Change your set and see whether the blood sugar comes down. You may need an antibiotic if an infection has occurred. It is best to change your sets every three days and avoid the problem entirely.

Running Out Of Insulin

Running out of insulin also can cause high blood sugars. Today's reservoirs hold 176, 200, 300 or 315 units of insulin. Many pumpers forget how quickly this insulin disappears. The following tips help in managing your insulin supply:

• Keep a bottle of rapid insulin and a syringe or an insulin pen available at all times in case you run out of insulin in your pump.

• Set the low reservoir alarm on your pump to alert when about half of your usual TDD is left in the pump. For instance, if your TDD is 50 units a day, set your alarm for about 25 units. When you hear the alarm, start planning how to deal with it.

• Keep a regular schedule for filling your reservoir and changing your infusion set and site. Choose a convenient time to change your set and site every second or third day, and have your pump remind you to do it at that time. Be careful not to do this near bedtime since you will not know if a problem develops during the next eight hours.

• If you have used more insulin than usual and don't have enough in your reservoir to last until your next scheduled change, you can conserve the insulin in your pump by using it only for basal delivery. Temporarily inject with a syringe or insulin pen for your boluses. Keep checking to be sure there is enough insulin left in your reservoir to provide the basal insulin you need.

• At least one pump has a hidden reserve that remains available for basal delivery. When the Smiths Medical Cozmo or CozMore pump reaches "zero insulin left," it actually has 10 units left that can be used only for basal insulin delivery. This is often enough to get you to the next scheduled infusion set change.

• If you run out of insulin and have no other insulin available, remember there are 10 to 20 units in your infusion line that can be accessed in an extreme emergency.

Contact The Manufacturer

If you have or suspect a problem with the pump itself, call the manufacturer for help. (The phone number can be found on the back of the pump.) The customer service representative can assist you in checking the pump. If a problem is found, they will send you a replacement and packaging to use to return your current pump. It is wise to have a vial of long-lasting insulin on hand and know how to use it if you have to rely on injections for a day or two. See Table 9.11 for how to replace your pump with injections.

Summary

Whenever your blood sugar is high, don't panic. You have time enough to think through what the cause might be before taking action. Could it be extra carbohydrate intake, too little bolus or basal insulin, an infection, or bad insulin? If these do not seem to apply, check for mechanical causes.

Do not continue to rely on pump therapy if your blood sugar remains high and you are unable to correct it after working on these issues. Anytime your blood sugar readings are over 250 mg/dl (13.9 mmol) twice in a row without a clear reason, take an injection of rapid insulin and test your blood sugar often until you are sure you have corrected the problem. Replace your reservoir and entire infusion set before relying on your pump again. Check for ketones and call your physician/health care team immediately if your ketones are moderate or high.

The wise pumper keeps all possible causes for an unexplained high in mind. It is important to quickly differentiate between whether a high blood sugar is due to a problem unrelated to delivery of insulin or whether you have a delivery problem with your site, infusion set, reservoir, or pump.

Frequent monitoring is the best way to detect a problem before it becomes serious.

The best and most beautiful things in the world cannot be seen or touched,
they must be felt with the heart.

Helen Keller

Solutions For Site And Skin Problems

A Teflon tube or metal needle placed through the skin, like a splinter or other foreign body, can cause irritation, discomfort, infection, or other problems beneath the skin. Infusion sets and adhesives, or more rarely insulin itself, can trigger an allergic reaction. Many pumpers rarely encounter a site or skin problem, while others have to pay close attention to avoid them.

This chapter discusses how to deal with site and skin problems

- Allergies
- Infections
- Bleeding
- Pump bumps
- Pump hypertrophy
- Scarring

Allergies

Your skin may not like every infusion set, plastic infusion line, tape or dressing you use to keep insulin flowing into your body. If a tape, adhesive, or tubing causes an allergic reaction, it is easy to diagnose because the itchy area, irritation, or redness forms a pattern with the same shape as the tape, dressing or infusion line that causes it. When an infusion set is the culprit, redness and irritation will occur at the point where the Teflon set enters the skin.

Allergies are unusual and usually start a few days or weeks after a particular tape or adhesive material is first used. Treatment involves switching to another brand of tape, dressing, or infusion set. A protective dressing like Skin Prep™ can also be used on the skin before applying a problematic tape or adhesive to provide a protective barrier between the skin and the offending material. If a Teflon or a metal infusion set is causing the allergy, a wide variety of infusion sets made by different manufacturers can be tried. Discuss changing to another product or using Skin Prep™ with your physician.

If an allergy to the plastic infusion line occurs, place Skin Prep™ or a compatible adhesive material under the infusion line as a barrier.

An insulin allergy starts as a localized reaction with itching and redness at the spot where the insulin is infused, usually within 5 to 15 minutes after insulin is given. Allergies to human insulin are extremely rare with today's highly purified insulins. Also rare are allergies for genetically altered varieties, such as Humalog, Novolog, or Apidra. Although rare, a serious systemic insulin allergy can trigger a widespread itching or possibly anaphylactic shock.

Infections

Many people with diabetes face a higher risk of infection because high blood sugar levels weaken the immune system. Most pump-related infections result from poor technique, such as breathing onto the infusion set, not washing the hands with soap and water before starting to change the set, touching the infusion needle or top of the insulin bottle, not using Opsite® IV Prep, Betadine™ Solution, or Hibiclens® on the skin, not using a bio-occlusive material, or leaving the infusion set at one site longer than 48 or 72 hours. To prevent infections, conscientiously use sterile technique, as described in Chapter 9. Assume an infection can happen and take care that it does not.

At the infusion site, watch for these signs of an infection:

- redness or inflammation
- pain
- warmth
- swelling

The first sign of an infection may be unexplained high blood sugars. Always check the infusion site if two unexplained high readings occur in a row to see if the infusion set has come out or if there is an infection. If signs of an infection are seen, contact your physician immediately. Early treatment with an antibiotic keeps a small infection from developing into an abscess, requiring surgery or hospitalization. Your physician will be happier calling in a prescription than having to lance an abscess or write hospital admission orders. Do not wait until it becomes a crisis.

If soreness or redness occurs at an infusion site, remove the set immediately and gently squeeze out any fluid underneath the skin. If bright red blood comes out, it is likely just a hematoma (bleeding under the skin). Change to a new infusion site using a new infusion set.

However, if the fluid is whitish, discolored, or appears to be pus, temporarily discontinue pump use until an antibiotic has been started by your physician. An infection may spread through the body to a new infusion site if you simply change your set and site. Remove the infusion set and start giving insulin by injection with a syringe or pen until an oral antibiotic has been used long enough for the site to clear. Do not use this site again until the inflammation and swelling have cleared. Once you restart on your pump, watch the new site to ensure an infection does not appear.

Nonfatal toxic shock has been reported from infusion site infections. One case was reported in a rebellious teenager, and another in a pumper who used only alcohol as a disinfectant and allowed several days to pass between infusion site changes.[89] Always treat site infections with care. If you are prone to skin infections, discuss with your physician having a prescription on hand for a broad spectrum antibiotic to use for early treatment. Fungal infections also may occur after prolonged use of sites.

Sterile technique and hygiene are your best insurance against infections.[90] To prevent infections and reduce the size of staph colonies, a common cause of site infection, on the skin, follow the steps in "Prepare Your Site" on pages 105 and 106.

Bleeding

Bleeding from a broken blood vessel occurs infrequently when an infusion set is placed through the skin. It may create a cosmetic problem or, at worst, require changing the set. Bleeding can occur in three areas and each requires different treatment.

On Top of the Skin

When an infusion set is inserted, it can nick a small blood vessel near the surface of the skin. This shows up as a blood stain under the tape or dressing. Surface bleeding can be ignored as long as the site is not inflamed, painful, enlarged, or threatening to discolor your wardrobe. Monitor this situation carefully to make sure it does not worsen. Even though this is not a critical situation, moving the infusion site does ensure that further bleeding will not occur.

Inside the Infusion Tube

Blood inside the infusion tubing near the needle means that bleeding is occurring at the tip of the infusion set. This dilutes the insulin the pump is delivering and decreases its action. A high blood sugar may be the first sign of this problem. Whenever you see blood inside the infusion tubing, immediately remove the infusion set and insert a new one at another location.

Under the Skin

Bleeding under the skin may cause a hematoma. The lump may feel uncomfortable or sore like a bruise. The skin may be normal in color or slightly red.

A pool of blood under the skin dilutes the insulin the pump is delivering, and a high blood sugar may be the first sign of this problem. The hard, enlarged lump under the skin is a pool of blood that invites bacteria to grow and multiply, thus increasing the risk for an infection or abscess.

Move the infusion site right away if you feel a lump under the skin. Firmly squeeze the lump to extract as much matter as you can. If the discharge comes out bright red, it is likely a simple hematoma, but if any other color is seen, it is more likely an abscess and may require an antibiotic. If you have any doubts or questions about whether a sore spot is a hematoma or an infection, call your physician or health care team immediately. Monitor the site carefully. Early treatment is always best.

Pump Bumps

A pump bump may sound like a dent found in your pump after you've dropped it, but it is instead a slightly red, raised, pimple-sized spot found at the infusion site after an infusion set is removed. The spot gradually disappears after you change to a new infusion site. What causes pump bumps is not clear, but theories include a reaction to the coating on the outside of the needle or catheter, or a reaction to preservatives and other trace chemicals found in insulin.

If you are concerned about pump bumps for cosmetic reasons, there are a couple of ways to reduce the chance of getting one. Cover the infusion site with IV Prep® and place an IV 3000 or other adhesive on the skin before inserting the infusion set. Take extra care to use sterile technique, and change the infusion site every 48 to 72 hours.

Pump Hypertrophy

When an infusion set is repeatedly placed into one area of the body, that area of the body will enlarge. Insulin causes cells, especially fat cells, to grow. This causes pump hypertrophy or enlargement when insulin is repeatedly placed under the skin in the same area of the body. Though not a medical problem, it may be a cosmetic concern. A simple solution is to rotate infusion sites through other parts of the abdomen, buttocks, or legs. Avoid the involved area for 3 to 4 weeks to allow healing to occur. Change infusion sites every three days whether there is a problem or not.

Scarring At The Infusion Site

If a certain area of your anatomy seems firm and unyielding to touch or has undergone surgery or an abscess in the past, there may be scarring. Luckily, the skin is our largest organ and there are many locations in which an infusion set can be placed. Poor absorption of insulin at infusion sites due to scarring occurs, but it receives an excessive amount of blame for control problems. When other sources for high blood sugars are carefully reviewed, scarring at the site rarely turns out to be the cause.

To determine whether tissue scarring may be the cause of high blood sugars, ask how soon after placing a new set did the high blood sugar start. If the blood sugar begins to rise soon after inserting a new set and remains high while that site is used, poor absorption becomes one of several possible causes. However, if the blood sugar rises eight or more hours later, look for another explanation for the high readings.

Exercise

Exercise sharpens the mind, tones the body, and strengthens the heart and lungs. It also combats depression, creates a sense of well-being, increases endurance, helps you resist stress and fatigue, and lowers body fat and cholesterol levels.

Exercise is important for anyone's health program, but especially those with diabetes. With planning, monitoring, and balancing of carbs and insulin, you can exercise with a renewed spirit and confidence, knowing that you are strengthening your body, improving your ability to manage your diabetes, and offsetting the risk of complications.

This chapter explains

- Benefits of exercise

- Things that affect the blood sugar during exercise: fuel sources, the insulin level, training status, duration, and intensity

- How to determine carb equivalents with ExCarbs to increase carb intake, reduce boluses or basals, or lower high readings

- Tips on blood sugar monitoring

- Ways to avoid exercise lows

- Reasons the blood sugar may rise after exercise: too little insulin, aerobic exercise, competition, and dehydration

- When is a blood sugar too high to exercise

- Exercise risks

Benefits

Exercise provides benefits to the heart and blood vessels and increases lifespan. The protection offered by exercise becomes especially important due to the higher risk for heart disease with diabetes. Researchers studying Harvard alumni found that lifespan increases steadily as exercise levels rise from burning 500 calories a week (couch potato) to 3,500 calories per week (physically fit).[91] The exercise needed to burn 3,500 calories is equivalent to walking three miles an hour for seven hours a week, bicycling 10 miles an hour for five hours a week, or running nine miles an hour for 2.7 hours a week.

Even fast walking by men with diabetes is associated with less heart disease and longer lifespan.[92] If burning 3,500 calories a week is too much, getting off the couch and exercising a small amount can

23.1 Let Your Goal Determine How You Exercise

Your Goal	Frequency	Intensity	Duration
Reduce Risk of Heart Disease and Illness	2-3 times a week	40% max. heart rate	15-30 min.
Get Physically Fit	4 times a week	70-90% max. heart rate	15-30 min.
Lose Weight	5 times a week	45-60% max. heart rate	45-60 min.

Use this formula to determine your maximum heart rate:
220 - your age = your maximum heart rate

© 2006 Diabetes Services, Inc.

be a major step to cardiovascular protection. Burning 1,000 calories a day, equivalent to walking a mile and a half, benefits the heart and may be more appealing for those who do not enjoy running marathons. Table 23.1 reviews the frequency, intensity, and duration of exercise required to reach different goals.

Regular exercise means less insulin is needed and blood sugars are easier to control. One research study of 30 people with Type 1 diabetes on frequent injections who exercised regularly found their A1c levels were lower (7.0% versus 7.9%) compared to 23 others on frequent injections who were sedentary.[93]

The amount of oxygen a person can breathe also depends on the blood sugar level. Research from Austria revealed that air flow through the lungs is reduced as much

23.2 How Your Blood Glucose Level Affects Performance

Blood Glucose	Effects Of Glucose And Insulin On Metabolism	Impact on Performance
< 70 mg/dl	Too much insulin and not enough glucose available to cells	Fatigue, poor performance
70 to 180	**Efficient fuel flow**	**Maximum performance**
> 180 mg/dl	If insulin level is OK, blood sugars come down	Performance may be reduced, exercise OK to do.
> 250 mg/dl	Insulin level determines whether glucose rises or falls (usually falls).	Fatigue, poor performance: check for ketones, consider taking bolus before exercise.

© 2006 Diabetes Services, Inc.

as 15 percent when the blood sugar runs high.[94] An oxygen deficit of this magnitude would certainly impede performance. Table 23.2 shows how the blood sugar level affects performance.

Things That Affect The Blood Sugar During Exercise

Carb intake and insulin reductions have to be tailored for a person's training level and the intensity and duration of exercise. These are some of the most important factors that affect the blood sugar during exercise and activity. Table 23.3 lists other things that will affect your blood sugar control during exercise.

23.3 Control During Exercise Depends On
• A recent history of good or poor control
• Recent low blood sugars
• Current insulin level
• Timing of the exercise relative to recent meals and injections
• Current blood sugar
• Length and intensity of the exercise
• Training level
• Whether exercise is aerobic or anaerobic
• Stress hormone release in competitive sports

Fuel Sources

The first fuel source available for exercise is the glucose already present in the blood. This limited supply is quickly followed by the release of glucose from muscle and liver glycogen stores. Although glucose and glycogen are easily accessible and rapidly released, the supply of these fuels in the body are limited.

For instance, during strenuous exercise, a normal glucose level in the blood can be depleted in about four minutes, compared to 30 minutes at rest.[95] The liver plays a critical role in supplying additional glucose by breaking down glycogen and releasing it as glucose into the blood. The liver's glycogen stores can be depleted after 20 to 30 minutes of very strenuous exercise.

Fat is the body's largest fuel reserve. Fat stores are about 2,000 times as large as glucose stores and are nearly impossible to deplete even in a thin person. To access internal fat stores for long periods of activity, the insulin level in the blood must fall.

The Insulin Level

The blood sugar is always directly affected by the insulin level, so it is not surprising that the insulin level is important to exercise and activity. When someone without diabetes starts a strenuous exercise like running a marathon, the blood insulin level drops to half of its pre-exercise level over the first 15 to 30 minutes.[96] During moderate exercise, about an hour passes before the same drop in the blood insulin level is seen.

23.4 How Your Insulin Level Affects Performance

Insulin Level	Level of Stress Hormones	Effect on Glucose and Fat Stores	Effect on Glucose	Effect on Performance
Low	Increased	Less glucose enters muscles, more release from glucose and fat stores	High or rising	Poor performance, possible ketosis
Ideal	**Normal**	**Glucose enters muscles, glucose and fat are released as fuel normally**	**Level**	**Optimal performance**
High	Decreased, until hypoglycemia begins	More glucose enters muscles, less release from glucose and fat stores	Low or falling	Poor performance, probable hypoglycemia

© 2006 Diabetes Services, Inc.

This natural drop in the insulin level as exercise begins allows

- Glucose to be released from glycogen stores in the muscle and liver
- Fat to be released and used as fuel
- New glucose to be created by the liver

The blood insulin level determines how much carbohydrate and fat can be accessed as fuel. When insulin levels are too high, more sugar enters exercising muscles from the blood, less is released from glycogen stores, and less fat is released to replace the dropping glucose level. The blood sugar will drop rapidly unless carbs are eaten, forcing the person to eat or drink carbs in order to balance the high insulin level.

On the other hand, when insulin levels are too low, an excess of glucose and free fatty acids are released into the blood, and glucose is less able to enter exercising muscles. This weakens performance and causes the blood sugar to rise. The right insulin level, neither too high or too low, prevents fuel delivery problems.

A person's best performance occurs when fuels are available during exercise to provide energy. Well-adjusted basal rates and boluses during and after long periods of activity allow the body to access more fat for fuel rather than having to rely on much smaller glucose and glycogen stores. The blood sugar becomes more stable once the insulin level is lowered enough that muscles can easily access internal stores of fat and glucose, but not so low that glucose can no longer be transported into muscle. Table 23.4 shows the impact that the insulin level has on stress hormones, glucose and fat stores, the blood sugar, and overall performance.

Training Status

Someone who is not trained requires as much as 25 percent more glucose for a particular exercise than someone who is trained. Training builds glycogen stores in the muscles involved in exercise so they can provide fuel locally when they are used again. A physically fit person has larger glycogen stores to draw upon and this usually dampens blood sugar fluctuations. If the blood sugar is falling, more glucose is available for release. When the blood sugar is rising, such as after a meal, more can be shifted into glycogen stores so the blood sugar is less likely to rise. Once basal rates and boluses are appropriately adjusted, the fit person has more stable readings.

If a sedentary person suddenly decides to engage in strenuous activity for a few hours, they will need more carbs and a greater reduction in insulin doses than the trained individual. A person who exercises different muscles than usual will also need more adjustments. For example, someone who runs regularly will experience a greater drop in blood sugar when they use different leg muscles, such as for a bike ride, even though the total energy they use may be the same. A greater than normal fall in the blood sugar will occur for several hours following a new activity as glycogen stores become enlarged in relatively untrained muscles. This enlarging of glycogen stores occurs after any new activity in case the person decides to do the same activity again.

The glycogen stores developed during routine exercise begin to disappear when an exercise is missed for three days or more. If a runner or biker has their normal schedule interrupted by weather or obligation, their muscles will undergo more glycogen rebuilding on their return to their exercise. They will experience a larger than normal fall in blood sugar in the first few days of restarting their normal exercise.

The less trained one is, the greater the insulin reduction that will be required. Those who have already set and adjusted basal and bolus doses accurately will find that smaller adjustments in these doses will be needed when they begin a daily exercise routine. When starting a new exercise or returning to your usual exercise after a few days, a larger reduction in boluses and basal rates is required.

The less trained you are for an activity, the more likely your blood sugar will go low and the greater the need to lower your insulin doses.

Intensity

Whether you walk or run a mile makes no difference in how much energy you use. Both consume the same number of calories, but where the calories come from differs. As exercise intensity increases, so does the amount of glucose that is needed as fuel. At rest, free fatty acids supply most of our fuel. During mild exercise like walking, energy is still largely obtained from fat, so the blood sugar is less likely to fall.

In a one-mile walk, about 20 percent of the calories consumed come from glucose while 80 percent come from fat. While running the same mile at a strenuous pace, as much as 80 percent of the calories come from glucose. When a higher percentage of glucose is used, the blood sugar is more likely to drop. Strenuous exercise requires more carb intake or a larger reduction in insulin doses than mild exercise even though a similar number of calories may be consumed.

The more strenuous an activity, the more likely your blood sugar will go low and the greater the need to lower your insulin doses.

Duration

Just as the length of a car trip affects the gallons of fuel consumed, duration of exercise affects the number of carbs consumed. Longer activities are more likely to cause the blood sugar to fall unless the insulin level is too low. For instance, a leisurely 30 minute walk has little impact on the blood sugar, but a 60 minute walk may require extra carbs or even a small reduction in insulin. In someone with a normal pancreas, when moderate or strenuous exercise extends beyond 40 to 60 minutes, the blood insulin level gradually falls so the body can preserve its limited stores of glucose and glycogen and switch to using more fat for fuel.

With diabetes, basal rates and boluses often need to be lowered when activities last longer than 45 to 90 minutes so the body can switch from using glucose to using fat as its primary fuel. If the insulin level is not reduced, less fat is available for fuel, and more carbs must be eaten to supply energy and prevent a low.

For example, a 150 pound person uses 3,350 calories during six hours of strenuous exercise. At the start of this exercise, a nondiabetic person will use glucose for 80 percent of the fuel they need. After three hours, about equal amounts of energy come from glucose and fat. After six hours, fuel use will have switched, with almost 80 percent of energy being derived from fat. Half the calories come from carbs that are eaten and glucose from internal glycogen stores, with the other half coming from fat. In someone with diabetes if the insulin level remains high, most of the 3,350 calories would have to be eaten to keep the blood sugar from falling. This is equivalent to almost two pounds of pure sugar or twenty 12-ounce cans of regular soda. Having a lower insulin level during long periods of exercise prevents low blood sugars as well as stomach aches.

The longer an activity lasts, the more likely your blood sugar will go low and the greater the need to lower your insulin doses.

Table 23.5 provides estimates for the grams of carb that are required for exercise at various personal levels of intensity and for various lengths of time. The number of grams are for each 100 lb. of weight and must be adjusted for an individual's weight. These estimates should be the maximum number required for the exercise. Fewer carb equivalents are often required. If more are required, carefully review whether your basal rates or boluses may be too high.

A normal blood sugar during and after exercise is the best indicator that you have an ideal balance between insulin doses and carb intake.

23.5 ExCarbs Needed For Exercise Per 100 lbs. Of Weight

Exercise Intensity

Duration (minutes)	1	2	3	4	5	6	7
0							
15	4	9	13	17	21	26	30
30	9	17	26	34	43	51	60
45	13	26	39	51	64	77	90
60	17	34	51	69	86	103	120
75	21	43	64	86	107	129	150
90	26	51	77	103	129	154	180
105	30	60	90	120	150	180	210
120	34	69	103	137	171	206	240
150	43	86	129	171	214	257	300
180	51	103	154	206	257	309	340
210	60	120	180	240	300	360	420
240	69	137	206	274	343	411	480

A = Carb Intake   B = Carb intake + bolus reduction
C = Carb Intake + bolus reduction + basal reduction

© 2006 Diabetes Services, Inc.

Determine Carb Equivalents With ExCarbs

One recommendation for how many carbs to consume during exercise is 15 to 30 grams every 30 to 60 minutes. Another estimate, based on body weight, says that intense activity requires about one half gram of carb per pound of body weight per hour.[97] This means that someone who weighs 120 lbs would normally require no more than 60 grams of carb per hour for strenuous exercise.

For more specific estimations of carb intake for various types of exercise, use ExCarbs. ExCarbs quantifies how many carbs an exercise will consume. For example, on a car trip, it is easy to determine how much fuel the car will need. Once you know how long a trip will take (duration), the car's average speed (effort or intensity), and how much fuel is used at that speed, you can closely calculate how many gallons of gas (energy) will be needed.

249

Estimating fuel need for exercise is similar. If someone weighs 150 pounds and runs 30 minutes (duration) at 7 miles per hour (effort or intensity), exercise physiologists know this run will consume 320 calories. If these calories came only from glucose, calculating the number of carbs needed would be simple. One gram of carb provides four calories, so 320 calories divided by 4 calories per gram equals 80 grams of carb.

However, the human body is similar to a hybrid car engine in that it uses two fuels. Internal stores of glucose and fat, as well as carbs that are eaten, can be used as sources of fuel during exercise. The ExCarb tables in this chapter estimate the number of carbs needed for exercise based on its intensity and duration in Table 23.5 or, alternately, for specific types of exercise in Table 23.6.

Exercise physiologists have determined how many calories are used in a variety of activities per 100 lbs. of weight. The intensity and duration of an exercise determines how much of the fuel burned will come from glucose compared to fat. The more intense an exercise, the greater the percentage of carbs that will be needed, while the longer an exercise lasts, the more fuel that must be supplied by fat. This allows a close determination of how many grams of carb will be consumed in different activities per 100 lbs. of body weight, as shown in Table 23.6.

The length of an exercise is easy to determine with a watch or clock, but intensity is specific to the individual. If two people are running side by side, one may be running at maximum intensity while the other is relaxed and carrying on an animated conversation. Intensity can be estimated with a 1 to 7 personal intensity scale. The number one is a slight increase in activity, such as a casual walk, while a seven would be all-out exercise, such as running hard while barely able to talk between deep breaths.

Lower numbers are given to activities that are relatively easy to do, such as casual walking. Middle numbers are given to things that make you breathe hard but you are able to do for some time, such as brisk walking or jogging. The highest numbers would apply to exercise that causes deep breathing but you can still carry on a conversation. Examples might be race walking or cross-country skiing.

Once you know how many ExCarbs your exercise will consume, you can replace them with more carb intake, with a reduction in basal rates or boluses, or to bring a high blood sugar down to your target.

ExCarbs allow you to balance exercise

1. By eating more carbs to maintain your current weight
2. By lowering bolus or basal doses to help with weight loss and more easily compensate for longer periods of exercise
3. By lowering an elevated blood sugar
4. By combining these

This ExCarb table shows the maximum grams of carbs required for one hour of specific exercises for people who weigh 100, 150, and 200 lbs. When insulin doses are appropriate, these should be the maximum needed per hour to prevent a low blood sugar.

Use ExCarbs As Carbs

The simplest way to balance exercise is to eat extra carbs. When carbs are eaten to replace the glucose consumed during activity, no carb bolus is needed to cover these carbs. To begin using ExCarbs, look up a planned exercise in Table 23.6 to determine how many carbs are likely needed for compensation. This number of carbs would usually be the maximum number you need to eat before, during and after the exercise to maintain control. Often less than these maximum amounts will be needed for those who are trained for the activity and have already reduced their insulin doses appropriately.

23.6 Ex Carbs: Grams Of Carb Per Hour Of Activity				
Activity		**Weight**		
		100 lbs.	**150 lbs.**	**200 lbs.**
baseball		25	38	50
basketball	moderate	35	48	61
	vigorous	59	88	117
bicycling	6 mph	20	27	34
	10 mph	35	48	61
	14 mph	60	83	105
	18 mph	95	130	165
	20 mph	122	168	214
dancing	moderate	17	25	33
	vigorous	28	43	57
digging		45	65	83
eating		6	8	10
golf (pull cart)		23	35	46
handball		59	88	117
jump rope 80/min		73	109	145
mopping		16	23	30
mountain climbing		60	90	120
outside painting		21	31	42
raking leaves		19	28	38
running	5mph	45	68	90
	8 mph	96	145	190
	10 mph	126	189	252
shoveling		31	45	57
skating	moderate	25	34	43
	vigorous	67	92	117
skiing	crosscountry 5mph	76	105	133
	downhill	52	72	92
	water	42	58	74
soccer		45	67	89
swimming	slow crawl	41	56	71
	fast crawl	69	95	121
tennis	moderate	23	34	45
	vigorous	59	88	117
volleyball	moderate	23	34	45
	vigorous	59	88	117
walking	3mph	15	22	29
	4.5 mph	30	45	59

(Do not cover these carbs with a bolus.)

For instance, if you weigh 150 pounds and take a one hour walk at 3 miles an hour, the ExCarb table shows that you will use 22 grams of carbs in your walk. This is equal to an average-size apple or a cup of milk plus a graham cracker. If you walk at the same pace for two hours rather than one, you will need 44 grams of carbohydrate, while if you walk only 30 minutes, 11 grams will be required.

If instead of walking, you run the same 3 miles at a speed of 8 m.p.h., you will need 53 grams of carbohydrate (145 grams times 22 min. ÷ 60 min.), even though it takes only 22 minutes to complete the run. This is more than twice the amount needed for the leisurely one-hour walk over the same ground! Though walking or running 3 miles requires the same total calories, a higher percentage of these calories comes from carbohydrates while running because it is more intense than walking.

During the first 30 minutes of moderately strenuous exercise, like running at 6 m.p.h., most of the carbs required come directly from glycogen stores in leg muscles. Only about 10 percent are immediately derived from the blood as glucose. Only this glucose has to be immediately replaced by eating carbs or by production and release of glucose from the liver. Even if insulin levels are high during a 30-minute run, only about 16 percent of the calories come from glucose in the blood. The rest of the glucose derived from glycogen stores can, in most instances, be replaced after the exercise, unless experience tells you otherwise.

During the first 30 minutes of exercise, local muscle glycogen contributes five times as much glucose as the blood. But as running continues beyond 30 minutes, more and more glucose begins to be drawn through the blood from sources other than local glycogen stores. The percentage of glucose coming from the blood gradually climbs to a maximum of about 40 percent during the first couple of hours. This makes it more and more necessary to eat or drink carbs to avoid a fall in blood sugar.

Immediate replacement of all the carbs used in exercise is not necessary. For instance, someone who weighs 150 lbs. and rides a bicycle at 10 m.p.h. for one hour will require about 48 grams of carbs. Replacement carbs can be eaten during and within a

23.7 Quick And Slow Carbs For Exercise

Not all carbs are the same. Different foods raise the blood sugar at different speeds. Knowing these speed differences can be useful.

Fast carbs are ideal for raising low blood sugars before or during exercise, and for exercise that consumes carbs rapidly. Fast carbs include glucose tablets, Sweet Tarts, honey, corn flakes, raisin bran, athletic drinks (Gatorade™, Power Ade™), dried or ripe fruits, and regular soft drinks.

Slow carbs help prevent a blood sugar drop during longer periods of activity. They can be eaten at the start of exercise and every 45 minutes thereafter. Slow carbs also help replenish glycogen stores after exercise. Slow carbs include PowerBars™, oatmeal, Swiss muesli, fruit,, ginger snaps, pasta al dente, brown rice, and many candy bars.

A trained marathon runner who is eating a high carb diet can run for about four hours before exhaustion sets in. However, when food high in fat and protein but low in carbohydrate is eaten, exhaustion begins in less than an hour and a half, long before the finish line.

Carbohydrate is needed to build muscle glycogen. Diets that are low in carbohydrate rob the muscles of the glycogen stores needed for maximum endurance and performance. To improve performance, many athletes "fuel up" glycogen stores in muscle cells by eating diets high in carbohydrate. This "carb loading" is often done the evening before a major exercise event but may be more effective when extra carbs are eaten within 30 minutes after any strenuous exercise.

couple of hours of the ride. This person could eat or drink 24 grams of carbs before and during the ride, and an equal number of grams within a couple of hours after the ride.

During exercise, the glucose derived from muscle glycogen does not need to be immediately replaced unless the insulin level is so high that glycogen stores are unable to release glucose. In this situation, eating becomes the only way to deliver fuel to exercising muscle and avoid a low.

The longer and more intense an exercise, the longer it takes to rebuild muscle glycogen. After a long period of activity, the blood sugar may fall for 24 to 48 hours as glucose is gradually removed from the bloodstream to rebuild depleted glycogen stores. When activity lasts longer than an hour, many of the carbs needed to compensate must be consumed in the hours that follow. Make sure to add uncovered carbs to the bedtime snack to prevent a nighttime drop for exercise during the day.

Use ExCarbs To Reduce Insulin

Eating extra carbs is the easiest way to handle shorter or less intense exercise, but as exercise becomes longer and more intense, a reduction in insulin doses becomes more necessary. How many units to reduce your insulin can be determined by dividing the ExCarbs an exercise requires by your carb factor. This converts grams of carb into equivalent units of insulin which can then be used to reduce basal rates or boluses.

If someone who weighs 150 lbs. will engage in one hour of moderate dancing, Table 23.6 shows that this will require about 25 grams of carb. If this person's carb factor is one unit for every 12 grams of carb, 25 grams divided by 12 grams per unit gives a maximum of 2 units that may need to be subtracted from bolus or basal doses. This person could also combine eating carbs and lowering insulin by choosing to eat 12 grams of free carbs and lower a bolus or basal rate by 1 unit.

Translate ExCarbs into an insulin reduction:

ExCarbs ÷ carb factor = units of insulin that could be reduced. For example, eat half the ExCarbs as carbs and use the other half to reduce bolus or basal insulin.

23.9 Carb And Insulin Adjustments To Balance Exercise Per 100 lbs. Weight

Exercise Duration	Exercise Intensity								
	Mild			Moderate			Intense		
	Carbs*	Bolus	Basal	Carbs*	Bolus	Basal	Carbs*	Bolus	Basal
15 min	+ 0 g	normal	normal	+ 0 g	normal	normal	+ 20 g	- 10%	normal
30 min	+ 10 g	normal	normal	+ 20 g	- 10%	normal	+ 40 g	- 20%	normal
45 min	+ 18 g	- 10%	normal	+ 30 g	- 20%	normal	+ 50 g	- 30%	normal
60 min	+ 25 g	- 15%	normal	+ 40 g	- 30%	normal	+ 60 g	- 40%	- 10%
90 min	+ 38 g	- 20%	normal	+ 55 g	- 45%	- 20%	+ 90 g	- 50%	- 20%
120 min	+ 50 g	- 30%	normal	+ 70 g	- 60%	- 20%	+ 110 g	- 70%	- 30%
240 min	+ 80 g	- 50%	- 10%	+ 120 g	- 60%	- 20%	+ 200 g	- 70%	- 40 %

These are only estimates and must be individually adjusted through testing.

*Important: The carb values above are for a person who weighs 100 lbs. If you weigh 200 lbs, you will need twice these amounts. If you have not trained for an activity, you may need slightly more than these amounts. Once you are trained, you may need substantially less.

A reduction in bolus or basal delivery during exercise allows fuel stores to be released from glycogen and fat, so that fewer carbs have to be eaten to provide fuel. This helps those who want to lose weight and those who participate in long periods of activity but do not want to consume the large portions of carbohydrate that would otherwise be required.

Whether you need to reduce basal, bolus, or both depends on the duration of the activity, its timing in relation to meals, and whether the exercise was planned. Keep in mind that these ExCarb reductions should be the maximum amount needed. Someone who is trained for a particular exercise will have already reduced their insulin doses and need less reduction than suggested by the ExCarb table. Remember also that some time will pass after basals or boluses are reduced before the insulin level in the blood begins to drop. Take a look at Table 23.9 for suggested changes in carb intake, carb boluses, and basal rates for different intensities and durations of exercise.

When exercise follows a meal, a carb bolus can be lowered to help reduce the insulin level. The carbs eaten in a meal work quickly to raise the blood sugar, so timing of the carb bolus is not critical. Ideally, the exercise would begin within an hour of the bolus so that the blood sugar does not rise too high before the exercise begins. A breakfast bolus can be reduced for exercise that starts after breakfast, but if you walk, run, or go to the gym before breakfast, you may need to eat carbs or try a temporary basal reduction to help handle this.

23.10 How Far Can Insulin Be Reduced For Exercise?

Can basals and boluses be totally eliminated if you exercise long enough? This may be possible for someone with Type 2 diabetes who retains adequate internal insulin production. With Type 1 diabetes, however, basal and bolus doses can only be lowered so far.

Consider what happens to insulin during maximum training in a marathon runner who does not have diabetes. Their blood insulin level drops no further than to about half of its original level. So with Type 1 diabetes, basal and bolus doses would normally be lowered no more than 40 to 50 percent for longer periods of intense exercise if the current basals and boluses are appropriate.

Insulin can be lowered only so far because some is always needed:

1. As basal delivery to enable glucose to enter cells and to keep internal stores of glucose and fat from being released in massive amounts, and ultimately prevent ketoacidosis, which results from this uncontrolled release

2. To cover some of the carbohydrates eaten in meals.

For strenuous exercise that lasts 60 minutes or longer, or moderate exercise lasting 90 minutes or longer, a reduction in the basal rate should be considered. Basal rates are ideally lowered one to two hours before an activity begins to allow enough time for the insulin level in the blood to begin to drop. After long, intense periods of exercise, both basal rates and boluses may need to be reduced for 24 to 48 hours afterward.

The blood insulin level will fall faster if the basal rate is completely stopped, but complete stoppage is generally not recommended. For several reasons, stoppage should never last longer than 60 to 90 minutes: to avoid ketosis, to avoid having the blood sugar spike afterward, and to lessen the risk of a clog in the infusion line. When basal reduction is used for long periods of exercise, a partial reduction that is 20% to as much as 50% lower than normal for long periods of strenuous exercise works the best.

Basal reductions are most effective when started well before the exercise begins. If an exercise is spontaneous or unanticipated, a short and sharp reduction in the basal rate can be considered. The basal rate is generally not lowered more than 40 to 50% for long periods of exercise, but a larger reduction, such as 75% for 60 to 90 minutes can be used to partially cover an hour of moderate or strenuous exercise before breakfast.

Example

Once you know how many ExCarbs are needed for an exercise, you can use your carb factor to translate some or all of these carbs into an appropriate insulin reduction. Let's say someone weighing 150 pounds wants to run for 30 minutes at 8 m.p.h.

Table 23.6 shows they will need about 72 grams of ExCarbs (145 grams per hour times a half hour) for this run. We can divide these carbs by their carb factor to find out how much insulin this exercise is equal to. Dividing 72 grams by this person's carb factor which is 16 grams per unit of insulin tells us that the run is equal to about 4.5

units of insulin (72 grams ÷ 16 carbs per unit = 4.5 units). Knowing the carbs and the equivalent insulin reduction required for the run, our runner can choose to eat extra carbohydrates, lower a meal bolus, or both. (A basal reduction would ordinarily not be used for a run that lasts only a half hour.)

Using only carbs, our runner could consume 24 grams

23.11 For Control During Exercise, Consider:

1. How long and hard you plan to exercise
2. Your current insulin level
3. How many carbs you need from Table 2356 or 23.6
4. Whether to apply your ExCarbs as extra carbs to eat, as reduced insulin doses, or as a combination of the two in table 23.9.*

*Never adjust insulin doses on your own without discussing the changes with your physician.

of carb before the run, 24 after the run, and the remaining 24 as needed later in the day. None of the extra carbs needed for the run would be covered with insulin, although fewer carbs would be needed if the insulin doses have been previously lowered for this as a regular run. If, instead, our runner chooses to only reduce carb boluses, one or two meal boluses close in timing to the exercise can be lowered by a total of 4.5 units. For a run an hour after breakfast, coverage for the carbs at breakfast could be reduced by 3 units with remainder taken out of boluses for lunch or midmorning snack.

A better combination would be to eat some carbs and reduce carb boluses. For example, our runner could reduce the breakfast bolus by 2 units (32 grams) and the lunch bolus by 1 unit (16 grams) for a total insulin reduction of 48 grams, so bolus reductions would cover 48 grams and the other 24 grams would be covered by carb intake.

Use ExCarbs To Lower A High Blood Sugar

Exercise can also be used to lower a high blood sugar. For example, Jeremy weighs 175 pounds, uses 50 units of insulin a day, and is generally in good control. He uses one unit for each 10 grams of carbohydrate and one unit for every 40 mg/dl above his target blood sugar of 100 mg/dl.

Let's say Jeremy finds his blood sugar is 180 mg/dl (9.6 mmol) before dinner and he wants to exercise to lower his blood sugar. He plans to eat 60 grams of carb for dinner and would usually take 6 units for dinner plus 2 units for the high blood sugar (80/40 = 2.0). To help lower the blood sugar, he plans to ride his bike at 10 m.p.h. for an hour after dinner. From Table 23.6, the ExCarbs for a 175 lb. person riding one hour at 10 m.p.h. is about 54 grams of carb.

These 54 grams of ExCarbs used by the exercise can be replaced by:

- eating 54 grams of carb not covered with a bolus during or after the exercise,
- giving 5.4 fewer units of insulin (54 grams of carb ÷ 10 grams per unit) in basal or bolus doses,
- or a combination of these.

Jeremy wants to lower his blood sugar by 80 mg/dl (4.4 mmol) with exercise. This would use 2.0 of the 5.4 units of blood sugar lowering capacity (80 mg/dl drop ÷ 40 mg/dl per unit = 2.0 units). The remaining 3.4 units could be converted into 20 free grams of carb eaten sometime after the bike ride (20 grams ÷ 10 grams per unit = 2.0 units), plus a reduction by 1.4 units in the normal carb bolus given for dinner. Instead of 6.0 units for 60 grams at dinner, Jeremy would give only 4.6 units. This total compensation of 1.4, 2.0, and 2.0 equals 5.4 units of insulin or 54 grams of carb needed for the bike ride.

Contrast this situation to a similar one that occurs before breakfast. The blood sugar is 172 mg/dl (9.6 mmol) before breakfast and the bike ride will occur after breakfast. When a high occurs on waking in the morning, the insulin level has been low overnight, so the liver is

23.12 Trust Your Own Experience

Never take a dose of insulin that seems inappropriate. If you usually take three units for your meal prior to the start of your exercise and your blood sugar control has been good, do not take more or less than this amount, even if a different dose is suggested by the ExCarbs system, the 500 Rule, or any other rule. Your own blood sugars and experience are always your best guide.

actually producing glucose. Because of this, the blood sugar may not drop as much as it would before dinner when the blood sugar started in a normal range at lunch if we assume that his basal rates are appropriate. When the liver is activated after several hours of higher readings overnight, the blood sugar may not come down as much as it will when the blood sugar had only been high for a short period.

Remember that the ExCarb estimates in Tables 23.5 and 23.6 should be the **maximum you need** for an exercise when your insulin doses are closely matched to your need. Fewer carbs or less insulin reduction than these amounts may be needed.

Tips On Blood Sugar Monitoring

Check your blood sugar often for optimum performance and to avoid highs and lows both during and after exercise. Use a continuous monitor, if possible, to know the direction and rate of change of your blood sugar before, during, and after exercise. For example, a blood sugar of 100 mg/dl (5.5 mmol) may be safe for exercise if the previous blood sugar was 70 mg/dl (4 mmol) but not if the previous blood sugar was 130 mg/dl (7.2 mmol). If your blood sugar is falling, you will need more carbs before and during your exercise. When you check your blood sugar, be sure to enter the reading into your pump to check your BOB. Excess BOB can cause your blood sugar to go low if you exercise. Extra carbs will be needed to avoid a low when you have excess BOB on board.

Ways To Avoid Exercise Lows

A low blood sugar during or soon after exercise is often difficult to recognize because hypoglycemia symptoms like tiredness and sweating could also be caused by the exercise. Warning signs that occur may go unnoticed due to the participant's focus on the activity or sport at hand. Water sports can be especially difficult because they mask sweating and shaking. Frequent blood sugar testing is the best way to exercise and keep readings in the target range.

Have quick-acting, high-carb snacks on hand to prevent or treat a low blood sugar. Be especially careful during and after exercise that is intense and for which you are not trained. Canoe trips, backpacking, skiing, horseback riding, spring cleaning, snow shovelling, home remodeling, heavy work in the garden, or even washing the car can create an unusually fast drop in the blood sugar if the exercise or activity is not done regularly. Infrequent activities that use the arm and shoulder muscles are especially likely to cause lows. A larger carb intake or greater insulin reduction is needed for any strenuous activity that is done infrequently.

Test often or use a continuous monitor after any long period of strenuous activity to avoid delayed lows. Strenuous exercise can cause a low up to 36 to 48 hours later and will be most likely to happen during the first night. Delayed lows are caused by the muscles and liver gradually removing sugar from the blood as they replenish the glycogen stores depleted during the activity. Delayed lows can be prevented by testing often, using a temporary basal rate reduction that night, and adding extra carbs at dinner and bedtime not covered by bolus insulin.

A low can also creep in when exercise conditions change. If you usually walk two miles on flat ground but decide to walk the same distance in hilly country, you will use more fuel climbing the grades. A strong headwind can increase fuel consumption by about one percent for each extra mile per hour of headwind (i.e., for a 10 m.p.h. headwind, increase carbs by 10 percent). Walking in dry sand or soft snow can double the amount of carbs you need compared to the same walk on firm ground.

23.13 Simple Tips For Exercise

For casual or light exercise
(i.e. casual walking, biking, softball)

- No adjustment to insulin
- Keep fast carbs and your meter and test strips with you.

For heavy or aerobic exercise
(i.e. tennis, baseball, football, jogging, swimming vigorously)

- Test your blood sugar before the exercise and every 30 minutes after you start
- If less than 120 mg/dl (6.7 mmol), eat 30 grams of carb before exercise.
- If between 120 and 200 mg/dl (6.7 to 11.1 mmol) eat 15 grams of carb.
- If over 200 mg/dl (11.1 mmol), don't eat anything but retest in 30 minutes.
- Test every 30 minutes and follow these tips each time you test.

Rather than occasional monitoring, many professional athletes with diabetes want to know the trend line of their blood sugar prior to, during, and after an athletic event. They want to know where their blood sugar is, what direction it is heading, and how quickly.

Athletes like Jay Leeuwenburg, former offensive lineman for the Cincinnati Bengals, would test his blood sugar every 20 to 30 minutes for about two hours before a football game, during the game as often as possible, and again for the same period after the game. Frequent testing allowed him to pick up the trend in his blood sugar and correct as needed with carbohydrates or insulin to keep his blood sugar as normal and level as possible. Post game readings helped him avoid unexpected highs and lows after his very strenuous exercise.

Trending, of course, will become easier as continuous blood sugar monitors become widely available. A continuous monitor lets you quickly determine the trend of your blood sugar.

Activities that have uneven pacing, like spring cleaning or playing football, can also cause problems in estimating carb need. With cleaning, it's hard to predict whether you will spend the next hour sorting through the closet for throwaways or moving furniture. In football, you could sit on the bench during the entire game or give your all on the field. Luckily, most activities do not suffer from this much unpredictability.

Why The Blood Sugar May Rise After Exercise

Usually, exercise lowers the blood sugar. However, there are times when the blood sugar rises after exercise. Let's review four of the most likely causes.

Too Little Insulin

Too little insulin is the most common reason for the blood sugar to rise after exercise. A common situation is when exercise starts first thing in the morning with an elevated fasting blood sugar of 150 mg/dl (8.3 mmol) or higher. The blood sugar later that morning may rise following exercise because the liver was producing excess glucose when the person awoke. This is indicated by the high fasting reading. A rise in the blood sugar in this situation suggests that the basal rate prior to waking is too low. If the same exercise is done on another morning when the fasting blood sugar is below 120 mg/dl (6.67 mmol), the blood sugar may stay level or fall.

If the ExCarb system does not seem to work, consider whether your current basals and boluses are properly set. If your insulin doses are too high and you have frequent lows in the afternoon, do not blame exercise for the several lows that follow when you start exercising at 4 p.m. without eating carbs or lowering the afternoon basal rate or lunch bolus. Blame it instead on the excessive insulin doses made worse by consuming too few carbs for the exercise.

Alternatively, someone with insulin doses set too low may wake up in the morning with a reading of 180 mg/dl (10 mmol) because the overnight basal rate is too low. If they then go jogging with this low insulin level, they should not be surprised to find the blood sugar has risen to 240 mg/dl (13.3 mmol) afterward. Again, the exercise is not to blame. The cause is the underlying lack of insulin that releases excess glucose from glycogen stores in the liver and muscles. Too little insulin makes it hard for glucose to move into muscles as fuel. The blood sugar would be better controlled by taking a small correction bolus before starting to jog. A much better approach, though, would be to make sure that your night basal rate is set accurately (see Chapter 11) so you avoid high morning readings all together.

Anaerobic Exercise

In short, intense anaerobic exercise, like running the 100-yard dash or power weight-lifting, glucose is almost the only fuel used. To provide this fuel, a rapid release of glucose into the blood occurs from internal glycogen stores, driven by a rise in adrenaline hormone levels. This hormone release during intense exercise can cause glucose production to rise seven or eight times higher than normal, while uptake of glucose into cells rises only three to four fold.[98] This mismatch causes the glucose level to rise in the blood. In contrast to less insulin needed for aerobic exercise, a rapid increase in the insulin level is required to accommodate the glucose mobilization that occurs during intense, anaerobic exercise.[91]

Unfortunately, the speed at which the insulin level in the blood has to change in situations like this cannot be mimicked by a pump. Although it is risky, those who participate in intense or anaerobic sports may need to adjust their insulin doses so they have a high insulin level at the start of an event (Discuss this with your physician ahead of time). Even this may not keep the blood sugar from rising. When participating in intense exercise, it is best to test frequently, keep good records, and use correction boluses as needed after the short event to correct any high readings that occur.

Strenuous or anaerobic activity raises the blood sugar when glucose is mobilized into the blood faster than it can be removed into cells by the current insulin level.

Competition

Large amounts of stress hormones can be released at the start of a competitive event, like a swim meet, a 10K run, or a century bike ride. Release of stress hormones causes release of large amounts of glucose in "fight or flight" situations. The person without diabetes quickly releases insulin into the blood to balance this glucose. In contrast, when someone with diabetes starts a competitive event, their blood sugar may rise rapidly even if their starting glucose is normal and the do not eat. Nervousness at the starting line suggests that stress hormones are at work.

Insulin adjustments are difficult for competitive exercise because rapid and unpredictable changes in the blood sugar may occur, along with the uncertainty about how many stress hormones have been released. When stress hormone release is likely, a small bolus prior to the event may help, but because the blood sugar is hard to predict, it is safer to bring down any high blood sugar that occurs after the event. Discuss this with your physician or health care team, and use insulin before your exercise only after testing has demonstrated that extra insulin is really needed.

Even with stress, extra insulin will not be needed for longer events if exercise eventually lowers the high blood sugar. Your personal experience with similar events is your best guide, along with frequent testing and good records.

Dehydration

A high blood sugar indicates you are already dehydrated. A high after exercise might be caused by too little insulin, but it may also be caused by dehydration. In hot, dry weather, a lack of fluids concentrates the blood and makes blood sugar readings appear higher than they are. If you think your insulin should be adequate and your pump appears to be working but your blood sugar is unusually high after a long and strenuous exercise, interpret the reading with caution. An apparent "high" reading may actually be dehydration. Drink ample fluids and retest your blood sugar 30 minutes later before deciding on how much correction bolus to give.

23.15 Easy Way To Measure Heart Rate/Pulse	
Feel your pulse at the wrist and count it for 10 seconds, then use this table to find beats per minute.	
10 second Pulse Count	**Beats Per Minute**
10	60
11	66
12	72
13	78
14	84
15	90
16	96
17	102
18	108
19	114
20	120
21	126
22	132
23	138
24	144
25	150
26	156
27	162
28	168
29	174
30	180

Staying hydrated is essential for turning glucose and fat into energy and for performance. Dehydration can also cause confusion and make it harder to recognize a low blood sugar. Frequent intake of fluid before, during, and after exercise prevents dehydration and loss of energy. Thirst begins only after you are already dehydrated, so drink fluids regularly during exercise before you become thirsty.

When Is A Blood Sugar Too High To Exercise?

High blood sugars impair performance during exercise in people with Type 1 diabetes. A high blood sugar likely means that some dehydration has already begun. A high blood sugar during exercise has been associated with a lower secretion of beta-endorphins and an increased RPE (a measure of difficulty) for leg and whole body effort. Exercise under these conditions likely leads to discomfort and stress.

If the blood sugar is 250 mg/dl (13.9 mmol) or above, exercise often is not recommended. If the insulin level is dangerously low at this time, exercise will cause the blood sugar to rise much higher. Although the insulin level cannot be directly measured, you can accurately guess it is low in many situations.

If a blood sugar were normal at bedtime but rises to 280 mg/dl (15.6 mmol) on waking because an infusion set became dislodged, the insulin level is likely to be very low and the person may even be in early ketosis. Exercising at this time will cause the blood sugar to rise and *put you at risk of ketosis* unless an injection is taken and enough time passes for the insulin to begin to lower the blood sugar.

Contrast this situation to one where the blood sugar is raised to 250 mg/dl (13.9 mmol) in preparation for a four-hour athletic event. ExCarbs covered by a reduced carb bolus before the event starts creating this high blood sugar, but the person can start the event confidently because the blood sugar will begin to drop shortly after the exercise starts. Even though the blood sugar is high, enough insulin is available to move glucose from the blood into exercising muscles.

Rather than raising the blood sugar this high, a better alternative is to reduce basal and bolus doses prior to the event so fewer carbs have to be eaten to exercise safely. With the insulin level lower at the start of the event, the starting blood sugar can remain at or near the normal range more safely. Additional carbs will be needed, but fewer than if the insulin level had not been lowered.

Exercise Risks

Existing medical problems must always be considered to avoid long-term consequences of exercise. Exercise carries certain risks for those who have nerve damage, eye changes, kidney disease, or a history of heart or blood vessel problems. Blood flow in involved muscles may increase 15 to 20 times above resting levels during strenuous exercise and cardiac output may increase fivefold. Increased blood flow and blood pressure move oxygen and fuel to muscles but also place extra strain on the heart. This could harm organs and blood vessels weakened by previous high blood sugars, high blood pressure, or high cholesterol.

With existing nerve damage, exercise presents special challenges. If feeling in the feet is reduced, the type and level of exercise has to be chosen carefully to prevent foot injuries because insensitivity to pain increases the risk of injury. Swimming or biking, which are non-weight-bearing activities, may be better choices than jogging. Proper footwear is essential for avoiding blisters or calluses that exacerbate the already high risk of foot problems.

Autonomic neuropathy involves damage to the nerves that control processes like digestion, heart rate, and blood vessel tone. It can create an artificially low heart rate and reduce blood flow to exercising muscle. With autonomic neuropathy, a heart rate monitor may not be an accurate way to measure exercise intensity. A gradual training program under supervision is strongly advised when autonomic neuropathy is present.

Autonomic neuropathy can be detected by changes that appear in an EKG or by measuring the change in blood pressure from a reclining to a standing position. If you suspect you have this disorder because you have had diabetes for a long time or have a history of poor control, discuss how to diagnose it with your physician.

Consider any risk you may have before beginning an exercise program, especially an exercises like heavy weight lifting or scuba diving that can significantly raise blood pressure. A gradual increase in training level or moderate goals may be required if blood vessel damage is a concern. Discuss your exercise plans with your physician before you start.

Summary

The need for insulin and carb adjustments before, during, and after exercise vary greatly from individual to individual. Although this chapter covers many aspects of control during exercise, these variations are complex and not completely understood. Some people may need to lower their boluses and basals only slightly for exercise, while others find that a large insulin reduction is the only way to control their blood sugars for the same exercise. For some, a breakfast bolus may not need to be lowered for morning exercise, but when they do the same exercise later in the day, they have to reduce their lunch or dinner bolus.

Be sure your insulin doses and carbohydrate intake are matched to your normal daily lifestyle before attempting to make adjustments for exercise. ExCarbs won't work if blood sugar control is not good when you are not exercising. Discuss your exercise program with your physician or health care team. Keep in mind your personal experience with similar exercise in the past.

The only way to determine your own response is to experiment, record your results, and discuss these with your physician. Remember, the ExCarb tables and the insulin adjustments that you make based on these tables are simply meant as a starting point to help you safely exercise and be active – your own experience is your ultimate guide! Experience will help you only if you look back over your records before deciding how to manage a particular situation.

Exercise Tips

- Test the blood sugar often: before, during, and 24 to 36 hours after exercise or use a continuous monitor for accurate insulin adjustments when you exercise.

- For performance and safety during exercise, keep the blood sugar between 70 and 150 mg/dl (3.9 to 8.3 mmol) and avoid dropping below 65 mg/dl (3.6 mmol) afterward. Proper insulin and carb adjustment help you do this.

- Vigorous exercise or heavy work may require major reductions in meal boluses of 50 percent or more before and after the exercise or activity. For example, if you normally take one unit for each 10 grams of carbohydrate, try taking one unit for every 20 grams while working or exercising hard.

- Correction boluses may also need to be lowered by 50 percent or more when given before or during long periods of moderate or strenuous exercise.

- For intense activities that last a day or two, such as a weekend backpacking trip, try a temporary basal rate that is 20 percent to 40 percent lower. Lower the basal rate before the activity begins and keep it somewhat lower for 24 to 36 hours after the activity ends.

- Basal rates rarely need to be lowered for short, random exercise.

- Some basal reduction may be needed when starting a new exercise training program or over time as your overall fitness improves.

- Before adjusting insulin for exercise, discuss these changes with your physician.

- Test your blood sugar often during and after exercise,

- Always carry fast carbs, like glucose tablets, SweetTarts™, or a sport fluid like Gatorade™ to rapidly correct low blood sugars.

- Stay hydrated. Always have water or a sport fluid available.

- For strenuous activities like triathlons, marathons, or century bike rides, tap the experience of other athletes with diabetes who have already encountered these challenges. Contact athletes who participate in your sport through the Diabetes Exercise and Sports Association at www.diabetes-exercise.org or (800) 898-4322.

- To lose weight with exercise, lower your basal rates and boluses so you need fewer carbs to meet your fuel needs. Keep your blood sugar well controlled and remember there is a limit to how far your insulin doses can be lowered.

Laughter is inner jogging.
Norman Cousins

Children And Teens

Kids and teens benefit from pump therapy even more than adults because of their greater need for precise dosing and flexibility. Small children are highly sensitive to insulin, and teens often face a strong Dawn Phenomenon that must be met with specific, well-timed dose adjustments. Children and teens both require an individualized approach to maintain control within the challenging and dynamic environment over the time in which their body is growing and developing.

When basal and bolus doses are carefully matched to carb intake, exercise, hormones, and changes in weight, the improved control enhances growth and school performance. The early years are also a time when healthy lifelong patterns need to be set. An insulin pump can make these tasks and challenges easier.

This chapter explains

- Why choose pump therapy
- Roles and responsibilities in care
- Setting the TDD, basals and boluses for kids and teens
- Special child and teen issues

Why Choose Pump Therapy

Blood sugar control is difficult in children who are smaller and more sensitive to insulin than adults, as well as impulsive in eating and activity. Some retain residual insulin production that either complicates insulin delivery or makes control easier. Recognizing the difficulty in matching insulin to need in children, the ADA recommends that goals for blood sugar targets and A1c be set higher in kids compared to adults, as shown in Table 24.1.

Parents and health care providers will want to consider pump therapy for any toddler or child who experiences frequent episodes of severe hypoglycemia or has wide fluctuations in their blood sugar. Intensive injection programs can be frustrating and difficult to manage in toddlers when they refuse to eat, are napping at shot time, or are ill. A pump makes these situations easier to handle by providing very precise insulin

A special thanks to Shannon Brow R.N., B.S., C.D.E. for her help and suggestions on this chapter.

24.1 ADA Goals For Glycemic Control			
	Toddler Preschoolers (0-6 yrs)	**School Age (6-12 yrs)**	**Adolescents/ Young Adults (13-19 yrs)**
A1c (%)	" 8.5 but ≥ 7.5	< 8	< 7.5
Preprandial plasma glucose	100-180 mg/dl (5.5-10 mmol)	90-180 mg/dl (5-10 mmol)	90-130 mg/dl (5-7.2 mmol)
Bedtime/overnight	110-200 mg/dl (6.1-11.1 mmol)	100-180 mg/dl (5.5-10 mmol)	90-150 mg/dl (5-8.3 mmol)

Diabetes Care. 2005; 28(suppl 1):S4-S36.

delivery without the problems of injections, and by tracking BOB in growing children and teens who eat and bolus frequently.

Kids and teens often learn to use a pump quicker than adults. Even so, kids and teens may object to pumping because it requires more planning, thought, attention, training, and finger sticks. Although lifestyle flexibility is increased on a pump, a child or teen may think the extra attention to detail means more responsibility and less spontaneity. Pump training and support are essential so that kids and teens accept pumping, and, in turn, feel better, and have better A1c's with an improved quality of life.

Parents are often willing to do their part in order to provide better control of their child's diabetes now and better health for their child in the future. However, a child who has not reached the age of reason or a teen with other issues to face can present major challenges to parents who already face the extra burdens of diabetes.

To encourage the acceptance of pumping, diabetes professionals need to discuss quality of life issues with the child or teen and family to ensure that pump therapy will improve their life. What are the limitations of multiple injection therapy. Is it frustrating to have to eat a snack before P.E. each day? Do meal times conflict with weekend soccer tournaments and little league games? Are there days when more carbs are desired but will require another injection? Does skipping meals or late meals create control problems? Do meals have to be eaten at the same time every day? Does an elevated blood sugar require tenths of a unit dosing which injections cannot do? Does sleeping in or going to bed late throw off the timing of the long-acting insulin?

These problems are often lessened by pump therapy. The flexibility, precision and discipline of pump therapy give a pump wearer more options that improve the quality of life. There are also some myths about how much pumping can improve diabetes problems. Parents and the child or teen have to be realistic about what a pump can do. Some common myths and realities ate listed in Table 4.3.

Overview Of Pump Therapy

A good approach to educating a child or teen about pump use is with an inter-disciplinary team headed by a physician and including a nurse or diabetes educator, a dietitian, and a social worker with expertise in diabetes and the physical and emotional needs of children and teens. Before starting on a pump, the child or teen will benefit from practicing MDI with a long-acting insulin to cover the body's basal need, plus a rapid insulin before meals and snacks to cover carbs and correct highs.

Training begins with a class or workshop on management skills and techniques taught by a diabetes educator and a dietitian. During this workshop, the child or teen learns to count carbs, dose insulin correctly, and record all the information needed to adjust insulin doses, carbs, and exercise. Any child or teen going on a pump needs at least one adult companion who is also trained in its use. The parent or primary care-giver must acquire the skills to set and test basal doses, calculate and give carb boluses, record data, analyze patterns, and troubleshoot when problems arise. In other words, the child or teen does not have to shoulder full responsibility at first, and the parent does not relinquish all control until maturity allows it.

Other caregivers may be trained by the diabetes educator or physician or the par-ent, child, or teen. Baby sitters, school nurses, camp nurses, and coaches need to know usual insulin doses, appropriate foods, the symptoms and treatment for hypoglycemia and hyperglycemia, and who to call for help. Diabetes supplies need to be provided in a bag for the school nurses and coaches and stored in the nurse's office or carried in a fanny pack by the child or teen.

Once essential skills are in place, the child or teen is ready to go on a pump. Children often have the motor skills to handle self-care on their own by age 10. Judg-ment and problem-solving come at a later age. Encourage self-care appropriate to the pumper's age and maturity. For example, allow a child to clean the skin with IV Prep and push the buttons on the pump while you supervise. After the child shows full proficiency in these skills, the parent may decide to check occasionally to make sure the technique is accurate. Table 24.2 shows suggested ages to recommend different self-management skills.

Roles And Responsibilities

It is wise to discuss the roles of parent and child or teen with your health care team. In general, the diabetes care team should provide thorough training and recom-mendations for the pump program. They will set up the basal rates, carb and correction factors, target ranges, and duration of insulin action and explain how to make the small adjustments needed. After the program is started, the same team must be available for frequent consultation, especially when the wearer is starting new insulin doses.

Problems with insulin doses for children and teens are not terribly different from those encountered by adults. The real difference is in the pumper's problem-solving skills. Very young children are incapable of self-care and older children may not be ready to analyze problems. Children and teens can be taught the basics, but they still require good supervision from a knowledgeable adult.

A parent needs to know how to verify that insulin doses are accurate and that they are being given. The child's blood sugar readings need to be regularly evaluated and issues must be discussed with an older child or teen in ways that produce positive outcomes. Recording carbs, blood sugars, and insulin doses and analyzing this data is needed to adjust the amount and timing of basal and bolus doses and carbs for the best results. Through all stages, a parent's compassion and readiness to forgive mistakes can be critical in steady improvement in a child or teen's improvement.

When doses are being adjusted, parents and health care professionals should be sure to have close phone availability and followup. Some diabetes centers use a system of faxed or emailed reports, similar to a log book or a *Smart Chart*.

24.2 When Is A Child Ready For Self-Care?

Children differ greatly in the age at which they can manage the self-care required on a pump. After acquiring a skill, relapses may occur, but the desire to manage the pump on their own is often reintroduced by the desire to stay overnight at a friends or go camping.

When is a child ready to:

insert an infusion set : average 12 years old

test blood sugar: average 10 years old

count carbs: 8, 9, or 10 years old

give a bolus: average 10 years old

determine a carb bolus: average 12 years old

Evaluating Outcomes

The overall goals for pump therapy for children and teens are similar to those for adults – less exposure to high glucose (a lower A1c) and less glucose variability (a lower SD). Meeting individual goals is also important. How well pump therapy is working depends on matching the original reasons a pump was chosen to a program that will accomplish this. For example, if the goal was for fewer hospital admissions, then one measure of success will be the reduction of hospitalizations.

Other measures of success are based on satisfaction and quality of life. Are the child or teen and the parents happy with the program? How often do they report complaints or problems with the pump, infusion set, and blood sugar tests? Does the child or teen proudly show their pump to friends and relatives? Has the child or teen benefitted medically, emotionally or socially? Has the child or teen's general confidence and competence grown in proportion to success with the pump?

Selecting Starting Doses For Kids And Teens

Setting basal and bolus doses is covered in Chapters 11, 12, and 13, but there are some differences when selecting basal rates and initial pump settings for children and teens. They require snacks in addition to meals to provide enough calories for growth and development. Depending on their growth cycle, a child may need to snack a little or a lot. How to best cover snacks needs to be individualized when setting doses.

Teens are notorious for inconsistent routines and random eating, with or without

24.3 Testing And Kids

When giving an injection or drawing blood from young children for monitoring, remember that their imagination can be vivid, and reassurance about their fears may be needed. Let them know that an infusion needle will not affect their heart or puncture a large blood vessel and cause bleeding, and that their bodies easily replenish the small amounts of blood removed for blood tests. Encourage them to ask questions so their fears are allayed.

diabetes. While a pump is the ideal tool for a varied or even erratic lifestyle, a teen will need to keep a consistent schedule for at least four weeks after the pump start to set insulin doses correctly. When schedules change, as at the start of school or vacation, basals and boluses often need to be retested and adjusted.

Hormonal changes at puberty can make this month's insulin program obsolete next month. During growth spurts and puberty, growth hormone and cortisol levels rise. This requires that insulin doses also rise. Covering teen hormones and growth spurts brings humility to the best diabetes clinicians. The most effective advice is to be prepared to adjust basal and bolus doses frequently to keep up with growth.

Setting The Total Daily Dose (TDD)

Chapter 10 has a full discussion for setting the TDD when switching from injections to a pump. Like adults, a child or teen's TDD is determined before basals and boluses, which are then calculated from Tables 10.4, 10.6, and 10.7.

Although a reduction in the TDD is generally recommended when starting on a pump, this may not be appropriate for a teen who has had inadequate blood sugar control before switching to a pump, or a child who has recently experienced a growth phase and now requires more insulin.

Basal/Bolus Balance

In the PedPump study conducted in Europe with 1,086 kids and teens between the ages of 1 and 18 on pumps, the participants had better blood sugar control and lower A1cs when boluses made up more than 50% of the TDD.[99] In this study, an average of 6.7 boluses were given a day to cover meals and snacks. Carb and correction boluses averaged 58% of the TDD. The high number and percentages of boluses found in this study may be replacing some basal delivery. The average duration of diabetes was only 4.7 years, so residual insulin production may also lessen the need for basal insulin.

Lower starting basal percentages, such as 40% of the TDD, can be tried for active children and teens who have residual insulin production, which usually includes those who have had diabetes less than five years. Prior to puberty, a high intake of carbohydrate and calories relative to weight necessitates a greater use of bolus insulin compared to basal. Teens, especially boys, often eat six high carb meals a day. Matching these snacks and meals with boluses creates good control. Alternatively, some teens do best when 60% or more of their TDD is basal due to their higher levels of circulating pubertal hormones.

Setting And Testing Basal Doses

Breast fed and bottle fed infants on a pump who feed every few hours will experience very small rises and falls in blood glucose levels. They may benefit from a slightly higher basal dose during the day to cover their carbs.

One way to cover lunches or afternoon snacks when a child or teen is forgetful about taking carb boluses is to raise the afternoon basal rate. A better way with today's pumps is to use reminders that can be set to remind the user to take a bolus or to warn if a bolus is not taken within a certain time period.

Children may have some Dawn Phenomenon, but teens often have a more pronounced one due to early morning surges of growth hormone and cortisol. Frequent nighttime blood sugar monitoring is necessary at first to determine whether the Dawn Phenomenon is present and its impact. After this initial testing phase, a blood sugar taken between 1:00 and 3:00 a.m. helps determine basal dose adjustments and should be done once every week or more often if nighttime hypoglycemia begins.

Raise or lower the basal in increments of 0.05 or even 0.025 units per hour unless a larger increase or decrease is obviously needed. Test the blood sugar every one to two hours during basal testing, if possible. See Chapter 11 for a full discussion of setting and testing basal doses.

24.4 Clever Pump Tricks

Prevent Afternoon Highs

A common problem among school age children and teens is a high blood sugar in the late afternoon or before dinner, usually caused when the child neglects to take prescribed boluses for after school snacks. A parent can often follow the paper trail of wrappers and containers in the trash, then compare these with the history of boluses actually delivered.

If afternoon highs are a problem for your child, review the bolus history regularly with him and give him guidelines for how much bolus to take for each snack, and even label each food container with how many grams it contains or the bolus dose it requires.

If forgetfulness is an issue, try using the bolus alarm, which will alarm when no bolus is given within a certain time period.

As an alternative, the afternoon basal can be raised to compensate for after-school eating if it is regular and continues through the weekend.

Setting And Testing Carb Boluses

Chapter 12 discusses setting and testing carb boluses and explains how to find the correct carb factor.

For children and teens, not all snacks need to be covered with a bolus. A small carb snack of 8 to 15 grams may not affect the blood sugar and not need for a bolus. Wether a particular bedtime snack needs to be completely covered will only be known after adequate testing. For instance, the first 10 to 20 grams in bedtime snacks may not need to be covered and more carbs might not be covered after an active day. This decision becomes easier after some experience about how the day's activity affects the overnight blood sugar.

Smart pumps allow different carb and correction factors to be set for different times of the day. These are especially convenient to reduce bedtime boluses and to reduce boluses when sports or other increased activities typically occur during the day.

Have the child or teen practice carb counting and bolus dosing. Be sure the child or teen calculates correctly several examples of counting and covering various carb amounts in meals and snacks. This ensures they understand how to determine bolus doses for a variety of foods and snacks.

Typically, boluses are given 10 to 20 minutes before meals when a meal's carb count and timing are known, but this may need to be tailored for specific situations:

Split boluses: Sometimes it is safer to bolus part of a meal now and the rest later. This is useful when you do not know how much food will be eaten or the time it will be served. This might happen during parties, restaurant dining, or all-you-can-eat buffets. It may also happen during holiday feasts, snacking on chips and salsa, or expecting to eat more than you really can, the "my eyes are bigger than my stomach" phenomenon. A child or teen should always keep in mind that using an extra bolus when food intake turns out to be more than expected is far better than having a high blood sugar later.

Combination or dual-wave boluses: Here, part of the entire bolus is given right away and the rest is delivered gradually over a period of time. If the carb amount turns out to be less than expected or not all of the food is eaten, the remaining part of the bolus can be cancelled. This helps picky eaters, low GI carbs, or foods like pizza that digest slowly because of their fat and protein content.

After-meal boluses: Though generally not recommended because it may cause postmeal highs, a meal bolus may be given immediately after a meal when a child is a picky eater or is ill and may not be able to keep food down.

Setting And Testing Correction Boluses

See Chapter 13 for steps to set and test correction boluses in adults. The procedure is similar in children and teens, but keep in mind that an active child or teen will lower high blood sugars faster through exercise than most adults.

Setting The Duration Of Insulin Action

How long a bolus affects the blood sugar after it is given is called its duration of insulin action. Setting this time accurately is critical for calculating carb and correction boluses that account for the Bolus on Board. Pages 43-47 discusses similarities and slight differences in how the duration of insulin action is set in children versus adults and Textbox 5.3 provides additional information.

Setting Blood Sugar Targets

The ADA has guidelines for blood sugar targets for the specific age groups of toddlers, school age kids and teens. These are shown in Table 24.1.

Special Control Issues

Growth And Growth Spurts

Growth spurts in children and teens will always challenge control. Small growth spurts are usually mixed with periods of more gradual growth through childhood. The onset of puberty also signals a time of rapid growth and blood sugar upheaval for teens. Hormones produced during puberty cause glucose to be released and impair insulin action, necessitating large increases in basal and bolus doses. An insulin pump allows teens and parents to make the rapid basal and bolus adjustments that are needed to keep up with changes in control during this transition time.

Children require about a half unit of insulin per pound of body weight each day, while teenagers can require up to one unit per pound. This need for extra insulin does not indicate that the teen's diabetes has become "worse." It is simply a physiological change caused by normal growth and the teenager needs to be told that frequently.

During the growth years and puberty, anticipate needing to increase basal and bolus doses every few weeks or months as the need becomes apparent. For some teens who encounter control problems during puberty, a pediatrician may recommend they take a prescription medication called metformin. Normally used in adults with Type 2 diabetes, metformin reduces the excessive amounts of glucose released from the liver when growth hormone levels are high. The use of metformin lowers glucose production to more normal levels, reduces the amount of insulin needed for control, and often makes the teen feel better. Discuss this with your child's doctor if your teen is having a difficult time with control. Teens will be glad to know their need for high insulin doses will taper off as they reach the late teen years. After puberty, their TDD may fall to half that used during puberty.

Good blood sugar control is necessary to realize full growth, especially height. This can be a motivator to the child or teen, particularly teenage boys, if they are made aware that short height can be one result of poor control during growth.

Menses

Some young women find their blood sugar is not affected by their cycle or their periods may be so random that there is little similarity from period to period. Others experience drastic changes in blood sugar levels a few days prior to the beginning and during the first day or two of their menstrual periods. High blood sugar levels that require higher basals and boluses often occur at this time. The need for insulin may drop dramatically after the first day and care must be used to avoid lows. A good practice is to test more often and record results prior to and during the period. Keep a record of menses and blood sugar levels to find patterns and discover how the cycle affects the blood sugar.

Many teens do not have regular, predictable cycles for several months after the onset of puberty. After the first period, it is wise to start recording dates of the periods even though they may be irregular so that any pattern in their effect on the blood sugar may be seen. With regular cycles and accurate records, their effect on the blood sugar can be anticipated and adjusted for. See page 168 for more information.

Considerations For Parents Of Infants And Toddlers

A cooperative effort between diligent, well-educated parents and their diabetes team is critical for success with a toddler. Education and evaluation should include carbohydrate counting, insulin needs, sick day management, and troubleshooting skills. What is learned at this time pays off for years in reassuring a parent that their child can be taken care of.

Basal and bolus doses in toddlers are much smaller, often in fractions of units, than those for older children. Doses must be carefully monitored by a team that is experi-

24.5 Grams of Carbs For Treating Lows In Children			
Age	**1-6 yrs**	**6-10 yrs**	**10 yrs -Adult**
Grams of Carbs	**5 - 10 grs**	**10 - 15 grs**	**15 - 20 grs**
Glucose Tabs 5 grams each	1 - 2 tabs	2 - 3 tabs	3 - 4 tabs
Glucose Tabs 4 grams each	1 - 2 tabs	3 - 4 tabs	4 - 5 tabs
Orange Juice 1/3 cup = 10 grams	1/4 - 1/2 cup	1/2 - 3/4 cup	3/4 - 1 cup
Apple Juice 1/3 cup = 10 grams	1/4 - 1/2 cup	1/2 - 3/4 cup	3/4 - 1 cup
Table Sugar 4 grams per tsp.	2 tsps.	3 tsps.	4 - 5 tsps.
Regular Soda 3 grs per oz.	2 - 3 ozs.	4 - 5 ozs.	5 - 6 ozs.
Lifesavers 3 grams each	2 - 3	4 - 5	5 - 7
Milk 8 ozs. = 12 grams	4 - 5 ozs.	6 - 7 ozs.	8 - 10 ozs.

Adapted from **Understanding Diabetes**, 10 ed., by H. Peter Chase, M.D., 2002

enced in working with small children. Basal delivery can be as low as 0.05 or 0.025 units per hour, and boluses as low as 0.05 unit, making precise dosing easier than ever before.

Ketoacidosis can result from a snag or clog in the infusion line, detachment of the infusion set, or any barrier to insulin delivery. There may be little outward sign of this, so frequent monitoring is essential for toddlers and children on pumps.

Toddlers and children often need to be tested while asleep. A convenient way to do this is to lift the blankets at the bottom of the bed and use a lancing device on one heel. This provides quick access for drawing blood and often does not awaken the child.

Parents and the diabetes care team should have realistic expectations for age appropriate goals regarding control. Infants and toddlers are unable to perceive and treat hypoglycemia or hyperglycemia, and an adult around them will have little success in sensing their glucose status. Therefore, setting a goal of 'tight control' or trying to achieve an A1c less than 7% may be dangerous. Instead, rely on safer measures of success: Is your child having fewer episodes of hypoglycemia? Are the fluctuations in blood glucose levels more controlled? Has your child's quality of life improved? Are you less fearful and anxious? Is your child growing and developing normally? If the answers to these questions are "Yes," pump therapy has proven to be a success. See Table 24.1 for ADA age-appropriate goals for control.

Babysitters And Daycare

Babysitters and daycare providers can be trained to deliver appropriate boluses and to recognize when a blood sugar reading indicates there is a problem. The parent or health care personnel should always directly supervise pump use and training. Simple worksheets with instructions can be created for the childcare provider regarding how to test the blood sugar, give boluses, and what to do if an infusion set becomes detached. With toddlers, carb boluses can be given after meals for those who may be finicky or unpredictable eaters.

Both written and verbal instructions should be given for when to immediately contact a parent, such as when the blood glucose is abnormally high or low, if the child is vomiting, or there is another critical issue. A parent must be accessible at all times. Any delay in response time can cause significant harm to a child as a result of ketoacidosis or severe hypoglycemia. A simple piece of advice for caretakers is that if something is wrong and they cannot test, always give fast-acting carbs. Stopping a low is more important than treatment of a high when waiting for help.

Special Issues For Children And Teens

This information may reduce a child or teen's concerns about these areas.

School

Key school personnel need to know about diabetes, the pump, the procedures typically followed, and what to do in case of emergencies. Many schools (in the US) have zero tolerance for medications and syringes. However, to receive federal funding schools must follow a 504 Plan that is an agreement between the parents of children and teens who have diabetes or other medical issues and the school they attend.

Sample 504 Plans are available at www.childrenwithdiabetes.com/504/. To minimize problems, the child or teen and parent should provide the school nurse, coach, teachers, and principal with printed materials about the insulin pump, and treatment of high and low blood sugars, including a 504 Plan. A diabetes educator or physician can also write a letter to the school concerning the child's diabetes.

Check with school officials about where the blood sugar can be tested and by whom. It greatly encourages good care if a child or teen is able to test their blood sugar wherever they are instead of having to go to a nurse's office. Although the school policy may require that all diabetes care be done in the nurse's office, this is open to the 504 Plan that is developed. Work out with school officials a health program that enables the child with diabetes to stay healthy while at school and to have the freedom other children and teens have with respect to outings and sports.

If an insulin pen is used at school as well as a pump, let the school administration know and have your physician write a letter to the school explaining why it may be needed if a pump problem occurs.

Keep your school kit filled and handy with these necessities:

- insulin
- insulin syringes and/or an insulin pen as backup
- spare infusion sets
- blood testing supplies
- ketone test strips or a Precision Xtra™ meter
- fast-acting carbs for lows
- crackers and cheese to cover exercise and activity

Physical Exercise

Activity levels during P.E. classes at school are never consistent. One day may be spent playing a vigorous game of soccer and the next day watching a movie. When vigorous exercise occurs, an additional snack of free carbs may need to be eaten at the beginning of class. A request to snack before exercise, if necessary, should be covered in the 504 plan. A snack can be available in a pocket or backpack. If no snack is available, the workout may need to be skipped.

If a sport has a practice session every day after school, reduce basal or bolus doses so that insulin levels are lower at that time. Eating carbs not covered by a carb bolus also works for practices. Practice sessions should be prepared for because lows and highs harm performance and may jeopardize a place on the team.

Athletics

Pumps are ideal for most athletes because adjustments in carbs, basal rates, and carb boluses are easily made on a pump, but it helps to have good guidance on fine-tuning the pump for success. A doctor may provide a reference to a coach who can help.

Chapter 23 provides guidelines about adjusting basal rates, boluses, and carb intake for various durations and intensities of exercise. Teens interested in or involved in exercise may want to join the Diabetes Exercise and Sports Association (www.diabetes-exercise.org or 1-800-898-4322). DESA holds an annual convention and regional conferences with information sharing, workshops, and group activities. Professional and amateur athletes with diabetes give inspiration and advice on competing in many types of events.

Fast Food And Chain Restaurants

Children and teens will often eat at fast food restaurants although we strongly discourage this while pump settings are being tested. To cover carbs from fast food restaurants with confidence, consult the nutritional information provided by these restaurants in their pamphlets. Excellent lists of the carb content in fast food and chain restaurant meals are in a book called **The Calorie King Calorie, Fat, and Carbohydrate Counter**. See Table 7.6 for more reference books and how to order. Chapter 7 on carb counting in this book provides helpful information on eating out.

A pizza may require an initial carb bolus to match part of the carbohydrate intake and then a delayed bolus to match the digestion of carbs slowed by the fat. Never be afraid to experiment with combination or dual wave doses and write down what works since the same food will probably be eaten again.

Although 3 to 5 grams of carbohydrate per teaspoon or packet of ketchup can usually be ignored, some condiments like barbecue sauce may contribute enough carbs to create problem readings. With vegetables like green beans, asparagus, lettuce, and other nonstarchy vegetables, carbs can be estimated by figuring that 1 cup of raw or 1/2 cup of cooked vegetables equals 5 grams of carb. Use this guideline to count carbs on vegetable plates and at salad bars.

Weight Gain

Improved control after starting on a pump may cause unwanted weight gain unless fewer calories are eaten than when the blood sugars were high and some carbs were not absorbed. The novelty of being able to eat anything and cover it with a bolus may encourage overeating. Also, with tight control more hypoglycemia may cause more carbs and calories to be eaten to raise the blood sugar to avoid a low. Pay attention to weight gain and work on adjusting insulin doses and food intake to avoid it.

Sleep-Overs

Apprehension about nights or weekends away from home may occur for parents and children. Having a sleep-over plan can help relieve some of this anxiety. It is difficult to predict which direction the blood sugar may go during a sleep-over. With the excitement and extra snacks, blood sugar levels may be higher than usual. On the other hand, being awake during usual sleep time with extra activity may cause lower blood sugar levels. The only way to know for certain is to test and be prepared to eat carbs to raise a low or to take an extra bolus if a high occurs. Always take your supplies if you stay overnight with a friend so that you are ready for anything.

Sleeping In

When first starting on a pump, it is better to follow a specific routine of waking, eating, and sleeping until the basal rates have been customized. The overnight basal rate needs to be set and tested to maintain a safe blood sugar through the night and into the morning before attempting to sleep late. Only when these rates have been tested can someone safely hit the snooze button and go back to sleep! Then when you wake up later than usual, you can enjoy a normal day without struggling to regulate out-of-control blood sugars.

Diabetes Camp

Diabetes camp is a great way to meet other children and teens with diabetes. The American Diabetes Association maintains a listing of camps throughout the U.S., as does Children With Diabetes at www.childrenwithdiabetes.com. These camps are great for helping you realize you are not alone with diabetes. Lifelong friendships can be developed, especially if you start young as a camper and attend for several years or become a junior counselor.

ID Tags

While wearing ID tags with diabetes has always been a good idea, it is even more important for someone on a pump. Ordinary ID tags may not appeal to many kids and teens, but newer tags include colorful sports bands complete with medical insignia. Some jewelry stores also make attractive bracelets and pendants. An ID card carried in a wallet is important, but you need clear identification that is visible to emergency personnel or helpful strangers. It's a good idea to have "diabetes," "insulin pump," any allergies, and a phone number on the ID bracelet or pendant. Don't leave home without it!

Special Issues For Teens

Acceptance

The physical, emotional and social demands of the teen years often lead to neglect of blood sugar testing, diet, carb counting and bolusing. Depression and denial may contribute to these behaviors. Work with your diabetes team by telling them what you have the most trouble with and how they can help you. They want to make your life easier if they can, but they have to understand your needs.

Work with your team to identify any specific causes of poor control and a plan to deal with them. Negotiate reasonable and specific goals, such as having no lows below

70 mg/dl (3.9 mmol) for two weeks, or no more than five readings above 250 mg/dl (13.9 mmol) in one week, and track how well you are meeting your goals. In turn, you will see fewer lows, feel better, and have more flexible meals and snacks.

Let your parents, friends, and diabetes team know how you are really doing. Try to involve your parents to help you stay on track. Confiding your struggles to your best friend may lead to some new approaches as well.

Driving

Always test your blood sugar before driving. Eat a snack of at least 15 grams of carbohydrate, such as 3 glucose tablets, before you put the keys in the ignition to ensure no low blood sugar occurs. Keep snack foods available in the car at all the times. On long trips, stop every hour and test the blood sugar. Always check BOB to see if you will go low from insulin action. Check your continuous monitor, and use a finger stick test when you need to confirm how low your blood sugar is.

Dating

To tell or not to tell is a personal decision. Friends and dates are often inquisitive about diabetes if they see a pump or see someone testing or counting carbs. This can serve as an "ice breaker" to start talking about and explaining diabetes. On the other hand, someone may feel more comfortable concealing their diabetes for awhile. Even if you do not want to reveal your diabetes at first, do not skip testing and taking your boluses. Excuse yourself and go to the restroom for these procedures, if necessary.

Alcohol

Drinking alcohol can have several adverse effects on diabetes. Alcohol prevents the liver from releasing glucose during hypoglycemia and may leave a pumper without the regulation that usually kicks in to raise the blood sugar out of a low. Drinking also impairs judgment and makes it difficult to recognize a low, as well as impeding the accuracy of carb counting and insulin dosing decisions.

Hypoglycemia symptoms are strikingly similar to those of intoxication. If you go low after drinking, the smell of alcohol may prevent someone else from recognizing the real problem and seriously delay treatment of hypoglycemia. You could be jailed rather than receive effective treatment. Alcohol and insulin should be mixed with care.

To make the best decisions about drinking, consider these tips:

- Know the laws in your state about drinking.
- Remember, you have the choice to say "No!"
- If you plan to drink, eat carbs first. Do not skip meals or snacks.
- Limit the amount of alcohol by drinking one or two drinks slowly or alternating alcoholic with nonalcoholic beverages.

- Usually wine, beer and straight alcohol like gin, or tequila do not need to be covered with a bolus. Mixed drinks, liqueurs, and margueritas have a higher sugar content and may need to be matched with a bolus.

- Never drink before you drive and never drive after drinking.

- Wear diabetes medical ID tags.

- Let friends know you have diabetes, how hypoglycemia might make you look or act, and that you can pass out from a low. Let them know a low cannot be slept off and you need medical attention if you are not responding appropriately for any reason.

- Test your blood sugar before going to sleep. For safety, eat an extra snack at bedtime after drinking alcohol.

Eating Disorders

With all the focus on food in diabetes care, it is not surprising that some teens with diabetes have eating disorders. This often occurs with young women who may have a distorted image of themselves and who want to lose inappropriate amounts of weight. They may discover a quick weight-loss technique by eating what they want while decreasing their insulin doses. Soon blood sugar, calories and ketones start to spill into the urine, resulting in weight loss but carrying with it an extreme risk for ketoacidosis in the short run, and a shorter and medically-challenged life in the long run.

Parents and diabetes professionals must stay aware of teens who are overly concerned about food and weight. These teens typically have poor glucose control because they do not calculate basal rates and boluses appropriately. For teens with these behaviors, psychological assessment and intervention are imperative.

If you are using any of these harmful weight-loss techniques or think that you have problems with food and weight, seek professional help. Untreated eating disorders are very dangerous and can be life threatening, especially with diabetes.

Pregnancy

Young women with diabetes need education about contraception. All commonly used hormonal contraceptives are safe, but often a low dose is used to offer protection with less effect on blood sugar levels. A series of unexplained low blood sugars in a young woman may be the earliest sign of pregnancy. Excellent blood sugar control in the weeks or months prior to conception and throughout pregnancy is critical for a healthy delivery. Refer to Chapter 26 for details.

Type 2 Teens

Teens with Type 2 diabetes who use insulin for blood sugar control can equally benefit from an insulin pump. Therapy for Type 2 starts with adequate exercise and appropriate eating through carb counting. An overnight basal rate from a pump can be matched to the Dawn Phenomenon and meals and snacks can be covered with boluses.

Type 2 teens on pumps are better able to reduce eating and match this with a smaller bolus, thus avoiding overeating. A pump also makes it easier to adjust insulin doses for planned and unplanned exercise or activity.

Summary

In the first years pump therapy was available, its value in the care of children and teens was not fully appreciated. This is no longer the case. Success and safety with proper pump use matched to the special needs of the young pumper occurs when the child or teen and their family are well-trained and properly supported. The well-being of the child or teen makes all the training and care worthwhile. A child or teen wearing a pump has the opportunity for excellent blood sugar control during the most challenging years of diabetes.

24.6 Differences In The Three Major Types Of Diabetes			
	Type 1	Type 1.5 / LADA	Type 2
Avg. age at start	12	46	61
Typical age at start	3-40*	20-70*	35-80*
% of all diabetes	10% (25%**)	15%	75%
Insulin problem	absence	deficiency	resistance
Antibodies	ICA, IA2, GAD65, IAA	mostly GAD65	none
Early treatment	insulin is vital, diet & exercise changes helpful	pills or insulin vital, diet & exercise changes helpful	pills helpful, diet & increased activity essential
Late treatment	insulin, diet, exercise (occasionally pills)	insulin, pills, diet, exercise	insulin, pills, diet, exercise

 * may occur at any age
** if all antibody positive cases are included, ie Type1 and Type 1.5   © 2003 Diabetes Services, Inc.

The early bird gets the worn and the early worm gets eaten.

Anon.

Pumps And Type 2 Diabetes

The benefits of an insulin pump are obvious with Type 1 diabetes, but most adults with Type 2 make equally good candidates when they need insulin to maintain control. Like Type 1s, they benefit from easy, precise, and convenient insulin delivery, reminders and data tracking.

This chapter explains

- Type 2 diabetes
- Insulin need in Type 2
- Type 1.5 diabetes often mistaken for Type 2
- Advantages of pumps in Type 2

Type 2 Diabetes

In Type 2 diabetes the blood sugar goes high because insulin is not efficiently moving blood glucose into cells. It is often part of a metabolic syndrome that includes a variety of problems: insulin resistance, high triglycerides, low levels of HDL or protective cholesterol, elevated blood pressure, and abdominal obesity. Type 2 is a progressive disease in which excessive insulin production tries to keep up with insulin resistance for the first few years but then gradually falls off as beta cells become exhausted.

As diabetes groups like the WHO, ADA, and AACE have faced a rising tide of Type 2 diabetes, glucose levels for diagnosis and treatment goals have fallen in an attempt to help people avoid complications. Suggested treatment goals in Type 2 diabetes include:

- A fasting plasma glucose of 110 mg/dl (6.1 mmol) or less
- Blood sugars of 140 mg/dl (7.7 mmol) or less 2 hours after eating
- An A1c of 6.5% or less

In the first years after a diagnosis, the blood sugar may be brought down to goal through lifestyle changes. However, many people fail in this effort because they have difficulty improving their diet, exercising regularly, and losing weight. When a person cannot control the blood sugar well enough to reach these goals, an oral medication is prescribed and increased or supplemented with other oral diabetes medications. New injectable medications, such as Symlin and GLP-1 inhibitors, may also be used for both weight loss and to lower blood sugar levels after meals. (See pages 181-183 for information.)

Insulin Need In Type 2 Diabetes

When control can no longer be maintained with medications like these, insulin is started. Type 2 diabetes is typically diagnosed about 10 years after it began, when half the insulin production has already been lost.[100] Excess insulin is often produced by the body in early stages of Type 2, but the stress of overproduction, along with the toxic effects of excess glucose and free fatty acids, eventually causes damage to beta cells and causes insulin output to fall. After diagnosis, beta cell insulin production continues to fall at about 4%

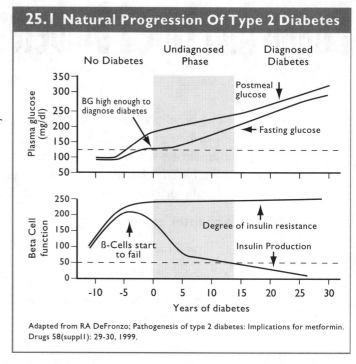

25.1 Natural Progression Of Type 2 Diabetes

Adapted from RA DeFronzo; Pathogenesis of type 2 diabetes: Implications for metformin. Drugs 58(suppl1): 29-30, 1999.

to 5% per year. Insulin replacement is most effective when started early where its use can slow damage to beta cells from stress and glucose toxicity.

Though rarely done, it is very helpful to give insulin for Type 2 at the first clinic visit when a blood sugar is high to overcome glucose toxicity and rapidly bring down the high reading. Sometimes an initial injection may be enough to gain blood sugar control.

Over half of those with Type 2 diabetes eventually require insulin using injections or a pump. Starting on insulin does not mean you have failed to control your diabetes. Rather, needing insulin results from a natural progression in Type 2 that we do not yet have the tools to stop (See Figure 25.1). Starting on insulin as soon as it is needed simply improves quality of life and health, and often prolongs beta cell productivity.

Over 20 million people in this country have Type 2 diabetes, but only about 34% use insulin. Many start on insulin only after their beta cells are already severely damaged. Early use of insulin appears to preserve some beta cell activity to make control easier.

Many diabetes specialists believe that use of insulin would rise to over 50% of those with Type 2 diabetes if their treatment were designed to provide true cardiovascular protection. New stringent goals to keep premeal blood sugars below 100 mg/dl (5.5 mmol) and postmeal readings below 135 mg/dl (7.5 mmol) are being attempted in an NIH study that will report its findings in about 2008. Called the ACCORD or Action to Control Cardiovascular Risk in Diabetes study, it is following 10,000 people with Type 2 diabetes.

The goal of the study is to find out how much impact on reduction of cardiovascular disease comes from improvements in blood sugar control, blood pressure control, and control of cholesterol levels. The goal for half of the participants is to get their average blood sugar into a normal range with an A1c below 6%. To achieve this, over half of the intensive control group are expected to require insulin. Watch for the results of this important study that is likely to show the benefits of improved control achieved through wider use of insulin.

Type 1.5 Diabetes Mistaken For Type 2

Adults diagnosed with diabetes at an age considered "too old" for the onset of Type 1 and who do not immediately require insulin for treatment are often told they have Type 2 diabetes. For many, this is a misdiagnosis. Their diabetes is actually a slow form of Type 1 diabetes, referred to as Type 1.5 or LADA (latent autoimmune diabetes in adults). One in every seven to ten people said to have Type 2 diabetes actually have antibodies that indicate they have Type 1.5. People with Type 1.5 number over 2 million people in the U.S. or double the million or so people with Type 1 diabetes.

Type 1.5 starts in adults as beta cells are slowly destroyed by antibodies. The only difference from Type 1 is that only one or occasionally two antibodies are involved, rather than three or more. The primary antibody involved in Type 1.5 is the GAD65 or glutamic acid decarboxylase antibody as shown in Table 24.6.

Type 1.5 differs from Type 2 in that insulin resistance is not usually involved. Type 1.5 starts about 15 years earlier at an average age 46 instead of 61, usually without excess weight, but often with a personal or family history of an autoimmune disease.[101] It should be suspected when an adult does not have other classic signs of Type 2 diabetes, such as high triglyceride or low HDL levels, abdominal obesity, or a family history of high blood pressure. Many people with Type 1.5 are not overweight, while others are, making a "visual" diagnosis difficult. As the population increases in weight, people with Type 1 and 1.5 can have traits of Type 2, such as excess weight, insulin resistance and cholesterol problems.

Correct diagnosis of Type 1.5 is important because insulin treatment will be required much sooner in Type 1.5 than Type 2 diabetes. If Type 1.5 is suspected, a GAD65 antibody test should be done. When GAD65 or islet cell antibodies are present, the decline in insulin production is faster and the person requires insulin earlier than in Type 2. In the UKPDS study, 94% of those with Type 1.5 diabetes required insulin six years after being diagnosed compared to only 16% of those with Type 2 diabetes and no antibodies.[100]

Those with Type 1.5 diabetes obtain the same benefits from a pump as those with Type 1. Because relatively low insulin doses are needed in early Type 1.5 while internal insulin production remains, a pump is better able to provide these precise doses and may also help preserve beta cell production. As beta cell production declines, small increases in basal and bolus delivery are more convenient on a pump.

Advantages Of A Pump In Type 2

Type 2 diabetes is often part of a metabolic syndrome with various health issues, including cholesterol problems, high blood pressure, and excess unperceived inflammation and oxidation. Use of insulin helps blood sugar control and some of these associated problems.

Many people with Type 2 diabetes resist using insulin. When they finally agree to start using it, they want a simple approach with as few injections as possible. For convenience and ease of use, they are often started on one or two injections of a premixed 70/30 insulin. This mixture of 70% slower background insulin and 30% rapid insulin is used to reduce the number of injections and simplify the calculation required for dosing. It attempts to cover background and meal needs, but doses are never be exact using this approach. The user is tied to eating to offset the activity of the rapid insulin every time they take the combined insulin to cover their background need.

A pump offers the convenience of a 70/30 insulin with a much more precise method of meeting insulin need. A pump uses only one type of insulin adjusted to provide a basal profile that matches background insulin need and easy bolusing for every snack and meal. It provides precise dosing without increasing the number of injections and improves the user's control. When insulin is needed, an insulin pump offers the most convenient and natural way to deliver the insulin that is lacking.

Although few studies have been done with people with Type 2 using pumps, the ones that exist suggest that people with Type 2 diabetes prefer pumps over multiple injections. One small study in 1993 found that people preferred pumps because they experienced less pain, fewer social limitations, less hassle, less life interference, and less burden. They also experienced more general satisfaction, flexibility, and convenience.[102] These positive aspects help Type 2s overcome their resistance to using insulin.

Short-term use of an insulin pump may prolong good control in early stages of Type 2 diabetes. In a French study, 82 people with Type 2, who were unable to control their blood sugars with a low calorie diet and maximum doses of Glucophage (metformin), were temporarily placed on insulin pumps for periods of 8 to 32 days.[103] Blood sugars were brought down to target in the few days they were on pumps, but what was more interesting was that the blood sugar stayed under control for several months after the pump treatment stopped! Brief use of an insulin pump appears to give an overworked pancreas a "vacation" and helps it again produce adequate amounts of insulin.

A Turkish study tried the same approach in people with newly-diagnosed Type 2 diabetes who did not respond to diet control. After two weeks on a pump, six of 13 patients were able to stay well controlled on diet alone for between 16 and 59 months, although four people required a second two-week treatment, and one required a third treatment.[104]

Helps Overcome The Metabolic Syndrome

Elements of the metabolic syndrome that affect many people with Type 2 can be dealt with more effectively by a pump. Better control improves sensitivity to insulin and reduces insulin resistance, while lowering the amount of insulin required to achieve control. A pump helps lower high triglyceride levels as rapid insulin is matched to the carbs in meals.[105,106] This lessens elevated cholesterol levels and reduces clotting which can be dangerously high in Type 2 diabetes and lead to heart problems.

Lowers High Morning Readings

In Type 2 diabetes, a high waking blood sugar is common, even when the person has gone to bed with a normal reading. The rise in blood sugar during the night occurs when the liver makes and releases glucose into the bloodstream. The liver does this because it cannot "sense" that the insulin level is low due to it own resistance to insulin. High glucose levels increase the resistance to insulin and make it even harder for the beta cells to keep up.

Oral medications may work for awhile at controlling the high morning blood sugar of a person with Type 2. But eventually, this problem requires the addition of insulin, usually in combination with oral medications. The insulin may be delivered with one or more injections, but a pump does the job better. Basal insulin from a pump can be precisely adjusted so that it is delivered in the exact amount and at the exact time it is needed during the night to prevent the liver's production and release of glucose.

Studies done in the early 1980's found that insulin levels in Type 2 needed to be increased by over 40% in the early morning to prevent high readings on rising.[107] This increase is about double that required to control the Dawn Phenomenon in Type 1 diabetes. This need for extra basal insulin in early morning hours is caused by insulin resistance and the release of free fatty acids that block insulin's effect. This is difficult to control with an injection of "flat" long-acting insulin. High morning blood sugars are always prevented better by the precise doses and exact timing of basal delivery on a pump.[105,106]

Decreases Weight Gain

Excess weight is common with Type 2 diabetes and insulin use can lead to weight gain. Someone with Type 2 often goes for years with high readings that flush excess calories into the urine. They may have adapted by eating an extra 500 to 1000 calories a day with no weight gain. When treatment with medications or insulin begins to lower the blood sugar level, these calories previously lost in the urine start to move into cells. Unless calorie intake is reduced as soon as blood sugar control improves, a rapid increase in weight will be seen.

Weight gain does not have to happen with improved control. The road to real blood sugar control lies in eating only what you need and adjusting your insulin to handle it. This does not cause weight gain. Less insulin is required on a pump to achieve control, resulting in less exposure to glucose and insulin. The data in a pump provides easy access to a history of carb intake and can even act as a coach for weight loss. Proper use of a pump means that all meals and snacks have to be taken into account, making "unconscious" eating less likely.

Weight loss is easier when the user does not need to eat to avoid lows. A lower calorie intake is easier on a pump that calculates and reduces carb boluses based on the number of carbs to be eaten. Choosing carbs from a carb database in a pump, a linked PDA or a smart phone also helps reduce calories and carbs.

Improves Control And Lowers A1c

An insulin pump improves control by stabilizing fasting blood sugars with precise overnight basals matched to need. Postmeal readings are lowered by using a variety of boluses, from extended to combination, that match insulin to carbs better. A carb data base and a carb factor put in the pump helps the pump give a recommendation for a carb bolus and tracks the history of how well control is maintained. Using this, successful insulin delivery is reproducible. The improved control also reduces complications.[104]

Medicare Pump Coverage

People with Type 2 or Type 1.5 who are eligible for Medicare are candidates for coverage for an insulin pump if they meet certain criteria. They can qualify for an insulin pump if they meet Medicare's definition of diabetes as shown by the C-peptide test or the beta cell autoantibody test. As shown in Table 25.2, Medicare's addition of the autoantibody test allows people with Type 1.5 or LADA to start on a pump when antibodies to GAD65 or islet cells are present. They can qualify before they lose all beta cell insulin production, which is indicated by a very low C-peptide level. Pump candidates must meet a second criteria that establishes the need for a pump based on the failure in some respect of MDI to provide good control, as shown in Table 25.3.

Pregnancy

Diabetes affects 10,000 pregnancies each year in women who have Type 1 diabetes prior to conception. An increasing number are also becoming pregnant with preexisting Type 2 diabetes as women develop Type 2 at younger ages and more become pregnant in their 30's and 40's.

Gestational diabetes (GDM) is an elevation of the blood sugar during pregnancy and affects 7% of all pregnancies or over 200,000 women a year in the U.S. GDM is a form of Type 2 diabetes that begins during pregnancy, often near the end of the second trimester or during the third trimester.

All of these women have a compelling reason for controlling their diabetes – to promote not only their own health but the health and wellbeing of the unborn baby. Insulin pumps are now used in pregnancies that involve all three forms of diabetes.

This chapter covers

- How blood sugar control affects complications
- Why blood sugar control is more difficult during pregnancy
- Testing for prediabetes and diabetes before pregnancy
- Preparing for pregnancy
- Pregnancy management in Type 1, Type 2, and GDM
- Gestational diabetes
- How to distribute carbs through the day with the Rule of 18ths
- Insulin adjustments during pregnancy
- Labor, delivery, and followup after delivery

Complications Found In Pregnancy

In addition to its normal benefits, glucose control becomes even more important during pregnancy. Only strictly controlled glucose levels can create the environment needed to produce a healthy baby. High blood sugars before conception and during

A special thanks to Lois Jovanovic, M.D. for her many contributions to improving pregnancy outcomes in pregnancy, many of which are included in this chapter.

the first eight weeks of pregnancy have been associated with serious birth defects. High levels in the second and third trimesters may result in fetal complications and problems during delivery or in the first few days afterward.

First trimester complications include

- Birth defects
- Spontaneous miscarriage

The risk for these complications increases in pre-existing Type 1 or Type 2 diabetes when blood sugars have been poorly controlled near the time of conception.

Second and third trimester complications include

- Premature delivery
- Delayed growth and development
- Large birth weight (over 9 pounds), often requiring a C-section

Problems for the child at birth include

- Injury during delivery
- Severe low blood sugars after delivery
- Seizures
- Respiratory distress syndrome
- Enlarged heart
- Low calcium level and tetany (jitters)
- Jaundice
- High red blood cell count (polycythemia)

These complications can arise due to poor control in Type 1, Type 2, or gestational diabetes. One complication resulting from high blood sugars during pregnancy is that the baby may not have fully developed lungs at birth even though it is full term and normal weight. Underdeveloped lungs may cause the baby to have respiratory distress or difficulty in breathing after delivery.

High blood sugars in the mother near the time of delivery can also cause severe hypoglycemia in the newborn baby after delivery. While in the womb during the third trimester, the fetus produces large amounts of insulin whenever the mother has a high blood sugar. If the mother's blood sugar is high near delivery, the baby will continue to produce excess insulin after delivery, triggering its own severe low blood sugars.

How Improved Control Affects Complications

Since 1949, blood sugar control has been directly linked to the survival of the infant. In that year, Priscilla White, M.D., reported from the Joslin Clinic in Boston that 18

26.1 Blood Sugar Goals During Pregnancy		
Time	**Whole Blood**	**Plasma**
Before meals and at bedtime:	60-90 mg/dl (3.3-5 mmol)	65-100 mg/dl (3.6-5.6 mmol)
1 hour after starting to eat:	<120 mg/dl (6.7 mmol)	<135 mg/dl (7.5 mmol)
2 a.m. to 6 a.m.:	60-90 mg/dl (3.3-5 mmol)	65-100 mg/dl (3.6-5.6 mmol)
Note: Keep your A1c at least 20% below the lab's upper limit of normal for nonpregnant women, i.e, in a normal range for pregnancy. You should know whether your meter is reading whole blood or plasma. © 2006 Diabetes Services, Inc.		

percent of the babies of mothers with diabetes were stillborn or died shortly after birth. She noted that "good treatment of diabetes" clearly improved the outcome.[108] In 1965, Jorgen Pedersen, M.D., studying pregnant women in Copenhagen, reported that women who had none of the Bad Signs in Table 26.2 had a 6.9 percent rate of fetal and neonatal deaths.[109,110] In contrast, in 130 pregnancies where one of these signs was present, the death rate rose to 31 percent.[111]

During the late 1960's and early 1970's, it became clear that the higher the average blood sugar level of the mother, the more likely a child would die near birth. By the early 1980's, the mother's blood sugar and the child's metabolic environment could be normalized through blood sugar testing at home. This helped to greatly reduce complications once the mother knew she was pregnant, but the problems caused by high blood sugars at conception still existed.

Around this time, birth defects emerged as a major cause of infant deaths in babies born to women with Type 1 diabetes.[112,113] In several studies that looked at this problem, birth defects were found to occur in 4% to 11% of infants born to women with Type 1 diabetes, compared to a rate of 1.2% to 2.1% in the general population.[114,115] Researchers and physicians realized that blood sugar levels need to be normalized prior to conception. The child's organs form rapidly during the first eight weeks after conception, often before a woman realizes she is pregnant.

26.2 Dr. Pederson's Bad Signs
Things to avoid in pregnancy:
1. Ketoacidosis
2. Preeclampsia toxemia of pregnancy: a combination of high blood pressure, headaches, protein in the urine, and swelling of the legs, usually occurs late in the pregnancy
3. Kidney infection
4. Neglect of prenatal care

Several researchers also noticed that higher A1c values during the first trimester were associated with more spontaneous miscarriages than were seen in nondiabetic women.[116,117] An A1c that is in the normal range or no higher than one percent above the upper limit of a normal range minimizes the risk of both birth defects and spontaneous abortions. Interestingly, one researcher found that women with diabetes who have excellent control throughout pregnancy actually have a lower rate of spontaneous abortion than nondiabetic women.[117]

26.3 Can Insulin Harm The Child?

Some women are concerned that injected insulin will harm the fetus. This cannot happen because the majority of the insulin does not pass through the placenta and the little bit of insulin that does pass is not biologically active. Glucose, on the other hand, passes easily through the placenta. As the child's own pancreas develops and begins producing insulin during the second and third trimester, the baby will try to lower any high blood sugar by producing insulin. Because insulin is a growth hormone, these excess amounts of insulin created by the baby adds excess and unneeded weight. Macrosomia (or "large body") develops and can make delivery difficult or dangerous for both mother and child.

The conclusion from these early studies was that maintaining normal blood sugars before and throughout pregnancy reduces the risk of complications. Women with Type 1 or Type 2 diabetes who plan to conceive should keep their blood sugar at the lower levels recommended for pregnancy before they conceive. This tightly controlled environment is needed prior to conception through delivery. The guidelines that follow provide a good way to maintain tight control during pregnancy.

Control Becomes More Difficult During Pregnancy – All Diabetes Types

Several factors contribute to making blood sugar control more complicated during pregnancy. During pregnancy, day-to-day blood sugar levels are naturally lower than prior to pregnancy, apparently to protect the fetus. Research shows that a normal waking blood sugar for a woman who is pregnant but does not have diabetes is 55 to 65 mg/dl (3 to 3.6 mmol) after an overnight fast. The blood sugar level is always less than 120 mg/dl (6.6 mmol) even one hour after eating a high carb meal. For good control and a healthy baby, A1c levels need to stay within a normal range throughout pregnancy. The A1c levels for pregnancy are 20 percent lower than the normal range for healthy adults.

These normal blood sugars during pregnancy come very close to a hypoglycemic range, as shown in Table 26.1. Control becomes complicated when morning sickness causes nausea and vomiting, and makes eating and insulin coverage difficult. Other factors that must be balanced are rising placental hormone release that raise the blood sugar and a gradual weight gain that requires additional insulin during the course of the pregnancy.

A pumps is better able to deliver the precise insulin doses required for tight control and makes it more convenient to give frequent boluses for frequent small meals that can greatly improve postmeal control while keeping track of BOB.

Preparing for Pregnancy – Type 1, Type 2

If you have Type 1 or Type 2 diabetes, you should have your blood sugar under good control before you try to conceive. If you have Type 2 diabetes and are using an oral medication, this should be discontinued prior to conception to avoid any possible effects on the fetus. A program for Type 2's using diet, exercise, and insulin, if needed, can be worked out with your physician to achieve optimal control before conception.

Until your blood sugar is controlled, use adequate birth control. Low dose birth control pills appear to be both safe and effective. Once your A1c is in the normal range, you are ready for pregnancy, and birth control can be discontinued.

Achieving optimal control before conception is necessary because the fetus begins to develop specialized organs and tissues from the time the egg is fertilized through the first three months of pregnancy. High blood sugars at this time interfere with cell division and can lead to DNA damage and birth defects. There is a 20 percent chance that the infant will develop complications or die if control was poor prior to conception and optimal control is achieved only in the second trimester.[118]

If you plan to become pregnant, follow a healthy food plan, exercise regularly, and supplement your diet with a prenatal vitamin. If you have any complication caused by diabetes prior to pregnancy, such as damage to the eyes, kidneys, or vascular system, there is a greater risk of complications in pregnancy for yourself and the baby.[119] This does not rule out a healthy pregnancy, but should be carefully considered before pregnancy begins.

Testing For Prediabetes or Diabetes Prior To Pregnancy

If you have a high risk of GDM (see Table 26.4) and are attempting to conceive, you should have a glucose tolerance test to determine if you have prediabetes (also known as glucose intolerance) or diabetes before conception. If these tests are positive, follow Preparing For Pregnancy – Type 1, Type 2 in the previous section. If these tests are negative, they should be repeated as soon as pregnancy is confirmed and, if again negative, repeated at 24 to 28 weeks of gestation.

These tests detect prediabetes if a fasting plasma glucose is equal to or above 110 mg/dl (5.8 mmol) and less than 126 mg/dl (7.0 mmol), or a random plasma glucose is equal to or above 140 mg/dl (7.8 mmol) and less than 200 mg/dl (11.1 mmol) at the two hour point during a 75 gram glucose tolerance test.

A diagnosis of diabetes is made if a fasting plasma glucose is equal to or above 126 mg/dl (7 mmol) or if the glucose is 200 mg/dl (11.1 mmol) or above two hours into a 75 gram oral glucose tolerance test (OGTT). A third way to diagnose diabetes involves the presence of diabetes symptoms plus a random plasma glucose equal to or above 200 mg/dl (11.1 mmol). A diagnosis can be made only if a second test on another day meets the same criteria on one of these tests. A diagnosis of prediabetes or diabetes warns that blood sugar levels are higher than normal and above optimal levels for pregnancy.

Gestational Diabetes

The most common form of diabetes during pregnancy is gestational diabetes mellitus (GDM), which is defined as glucose intolerance that is first recognized during pregnancy. It typically develops late in the second trimester or early in the third trimester of an otherwise normal pregnancy due to the increasing demand for insulin production at this time. Gestational diabetes puts both the mother and baby at risk for serious complications during the pregnancy if not managed carefully.

Gestational diabetes is usually a form of early Type 2 diabetes uncovered by the increased insulin requirement that occurs during pregnancy. A mother with GDM faces a high risk of developing Type 2 diabetes later in life.

26.4 High Risk Factors For GDM
• Women who are > 25 years of age
• Overweight or obese
• Family history of diabetes
• History of abnormal glucose metabolism
• History of poor obstetric outcome
• A member of an ethnic/racial group with a high prevalence of diabetes (e.g., Hispanic American, Native American, Asian American, African American, Pacific Islander)
• Family history of Type 2 diabetes

Blood sugar elevation during pregnancy can also result from early Type 1.5 diabetes defined on page 287. If a woman with GDM also has GAD65 antibodies, she has Type 1.5 diabetes where the need for insulin therapy is seven times as likely compared to Type 2 diabetes.[120] In most cases, glucose regulation returns to normal after delivery, but the underlying problem often persists and needs to be addressed through lifestyle changes.

Screening For GDM

An accurate diagnosis of gestational diabetes is important to reduce health risks to the mother and baby, especially to prevent having a large baby, called macrosomia. Macrosomia often necessitates a C-section and causes problems for the newborn. Pregnant women who are at high risk of GDM should be tested at the first prenatal visit.

When a pregnant woman does not have high risk characteristics, the current recommendation is that she be screened for GDM with a shortened glucose tolerance test. This is routinely done in all pregnant women between the 24th and 28th weeks (the sixth month) of pregnancy. All pregnant women should be screened for GDM because traditional risk factors have a low probability of predicting who will develop GDM, especially during the first pregnancy.[121] It is important to use both fasting and glucose tolerance tests to detect GDM because an elevation of either one may be the only clue that GDM is present.

Fasting hyperglycemia may be particularly important. One research study involving over 145,000 births in Dallas, Texas, found that a fasting plasma glucose of 105 mg/dl (5.8 mmol) or higher was over three times as likely to be associated with fetal malformations compared to women without diabetes and surprisingly to women who did have

GDM but whose fasting value was below 105 mg/dl. Women who had diabetes prior to pregnancy were at the highest risk of fetal malformations at 6.1%, followed by those with GDM and an elevated fasting plasma value at 4.8%, then women without diabetes at 1.5%, and finally those with GDM and a low fasting plasma glucose value at 1.2%.[122]

Be aware that serum and plasma glucose values of labs and most meters are 10% to 15% higher than whole blood values. A few home blood sugar meters measure whole blood, although most translate it into a plasma equivalent. Table 26.1 shows appropriate target blood sugar values for pregnancy using both plasma and whole blood values.

The first glucose test that is done should determine whether diabetes is already present. A fasting plasma glucose with a reading over 126 mg/dl (7 mmol) or any random glucose higher than 200 mg/dl (11.1 mmol) provides half the testing required to diagnose diabetes. If one of these tests is positive, there is no need to do a glucose challenge test because diabetes exists. A second confirmatory test is normally done at the lab on another day but can be replaced by a test in the clinician's office or by home monitoring results to speed initial treatment and rapidly normalize glucose levels.

If the glucose results are not high enough on these tests to warrant a diagnosis of diabetes, further evaluation should be done with one of these two approaches:

ADA One Step Approach

Here an oral glucose tolerance test (OGTT) uses 100 grams of glucose. Criteria for diagnosis of GDM using the 100 gram OGTT are shown in Table 26.5. If the blood sugar is equal to or higher than two of these values, a diagnosis of GDM is made. This one step approach may be cost-effective in high-risk populations, such as Native Americans.

ADA Two Step Approach

Here two steps are used. An initial screening is performed by measuring the plasma glucose one hour after a 50 gram glucose load which is called a glucose challenge test or GCT. A glucose threshold of 140 mg/dl (7.8 mmol) or higher will pick up 80% of women who have GDM, while a value of 130 mg/dl (7.2 mmol) or higher will pick up 90%. The problem with using the lower value, however, is that it gives more false positives than the higher value and many women without GDM are reported as having it. A diagnostic OGTT is then performed on the women who exceed these threshold values on the GCT.

Regardless of the approach used, a diagnosis is based on an OGTT. This three hour glucose challenge is done in the morning after an 8 to 14 hour fast and after at least three days of unrestricted eating that includes plenty of carbohydrate. On the morning of the test, the woman has a drink containing 100 grams of glucose. If two or more of the glucose results exceed the values in Table 26.5, a diagnosis of GDM can be made.

Pregnancy Management Program – All Diabetes Types

Regardless of whether you have Type 1, Type 2, GDM, or marginal glucose control values during testing, you will want to make every effort to keep your blood sugar

26.5 Screening And Diagnosis Of Gestational Diabetes (GDM)

When a test is done, a blood sugar above the threshold indicates GDM.

ADA Screen	Fasting	1 hr	2 hr	3 hr
Screen with 50g GCT*	–	>140 mg/dl* (7.8 mmol)	–	–
ADA 1 Step				
Diagnose with 100g OGTT	>95 mg/dl (5.3 mmol)	>180 mg/dl (10 mmol)	>155 mg/dl (8.6 mmol)	>140 mg/dl (7.8 mmol)
ADA 2 Step				
Screen with 50g GCT	–	>140 mg/dl (7.8 mmol)	–	–
Diagnose with 100g OGTT	>95 mg/dl (5.3 mmol)	>180 mg/dl (10 mmol)	>155 mg/dl (8.6 mmol)	>140 mg/dl (7.8 mmol)
Alternative 1 Step				
Diagnose with 75g OGTT	>95 mg/dl (5.3 mmol)	>180 mg/dl (10 mmol)	>155 mg/dl (8.6 mmol)	–

GCT = glucose challenge test; OGTT = oral glucose tolerance test
* Two research studies have used this as a cost-effective diagnostic tool. One study used the 50g GCT screening test at 16 weeks and found values above 135 mg/dl (7.5 mmol) to be a sensitive diagnostic tool.

throughout pregnancy within the normal targets shown in Table 26.1. You need to manage your diabetes in the following ways:

- Frequent blood sugar and A1c tests to determine your exact level of control
- An eye exam for retinopathy
- A 24-hour urine collection for creatinine clearance, total protein, and microalbumin to assess the health of your kidneys, done each trimester
- An evaluation of your cardiovascular system
- A detailed diet program, using the Rule of 18ths in Table 26.8 or a similar plan
- A regular exercise program

Blood Sugar Monitoring

As weight is gained during pregnancy, the need for insulin rises. In order to adjust insulin to need in Type 1 diabetes, you must maintain a very strict regimen of glucose monitoring. Check at least eight times a day, before each meal, an hour after each meal, at bedtime, and at 2 a.m., to alert yourself and your health care team quickly to any increased need for insulin. Table 26.6 shows the typical rise in insulin requirements throughout pregnancy for women with Type 1 diabetes.

The tests done at one hour after eating should be the highest blood sugar readings of the day with a desired target at this peak of less than 130 mg/dl (7.2 mmol) on a plasma meter or below 120 mg/dl (6.7 mmol) on a whole blood meter. A test result in the lower end of the target range could indicate you should eat more carbs to avoid a low blood sugar.

For women with Type 2 and GDM, testing the blood sugar four to seven tests a day is required to reduce exposure of the fetus to elevated glucose readings. Readings done while fasting and one hour after each meal are the most important times to test and are considered the minimum testing required to ensure adequate glucose control during pregnancy. Tests before meals and at bedtime are also very helpful. Adjustments in insulin, diet, and activity are made based on how well the blood sugar targets are being met.

The last three months of the pregnancy when the baby can produce its own insulin is an especially critical time to test. The baby will overproduce insulin if the mother's blood sugar is higher than normal for pregnancy. The mother's excess glucose easily crosses the placenta, but the excess insulin which the baby makes to counter it cannot. Instead, it causes unwanted weight gain in the baby. This often makes a C-section necessary for delivery and creates other problems for the child after delivery.

26.6 Typical Rise In Total Daily Insulin Doses By Trimester For Type 1 Diabetes

If your weight is:	At this trimester:			
	Pre	1st*	2nd	3rd**
100	27 u	32 u	36 u	41 u
120	33 u	38 u	44 u	49 u
130	35 u	41 u	47 u	53 u
140	38 u	45 u	51 u	57 u
160	44 u	51 u	58 u	65 u
180	49 u	57 u	65 u	74 u
200	55 u	64 u	73 u	82 u

In contrast to Type 1 diabetes, the TDD for women with Type 2 diabetes and recently diagnosed gestational diabetes varies greatly.

* From week 7 to 12, the need for insulin may decrease about 9%.
**In the last 4 weeks, the need for insulin may decrease slightly.

Adapted from Jovanovic L, et al. Am J Med. 71: 925-927, 1981

Other Pregnancy Tests

Certain tests are essential for all women with diabetes and pregnancy:

- Monitoring of ketones at home with a urine test first thing in the morning is essential to detect whether there are too few calories or carbohydrates in the diet.

- Blood pressure measurement at home and at each clinic visit is essential to detect a severe disorder called preeclampsia or toxemia of pregnancy. This is a combination of very high blood pressure, swelling, and protein in the urine that starts in middle to late pregnancies about 5% of the time.

- A sonogram done early in the third trimester can assess the size of the fetus and warn of macrosomia.

Medical Nutrition Therapy (MNT) And Carbohydrate Adjustments

Medical nutrition therapy (MNT) should be started by all pregnant women with diabetes after nutritional counseling by a registered dietitian. Food eaten during pregnancy needs to be consistent with ADA guidelines and include adequate calories and nutrients for the pregnant woman based on her weight, height, and activity.

Eating a balanced diet every day is important for a pregnant woman with diabetes. The fetus continually removes glucose from the mother's blood for its growth, so it is important that the mother eat many meals and snacks throughout the day. More frequent eating also allows the amount of carbs at individual meals to be reduced for better glucose control through the day.

During pregnancy, a diet made up of 40 percent carbohydrate, 40 percent fat, and 20 percent protein is generally recommended. Again, spreading the carbohydrate portion throughout the day makes blood sugar control easier.

One way to spread carbohydrates is to use the "Rule of 18ths" shown in Table 26.7. With the help of your dietician, estimate your total daily caloric need. Then distribute the carbohydrate portion throughout the seven meals or snacks of the day (see Table 26.8) based on the number of 18ths of total carbs needed at each time.

As an example, if you require 1800 calories per day, eat 180 grams of carbohydrate (1800 calories times 40% of calories as carbs divided by 4 calories per gram of carb). This total of 180 grams divided by 18 (Rule of 18ths) equals 10 grams per 18th. According to Table 26.8, your breakfast with two 18ths would include 20 grams of carb.

Breakfast carbs are kept low compared to other meals of the day because most women with Type 1 diabetes

26.7 Carb Distribution With The Rule Of 18ths		
Meal or Snack	**Portion Of The Day's Total Carbohydrate:**	**Percent Of Total Daily Carbs**
Breakfast	2/18	11.0%
Midmorning Snack	1/18	5.5%
Lunch	5/18	27.5%
Midafternoon	2/18	11.0%
Dinner	5/18	27.5%
After-Dinner Snack	2/18	11.0%
Bedtime Snack	1/18	5.5%

26.8 Rule Of 18ths: Grams of Carb Per Meal Based On Total Calorie Need

Meal	Carbs as 18ths	Total Calories Per Day							
		1600	1800	2000	2200	2400	2600	2800	3000
Breakfast	2/18 =	19 g	20 g	22 g	24 g	26 g	29 g	30 g	34 g
Morning Snack	1/18 =	9 g	10 g	12 g	14 g	14 g	14 g	16 g	17 g
Lunch	5/18 =	44 g	50 g	55 g	60 g	66 g	72 g	78 g	82 g
Afternoon Snack	2/18 =	18 g	20 g	22 g	24 g	27 g	30 g	31 g	82 g
Dinner	5/18 =	44 g	50 g	55 g	60 g	66 g	72 g	78 g	34 g
Evening Snack	2/18 =	18 g	20 g	22 g	24 g	27 g	29 g	31 g	82 g
Bedtime Snack	1/18 =	9 g	10 g	12 g	14 g	14 g	14 g	16 g	34 g
Total Carbs/Day =		160 g	180 g	200 g	220 g	240 g	260 g	280 g	300 g
40% of Total Cal/Day =		640 cal	720 cal	800 cal	880 cal	960 cal	1040 cal	1120 cal	1200 cal

have at least a mild Dawn Phenomenon and are more resistant to insulin at the beginning of the day. Women with Type 2 and gestational diabetes often have insulin resistance which can also cause high morning readings. Keeping carb intake low until noon helps in dealing with this. Staying away from high glycemic foods that spike the blood sugar is a good idea at all times. Check glycemic index rankings and select foods that rank 60 or below on the index.

Your caloric need will rise during pregnancy, usually adding between 500 to 1,000 extra calories per day by the end of the nine months. These calories supply fuel for your higher metabolic rate and your required weight gain. The distribution of carbohydrates changes along with the calorie change. Table 26.8 provides guidance for distributing the carb portion of these calories.[123]

Exercise

Increased exercise is a critical part of blood sugar control during pregnancy. An ideal way to do this is to walk for 15 to 20 minutes after each meal. When this can be done, postmeal blood sugars are greatly improved. A total of 45 to 60 minutes of walking a day is ideal during pregnancy. Starting or continuing an exercise program is highly recommended to improve control of blood sugar, blood pressure, weight and circulation during pregnancy.

Insulin Therapy

If you have well-controlled Type 1 diabetes when you become pregnant, you can begin adjusting your normal basal doses and boluses through the pregnancy. If you are not in good control, you'll need expert guidance to maintain a healthy pregnancy.

Insulin requirements rise steadily throughout pregnancy and will usually double by the last month.[124] The rising need for insulin is caused by several factors, including weight gain, increased caloric intake, creation of new tissue, and an increase in hormones made by the enlarging placenta. The action of placental hormones, especially estrogen, cortisol, and human placental lactogen, conflict with the action of insulin. Each woman's experience varies, so an insulin program must be tailored to each individual's need.

However, there are two periods during a pregnancy when a reduction in insulin may be needed. The first period occurs in Type 1 diabetes during a five week interval between weeks 7 and 12 of gestation. In one clinic's experience, after an initial rise in insulin doses of 18% between weeks 3 and 7, a significant drop in insulin requirement averaging 9% was seen in weeks 7 through 12.[125]

The reason for this insulin change is not clear, but it may be caused by an initial increase in doses to correct past hyperglycemia followed by improved sensitivity as a result of the better control. It may also be caused by a decline in progesterone secretion at this time. The fall in insulin need early in pregnancy was first noted by physicians in the 1950's who found that unexpected, sudden hypoglycemia in women with Type 1 diabetes was often the first sign of pregnancy.

The second exception to a general rise in insulin need as pregnancy progresses occurs in the last four weeks. At this time, the fetus starts to draw more glucose from the mother's blood for its own use, causing the mother's insulin need to fall slightly.

If a decreased need occurs, basal rates and boluses may need to be reduced. A reduced overnight basal and a larger bedtime snack may be required to keep the blood sugar from dropping during the night at this time. Reduce your carb boluses as needed if you are unable to eat substantial meals because of your enlarging uterus.

Caution: If you experience a drop in your need for insulin that does not occur at these times and is not caused by another obvious reason, contact your obstetrician for consideration of immediate delivery.

Insulin Pump Therapy

With Type 1 diabetes, the flexibility of an insulin pump works well for maintaining control as the need for insulin constantly rises, especially in the last four months of pregnancy. During pregnancy with Type 1 diabetes, basal insulin delivery usually makes up 50 to 60% of the TDD and will usually remain near the starting percentage through the pregnancy.

In GDM and Type 2 diabetes where significant insulin production remains, control can often be achieved with two or three injections a day, although some may benefit from the precise delivery of a pump. In the presence of insulin resistance, 70% or more of the TDD may be needed for basal insulin, with the rest for meal boluses.

Correction boluses should be used whenever they are needed, whether by injection or by pump, to bring down a high blood sugar. This should be done quickly so that the fetus is not harmed. If the blood sugar continues to rise above your targets, it is time to raise your basal and bolus doses. An increase in the TDD is usually required every 5 to 15 days through most of the pregnancy. See Table 26.6 for the typical rise in TDD. A graphic charting system like *Smart Charts* or a comprehensive logbook should be used during pregnancy to track everything that may affect your control.

Insulin Choices

ADA guidelines currently say human Regular insulin should be used during pregnancy. Rapid analog insulins are structurally different from human insulin and are not yet approved for use. The FDA requires all insulins to be carefully studied to detect unwanted changes during the rapid cell division and organ development of pregnancy, especially during the critical first three months. One measure of cell change is whether those using an analog insulin have any more retinopathy compared to existing insulins, and no difference has been detected in studies involving large numbers of users.

Humalog (lispro) has been available since 1997 and used by many women during the time in which they conceived and through the subsequent pregnancy. To this point, research studies have found no detrimental effects on the fetus from using Humalog in Type 1 or Type 2 diabetes.[126-129] Several studies have concluded that use of Humalog in pregnancy results in outcomes that are comparable to other large studies of diabetic pregnancy. Though not approved for use in pregnancy, many clinicians prefer to use a rapid insulin in Type 1, Type 2 and GDM to improve postmeal glucose control.

Oral Diabetes Medications

Oral diabetes medications are not FDA approved for use in pregnancy. If you have Type 2 diabetes or GDM, you may be controlling your diabetes with diet and medication. With pregnancy, diabetes medications are usually replaced immediately with insulin, since some oral agents may have a negative effect on the fetus. If your diabetes is diet-controlled, your blood sugar should be monitored carefully at home and in the clinic with the goal of staying within the targets in Table 26.1. Insulin will be started when the blood sugar rises above the target level required for a healthy pregnancy.

One study of the diabetes medication glyburide showed it could achieve tight control in a head to head study with insulin. The study involved over 400 women with gestational diabetes who were not able to achieve blood sugar control with MNT alone, but started after conception. No differences were found in control or outcomes between the two groups.[130] However, a full scale clinical trial at various locations will need to be done to confirm this study. Glyburide has not yet been approved for use in pregnancy.

Older sulfonylureas are known to cause fetal damage and are avoided. Prolonged hypoglycemia lasting four to ten days has been seen after delivery in women receiving other sulfonylureas, so glyburide should be discontinued at least 2 weeks before delivery if used.

Many women of child-bearing age with Type 2 diabetes or PCOS have been treated with metformin to improve fertility, so pregnancy may occur while the metformin is still being used. Generally an excellent diabetes medication, one issue that arises with metformin's use is that it can lower levels of folic acid and vitamin B12 in the blood. Folic acid intake is generally low in the diet. A lack of folic acid during pregnancy can cause spina bifida and other neural tube defects in the child. Loss of folic acid and vitamin B12 can also raise homocysteine levels in the blood, a risk factor associated with an increased risk of heart disease. Malabsorption of vitamin B12 caused by metformin appears to be corrected by taking a calcium supplement.[131] Women of child-bearing age on metformin would be wise to take a calcium supplement along with their prenatal vitamin that contains 400 mg. of folic acid.

When To Start Insulin – Type 2, GDM

Ten to fifteen percent of women with gestational diabetes require insulin to control high blood sugars. Starting insulin doses depend on how much insulin the woman is producing, how high the blood sugar is, the current weight, and when during pregnancy insulin is started.

Insulin is needed as soon as the blood sugar rises above a normal range for pregnancy. For women with Type 2 diabetes or GDM, the American Diabetes Association recommends adding insulin therapy to medical nutritional therapy and exercise when fasting home monitoring values are above 95 mg/dl (5.3 mmol) in whole blood glucose or above 105 mg/dl (5.8 mmol) in plasma glucose, or one hour postprandial values are above 140 mg/dl (7.8 mmol) in whole blood or above 155 mg/dl (8.6 mmol) in plasma.

These values recommended for starting insulin by the ADA are higher than the glucose values seen during a normal pregnancy. Some pregnancy specialists recommend that insulin be started as soon as home blood glucose tests (plasma values) are greater than 100 mg/dl (5.6 mmol) fasting, or above 130 mg/dl (7.2 mmol) one hour after a meal.[122] Home glucose values are more indicative of actual control and are easier to obtain during the pregnancy than tests done in a medical office.

Another reason to begin insulin therapy is when a fetal ultrasound at 29 to 33 weeks shows the fetal weight to be greater than the 70th percentile. Insulin is started for this reason regardless of the mother's glucose levels.[132] When macrosomia is controlled, the need for a C-section becomes less likely. Gestation should last 38 weeks when possible, but not go beyond 38 weeks because longer pregnancies increase the risk of macrosomia and do not decrease the risk of a C-section.

Use Of Insulin With Nausea In Type 1 And Type 2

Nausea and vomiting often occur in the first trimester and become a concern when a pregnant woman with diabetes cannot eat because she is nauseated. Keep in mind that when a woman is nauseated basal delivery is still required to keep the blood sugar from rising. No carb bolus is needed if nothing is eaten, unless the blood sugar is high.

If nausea occurs often, as it will in some pregnancies, part of the carb bolus can be

26.9 Glucagon: How Much Do You Need?

Each 0.15 mg of glucagon or 1/6 of a standard dose raises the blood sugar 30 mg/dl! Avoid taking too much glucagon as this raises the blood sugar too high and may cause nausea.

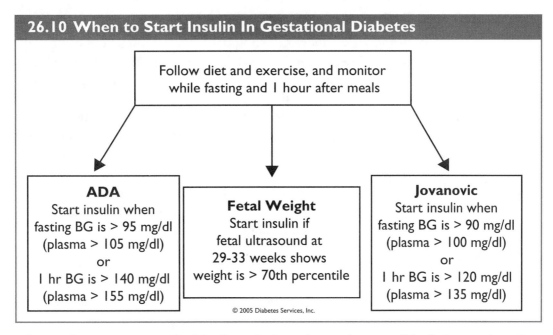

26.10 When to Start Insulin In Gestational Diabetes

Follow diet and exercise, and monitor
while fasting and 1 hour after meals

ADA
Start insulin when
fasting BG is > 95 mg/dl
(plasma > 105 mg/dl)
or
1 hr BG is > 140 mg/dl
(plasma > 155 mg/dl)

Fetal Weight
Start insulin if
fetal ultrasound at
29-33 weeks shows
weight is > 70th percentile

Jovanovic
Start insulin when
fasting BG is > 90 mg/dl
(plasma > 100 mg/dl)
or
1 hr BG is > 120 mg/dl
(plasma > 135 mg/dl)

© 2005 Diabetes Services, Inc.

taken and eating attempted. If food can be kept down, the rest of the bolus can be taken as soon as the meal is finished.

If food or caloric drinks won't stay down but a meal bolus has been taken, a partial dose of glucagon can be injected to quickly raise the blood sugar. Usually, one third to one half of a standard one milligram glucagon kit is all that is needed to prevent a low blood sugar. Glucagon should be kept available for both severe lows and for when a carb bolus has been taken but nausea prevents eating. Glucagon makes the liver release some of its stored glucose to raise the blood sugar to a safe level.

Prevention Of Ketoacidosis In Pregnancy

With Type 1 diabetes, the greatest threat to the fetus and the mother are high blood sugars that lead to ketoacidosis. If the mother develops severe ketoacidosis, there is a 95 percent probability that the fetus will die. The following precautions help to avoid ketoacidosis:

• Test the blood sugar frequently to ensure that control is constant

• Take a correction bolus to lower any blood sugar over 160 mg/dl (8.9 mmol)

• Check for ketones each morning and when the blood sugar is above the target level

• Give NPH insulin by injection at bedtime equal to 30% of the entire day's normal basal delivery. For instance, if the basal rate makes up 30 units per day, give 9 units of NPH at bedtime. Lower the night basal rate at the same time, giving 40% of the current basal starting at bedtime for the next 10 hours. A drawback to NPH is its variability in action. Although there is less experience with Lantus and Levemir and they are not approved for use in pregnancy, they do offer a more consistent activity. They are used by some clinicians for this reason to replace about half the basal delivery.

Labor And Delivery

During active labor at the hospital, muscle contractions can be equivalent to strenuous exercise. This reduces insulin need dramatically. The goal is to maintain blood glucose levels between 60 and 100 mg/dl (3.3 and 5.6 mmol). If you have Type 1 diabetes, you might attain this level of control by reducing your basal doses quickly and discontinuing all boluses during labor. Hospital personnel find it far easier, however, to disconnect the pump and start an intravenous line to give insulin as needed to lower the blood sugar or to give glucose to raise it. The blood sugar should be monitored closely to ensure that the intravenous line is controlling the blood sugar.

Women who have pre-existing Type 2 diabetes or GDM generally discontinue both basal delivery and carb boluses when active labor begins. If insulin or glucose is needed, they can be given through the IV line.

After Delivery

After delivery, the hormones from the placenta that antagonized insulin are no longer present. Insulin requirements drop rapidly right after delivery. Most women with GDM who required insulin during their pregnancy no longer need it. Women with GDM may continue to have diabetes and need some type of treatment, but often they return to impaired glucose tolerance, impaired fasting glucose, or to normal blood sugars. However, about half of women with gestational diabetes will develop Type 2 diabetes within the next 20 years.

A reduced demand for insulin after delivery, together with the prolonged "exercise" of labor, may dramatically reduce insulin need, even in Type 1 diabetes, for a day or two. If a woman has had a C-section, her eating will be limited for the next two to three days, which also limits insulin need. In a few days, the woman with Type 1 will be back to her pre-pregnancy insulin requirements if weight gain during pregnancy has been minimal.

Breast Feeding –Type 1, Type 2

Breast feeding benefits the baby's immune system, but may lower insulin requirements below those used prior to conception because some glucose is diverted into breast milk. Adjust your calorie intake to match the child's breast-feeding habits. If the baby consumes most of its calories at bedtime or in the middle of the night, you must do the same. Many Type 1 women with this breast-feeding pattern need only a low basal rate to cover eating in the evening hours.

Care Following Delivery

In GDM, tests are performed six weeks after birth to determine whether the mother's blood sugar has returned to normal. The criteria for a diagnosis of diabetes at this time are the same as for diagnosing the general population. See Testing For Prediabetes Or Diabetes Before Pregnancy on page 285. Women with a diagnosis of prediabetes or diabetes should be counseled on diet, exercise and medications to treat the condition.

Babies born to women with GDM should be followed closely to prevent the development of obesity or abnormal glucose tolerance.

Wrap Up

Now that you've worked through **Pumping Insulin**, you have the information and skills to begin to control your blood sugars on a pump. You know good control makes you feel better and and reduces the risk of complications in the long run. You've got the knowledge and motivation needed to take control of your diabetes, but what else do you need?

The information you've worked hard to get is never enough by itself. It has to be supplemented with hands on experience, perseverance, doing the same or similar thing over and over again until you have better results. Setting basal and bolus doses, counting carbs and matching them with carb boluses, testing blood sugars, correcting highs, avoiding lows and recording these details in a useful way are all part of the mix.

One thing we can guarantee you will need is patience. Life has a way of changing and your blood sugar control will change with it. Once you attain reasonable control, it may last weeks, months, years or only a short time before it's highs and lows all over again. You may have no idea why your good control is gone. Just go back, troubleshoot and problem solve and make some changes and test until you see improvements again. Once you succeed through science or luck, you will have the confidence to try again.

If you draw a blank, seek help from a trained health professional who can spot important details and patterns in your charts that you may miss. You are responsible for collecting and recording the information related to your blood sugars, but you don't have to solve all your problems alone. Develop a good relationship with a knowledgeable and supportive health care team to speed your success.

We hope you're encouraged by the new smart features in pumps and get involved in learning how to use them to their fullest capacity. They make pumping easier and safer. Future developments in pumps, meters, continuous monitors and blood sugar lowering drugs are happening very quickly to improve your blood sugar control and quality of life.

Another helpful aid in many communities is a support group. Here you'll meet other pumpers, their families and friends, local health care providers, researchers and sales reps from companies that provide pumps and associated products. This supportive community allows everyone an opportunity to catch up on the latest news in diabetes drugs, devices and treatments. People share advice and information, help each other accept diabetes and deal with it more effectively, and understand its rewards and difficulties.

If no pump support group exists near you, start one. You need no agenda, just the desire to know and share your experience with other people wearing insulin pumps to control diabetes.

We hope the information in this book helps you move toward your goal. We learned a great deal in writing it. Thanks for being such an engaging and hardworking audience to address. We keep you in mind as we write so that the concepts we present fit your needs and are clear and understandable. We offer our wholehearted support for your success in using your pump to improve your blood sugars and health. You've already come far, simply by engaging in this process. Our best to you on your adventure.

Counting Carbs With A Scale & Carb Percentages

Few foods, other than table sugar and lollipops, are totally carbohydrate. The carb percentages on the following pages give the amount of carbohydrate in 1 gram of that food. To find out how much carbohydrate you are eating in a particular food, do a simple calculation:

1. Weigh the food you want to eat on a gram scale to get its total weight, or check the label to find its weight in grams.

2. Find your food and its carb percentage in the tables that follow.

3. On a calculator, multiply the food's weight in grams by its carb percentage.

4. Your answer gives the number of grams of carb you are eating.

Example: Let's say you place a small apple on a gram scale and find that it weighs 100 grams. You look up its carb percentage and find that it is 0.13. You then multiply 100 grams by 0.13 to get the carbohydrate you will be eating:

100 grams of apple X .13 = 13 grams of carbohydrate

Additional Information

Carb percentages give the actual concentration of carbohydrate in foods. For instance, apples are 13% carbohydrate (most of their weight is water); raisins are 77% carbohydrate by weight, and bagels contain 56% carbohydrate by weight. Both apple juice and regular sodas are 12% carbohydrate, although the carbohydrate in apple juice is higher in fructose, while a regular soda has more of its carbohydrate as sucrose or sugar.

Cranberry juice is even richer in carbohydrate at 16%, while grapefruit juice contains only 9% by weight. A 6-oz. glass of cranberry juice will therefore contain almost twice as much carbohydrate as an identical glass of grapefruit juice. Because it contains more carbohydrate, the glass of cranberry juice can raise the blood sugar nearly twice as far as the same amount of grapefruit juice. It will also require almost twice as much insulin to cover it.

Carb Percentages For Various Foods Cont.

Juices

apple cider	.14	frozen	.09	orange-apricot	.13
apple juice	.12	grapefruit-orange: canned	.10	papaya	.12
apricot	.12	frozen	.11	pineapple: canned	.14
apricot nectar	.15	lemon	.08	frozen	.13
cranberry	.16	lemonade, frozen	.11	prune	.19
grape: bottled	.16	orange: fresh	.11	tomato	.04
grape: frozen	.13	canned, unsweet	.10	V-8	.04
grapefruit: fresh	.09	canned, sweet	.12		
canned	.07	frozen	.11		

Dressings, Sauces, Condiments

bacon bits	.19	olives	.04	soy sauce	.10
BBQ sauce	.13	pickles, sweet	.36	spaghettie sauce	.09
catsup	.25	salad dressings: blue cheese	.07	steak sauce	.09
cheese sauce	.06	ceasar	.04	sweet & sour sauce	.45
chili sauce	.24	diet	.22	tartar sauce	.04
hollandaise sauce	.08	French	.17	tomato paste	.19
horseradish	.10	Italian	.07	Worcestershire sauce	.18
mayonnaise	.02	Russian	.07		
mustard	.04	pickle relish, sweet	.34		

Fruit

apple	.13	dried	.62	pears: fresh	.15
apple sauce	.10	fruit cocktail, in water	.10	canned in water	.09
apricots: fresh	.13	grapes: concord	.14	persimmons: Japanese	.20
canned in water	.10	european	.17	native	.34
canned in juice	.14	green, seedless	.14	pineapple: fresh	.14
dried	.60	grapefruit	.10	canned in water	.10
banana	.20	kiwi	.15	canned in juice	.15
blackberries	.12	lemons	.09	plums: fresh	.13
blueberries	.14	limes	.10	canned in water	.12
cantalope	.08	mangoes	.17	prunes: dehydrated	.91
cherries: fresh, sweet red	.16	nectarines	.17	dried, cooked	.67
fresh, sour red	.14	oranges	.12	raisins	.77
canned in water	.11	papayas	.10	rasberries, fresh	.14
maraschino	.29	peaches: fresh	.10	strawberries, fresh	.08
cranberry sauce, sugar	.36	canned in water	.08	tangerines	.12
dates, dried and pitted	.74	canned in juice	.12	watermelon	.06

Carb Percentages For Various Foods Cont.

Vegetables

artichoke	.10	cooked	.07	potatoes: baked	.21
asparagus	.04	cauliflower: raw	.05	boiled	.15
avocado	.05	cooked	.04	hash browns	.29
bamboo shoots	.05	celery	.04	French Fries	.34
beans: raw green	.07	chard, raw	.05	chips	.50
cooked green	.05	coleslaw	.12	sweet	.24
beans: kidney, lima, pinto,		corn: canned	.06	pumpkin	.08
red, white, baked	.21	steamed, off cob	.19	radishes	.04
beans sprouts	.06	sweet, creamed	.20	sauerkraut	.04
beets, boiled	.07	cucumber	.03	spinach: raw	.04
beet greens, cooked	.03	eggplant, cooked	.04	cooked	.08
broccoli	.06	lettuce	.03	soybeans	.11
brussel sprouts, cooked	.11	mushrooms	.04	squash: summer, cooked	.03
cabbage: raw	.05	okra	.05	winter, baked	.15
cooked	.04	onions	.07	winter, boiled	.09
Chinese, raw	.03	parsnips	.18	tomatoes	.05
Chinse, cooked	.01	peas	.12	turnips	.05
carrots: raw	.10	peppers	.05		

Cold Cereals, Dry

All Bran™	.78
Cheerios™	.70
Corn Chex™	.89
Corn Flakes™	.84
Frosted Flakes™	.90
Fruit and Fiber™	.78
granola	.68
Grapenuts™	.83
NutriGrain™	.86
Product 19™	.77
Puffed Wheat™	.77
Raisin Bran™	.75
Shredded Wheat™	.81
Special K™	.76
Rice Chex™	.86
Rice Krispies™	.88
Total™	.79
Wheaties™	.80

Combination Dishes

beef stew	.06
burrito	.24
chicken pie	.17
chili: with beans	.11
no beans	.06
con carne	.09
coleslaw	.14
enchilada	.18
fish and chips	.18
fish sticks	.37
hot dog	.18
lasagna	.16
macaroni and cheese	.20
pizza	.28
potato salad	.13
spaghetti with meat sauce	.15
tossed salad	.05
tuna casserole	.13

Sandwiches

BLT	.19
chicken salad	.24
club	.13
egg salad	.22
hot dog with bun	.26
peanut butter and jelly	.50
tuna salad	.24

Soups

clam chowder	.07
cream of mushroom	.04
tomato	.09
vegetable beef	.04
bean w/ pork	.09
chicken noodle	.07
chicken w/ rice	.07

Carb Percentages For Various Foods Cont.

Desserts and Sweets

apple butter	.46	lollipops	.99	ice cream: plain	.21
banana bread	.47	peanut brittle	.73	cone	.30
brownie	.71	gum drops	.99	bar	.25
brownie with nuts	.50	chocolate syrup	.65	ice milk	.23
cakes: angel food	.60	cookies: animal	.80	jams	.70
chocolate	.55	chocolate chip	.73	jellies	.70
coffee	.52	fig bar	.71	pies: apple	.37
fruit	.57	gingersnap	.80	blueberry	.34
pound	.61	oatmeal & raisin	.72	cherry	.38
sponge	.55	vanilla wafers	.74	lemon meringue	.47
white	.63	danish pastries	.46	pecan	.57
candies: caramel	.76	doughnuts: cake	.52	pumpkin	.23
fudge with nuts	.69	jelly filled	.46	preserves	.70
hard	.96	fruit turnovers	.26	pudding, chocolate	.23
jelly beans	.93	honey	.76	sherbert	.32

Breads and Grains

bagel	.56	couscous	.33	brown	.23
barley, cooked	.28	English muffin	.51	white	.25
biscuits	.45	French toast	.26	rolls	.60
bread: italian	.50	lentils	.19	spaghetti: plain	.26
rye	.47	macaroni: plain	.23	with sauce	.15
wheat	.47	cheese	.20	toast	.70
white	.49	muffins	.45	tortillas: corn	.42
bread crumbs	.74	noodles	.25	flour	.58
bread sticks	.75	pancakes & waffles: dry mix	.70	wheat flour	.76
buns	.50	prepared	.44		
corn starch	.83	rice, cooked	.24		

Alcoholic Beverages | ### Beverages | ### Hot Cereals, Cooked

beer: regular	.04	carbonated soda	.12	corn grits	.11
light	.02	chocolate milk	.11	Cream of Wheat™	.14
champagne	.01	eggnog	.08	Farina™	.11
liqueurs	.30	flavored instant coffee	.06	oatmeal	.10
wine: dry	.04	milk	.04	Roman Meal™	.14
sweet	.12	punch	.11	Wheatena™	.12

Carb Percentages For Various Foods Cont.

Snack Foods

almonds	.19	saltines	.70	popcorn, popped, no butter	.78
cashews	.26	marshmallows	.78	with butter	.57
cola	.10	mixed nuts	.18	potato chips	.50
corn chips	.57	onion dip	.10	pretzels	.75
cheese	.58	peanut butter	.17	sunflower seeds, no shell	.19
crackers: graham	.73	peanuts	.20	walnuts	.15
round	.67	pecans	.20		
rye	.50	pistachios	.27		

Dairy

cheese: cottage	.03	ice cream: choc	.28		
ricotta	.05	vanilla	.22		
cheddar	.01	milk	.05		
		yogurt	.08		

References

[1] M.R. Graff, R.R. Rubin, and E.A. Walker: How diabetes specialists treat their own diabetes: findings from a study of the AADE and ADA membership. *Diabetes Educ* 26(3): 460-467, 2000.

[2] Pickup JC, White MC, Keen H, Parsons JA, and Alberti KG: Long-term continuous subcutaneous insulin infusion in diabetics at home. *Lancet* 2, 8148: 870-873, 1979.

[3] J, Weissberg-Benchell, J. Antisdel-Lomaglio, and R.W. Seshadri: Insulin pump therapy: a meta-analysis. *Diabetes Care* 26(4):1079-87, 2003

[4] D. Fedele et. al.: Influence of continuous insulin infusion (CSII) treatment on diabetic somatic and autonomic neuropathy. *J Endocrinol Invest* 7: 623-628, 1984.

[5] A.J. Boulton, J. Drury, B. Clarke, and J.D. Ward: Continuous subcutaneous insulin infusion in the management of painful diabetic neuropathy. *Diabetes Care* 5: 386-390, 1982.

[6] G. Viberti: Correction of exercise-induced microalbuminuria in insulin-dependent diabetics after 3 weeks of subcutaneous insulin infusion. *Diabetes* 30: 818-823, 1981.

[7] K. Dahl-Jorgensen et al.: Effect of near normoglycemia for two years on progression of early diabetic retinopathy, nephropathy, and neuropathy: the Oslo study. *BMJ* 293: 1195-1201, 1986.

[8] T. Olsen et. al.: Diabetic retinopathy after 3 years' treatment with continuous subcutaneous insulin infusion. *Acta Ophthalmol* (Copenh) 65: 185-189, 1987.

[9] H.L. Eichner et. al.: Reduction of severe hypoglycemic events in Type I (insulin dependent) diabetic patients using continuous subcutaneous insulin infusion. *Diabetes Research* 8: 189-193, 1988.

[10] E. Chantelau, M. Spraul, I. Muhlhauser, et. al.: Long-term safety, efficacy and side-effects of continuous subcutaneous insulin infusion treatment for Type I (insulin-dependent) diabetes mellitus: a one center experience. *Diabetologia* 32: 421-426, 1989.

[11] H. Beck-Nielsen, B. Richelsen, C. Hasling, et. al.: Improved in vivo insulin effect during continuous subcutaneous insulin infusion in patients with IDDM. *Diabetes* 33: 832-837, 1984.

[12] A.O. Marcus: Patient selection for insulin pump therapy. *Practical Diabetology* (November, 1992) 12-18.

[13] B. Guerci, L. Meyer, et al: Blood glucose control on Sunday in IDDM patients: intensified conventional therapy versus contiuous insulin infusion. *Diabetes Res Clin Pract* 40: 175-180, 1998.

[14] C. Binder et al.: Insulin pharmacokinetics. *Diabetes Care* 7: 188-199, 1984.

[15] I.B. Hirsch, B.W. Bode, S. Garg et.al: Continuous subcutaneous insulin infusion (CSII) of insulin aspart versus multiple daily injection of insulin aspart/insulin glargine in type 1 diabetic patients previously treated with CSII. *Diabetes Care* 28(3): 533-538, 2005.

[16] T. Lauritzen et al.: Pharmacokinetics of continuous subcutaneous insulin infusion. *Diabetologia* 24: 326-329, 1983.

[17] The Diabetes Control and Complications Trial Research Group: The effect of intensive treatment of diabetes on the development and progression of long-term complications in insulin-dependent diabetes mellitus. *N Engl J Med* 329: 977-986, 1993.

[18] N. Weintrob, A. Schechter, et. al.: Glycemic patterns detected by continuous subcutaneous glucose sensing in children and adolescents with type 1 diabetes mellitus treated by multiple daily injections vs continuous subcutaneous insulin infusion. *Arch Pediatr Adolesc Med.* 158: 677-684, 2004.

[19] S.M. Willi, J. Planton, L. Egede, S. Schwarz: Benefits of continuous subcutaneous insulin infusion in children with type 1 diabetes. *J Pediatr* 143: 796-801, 2003.

[20] R. Linkeschova, M. Raoul, U. Bott, M. Berger, M. Spraul: Less severe hypoglycaemia, better metabolic control, and improved quality of life in Type 1 diabetes mellitus with continuous subcutaneous insulin infusion (CSII) therapy; an observational study of 100 consecutive patients followed for a mean of 2 years. *Diabet Med* 19: 746-751, 2002.

[21] H. Hanaire-Broutin, V. Melki, S. Bessieres-Lacombe, J.P. Tauber: Comparison of continuous subcutaneous insulin infusion and multiple daily injection regimens using insulin lispro in type 1 diabetic patients on intensified treatment: a randomized study. The Study Group for the Development of Pump Therapy in Diabetes. *Diabetes Care* 23: 1232-1235, 2000.

[22] N. Sulli and B. Shashaj: Continuous subcutaneous insulin infusion in children and adolescents with diabetes mellitus: decreased HbA1c with low risk of hypoglycemia. B. *J Ped Endocrinol Metab* 16: 393-399, 2003.

[23] Bode BW, Steed RD, and Davidson PC: Reduction in severe hypoglycemia with long-term continuous subcutaneous insulin infusion in type 1 diabetes. *Diabetes Care* 19: 324-327, 1996.

[24] I.B. Hirsch, R. Farkas-Hirsch and P.D. Cryer: Continuous subcutaneous insulin infusion for the treatment of diabetic patients with hypoglycemic unawareness. *Diabetes Nutr Metab* 4: 1-3, 1991.

[25] R. Farkas-Hirsch and I.B. Hirsch: Continuous subcutaneous insulin infusion (CSII): A review of the past and its implementation for the future. March/April, 1994 issue of *Diabetes Spectrum*.

[26] C.G. Fanelli, L. Epifano, A.M. Rambotti, S. Pampanelli, A. DiVincenzo, F. Modarelli et. al.: Meticulous prevention of hypoglycemia normalizes the glycemic thresholds and magnitude of most of neuroendocrine responses to, symptoms of, and cognitive function during hypoglycemia in intensively treated patients with short-term IDDM. *Diabetes* 42: 1683-1689, 1993.

[27] M.J. Castillo, A.J. Scheen, and P.J. Lefebvre: The degree/rapidity of the metabolic deterioration following interruption of a continuous subcutaneous insulin infusion is influenced by the prevailing blood glucose level. *J Clin Endocrinol Metab.* 81(5): 1975-1978, 1996.

[28] R.S. Mecklenburg et al.: Acute complications associated with insulin infusion pump therapy. *JAMA* 252: 3265- 3269, 1984.

[29] J.J. Bending et al.: Complications of insulin infusion pump therapy. *JAMA* 253: 2644, 1985.

[30] R. Renner: Therapy of Type 1 diabetes with insulin pumps; *Diamet*, June, 1991.

[31] The DCCT Research Group: The effect of intensive treatment of diabetes on the development and progression of long-term complications in insulin-dependent diabetes mellitus. *NEJM* 329: 977-986, 1993.

[32] D. M. Nathan, P. A. Cleary, B. Zinman, S. M. Genuth, J.M. Lachin, J.C. Backlund and the DCCT/EDIC Research Group: Effect of Intensive Diabetes Management on Cardiovascular Events in the DCCT/EDIC (Diabetes Control and Complications/Trial Epidemiology of Diabetes Interventions and Complications) presented at the American Diabetes Association 65th annual scientific sessions, June, 2005.

[33] UK Prospective Diabetes Study Group: Association of glycaemia with macrovascular and microvascular complications of type 2 diabetes (UKPDS 35) *BMJ* 321: 405-412, 2000

[34] M. Shichiri, H. Kishikawa, Y. Ohkubo, N. Wake: Long-Term Results of the Kumamoto Study on Optimal Diabetes Control in Type 2 Diabetic Patients, *Diabetes Care* 23(2): , 2000

[35] UK Prospective Diabetes Study Group (UKPDS): Complications in newly diagnosed type 2 diabetic patients and their association with different clinical and biochemical risk factors. Diabetes Research. Tivot-Kimpton Publications. 1998.

[36] D.M. Nathan, P.A. Cleary, M.S. Jye-Yu, M.S. Backlund, S.M. Genuth, J.M. Lachin, T.J. Orchard, P. Raskin, and B. Zinman: Intensive diabetes treatment and cardiovascular disease in patients with type 1 diabetes. *N Engl J Med.* 353 (25): 2643-2653, 2005.

[37] LP Aiello, SE Bursell, A Clermont, E Duh, and GL King: Vascular endothelial growth factor-induced retinal permeability is mediated by protein kinase C in vivo and suppressed by an orally effective beta-isoform-selective inhibitor. *Diabetes* 46: 1473-80, 1997.

[38] SE Bursell, C Takagi, et al.: Specific retinal diacylglycerol and protein kinase C beta isoform modulation mimics abnormal retinal hemodynamics in diabetic rats. *Invest Ophthalmol Vis Sci* 38: 2711-20, 1997.

[39] M Kunisaki, SE Bursell, F Umeda, H Nawata, and GL King: Prevention of diabetes-induced abnormal retinal blood flow by treatment with d-alpha-tocopherol. *Biofactors* 7: 55-67, 1998.

[39a] A. Himmelmann, J Jendleet. al.: The Impact of Smoking on Inhaled Insulin *Diabetes Care* 26: 677-682, 2003

[40] M Lu, M Kuroki, S Amano, et al.: Advanced glycation end products increase retinal vascular endothelial growth factor expression. *J Clin Invest* 15: 1219-24, 1998.

[41] E. Van Ballegooie, J.M. Hooymans, Z. Timmerman, et. al.: Rapid deterioration of diabetic retinopathy during treatment with continuous subcutaneous insulin infusion. *Diabetes Care* 7:236-242, 1984.

[42] D. Dahl-Jorgensen, O. Brinchmann-Hansen, K.F. Hansen, et. al.: Transient deterioration of retinopathy when multiple insulin injection therapy and CSII is started in IDDM patients. *Diabetes* 33(1): 4A, 1984.

[43] M. Kotoula, G. Koukoulis, E. Zintzaras, C. Karabatsas, and D. Chatzoulis: Metabolic control of diabetes is associated with an improved response of diabetic retinopathy to panretinal photocoagulation. *Diabetes Care* 28: 2454-2457, 2005.

[44] J.C. Javitt, L.P. Aiello, Y. et al: Preventive Eye Care in People with Diabetes Is Cost-Saving to the Federal Government: Implications for Health Care Reform. *Diabetes Care* 17(8): 909-917, 1994.

[45] J.C. Javitt, L.P. Aiello, Y. et al: Detecting and Treating Retinopathy in Patients with Type I Diabetes Mellitus: Savings Associated with Improved Implementation of Current Guidelines. *Ophthalmology* 98(10): 1565-1573, 1991.

[46] M. Brownlee: Banting Lecture 2004: The Pathobiology of Diabetic Complications, A Unifying Mechanism *Diabetes* 54: 1615-1625, 2005.

[47] Y.I. Lin, L. Seroude, S. Benzer: Extended life-span and stress resistance in the Drosophilia mutant methuselah. *Science* 282: 943-946, 1998.

[48] R. Derr, E. Garrett, G.A. Stacy, C.D. Saudek: Is HbA(1c) affected by glycemic instability? *Diabetes Care* 26: 2728-2733, 2003.

[49] ACE Consensus Development Conference on Guidelines for Glycemic Control. *Endocr Pract. Suppl.*, Nov/Dec 2001.

[50] American Diabetes Association: Standards of Medical Care In Diabetes. *Diabetes Care* 28 (Suppl 1): S11, 2005.

[51] A.Risso, F. Mercuri, L. Quagliaro, G. Damante, A. Ceriello: Intermittent high glucose enhances apoptosis in human umbilical vein endothelial cells in culture. *Am J Physiol Endocrinol Metab.* 281(5): E924-30, 2001.

[52] L. Quagliaro, L. Piconi, R. Assaloni, L. Martinelli, E. Motz, A. Ceriello: Intermittent high glucose enhances apoptosis related to oxidative stress in human umbilical vein endothelial cells: the role of protein kinase C and NAD(P)H-oxidase activation. *Diabetes* 52: 2795-2804, 2003.

[53] J. Beyer et. al.: Assessment of insulin needs in insulin-dependent diabetics and healthy volunteers under fasting conditions. *Horm Metab Res Suppl* 24: 71-77, 1990.

[54] R.S. Beaser, R.S. Clements et al: Upgrading Diabetes Therapy: What Every Primary Physician Needs To Know. *Novo Diabetes Care*, pg. 5, 1994.

[55] W. Bruns et. al.: Nocturnal continuous subcutaneous insulin infusion: a therapeutic possibility in labile Type I diabetes under exceptional conditions. Z. *Gesamte Inn Med* 45: 154-158, 1990.

[56] K. Haakens et. al.: Early morning glycaemia and the metabolic consequences of delaying breakfast/morning insulin. A comparison of continuous subcutaneous insulin infusion and multiple injection therapy with human isophane or human Ultralente at bedtime. *Scand J Clin Lab Invest* 49: 653-659, 1989.

[57] G. Perriello, P. De Feo, E. Torlone, et. al.: The Dawn Phenomenon in Type I (insulin-dependent) diabetes mellitus; magnitude, frequency, variability, and dependency on glucose counterregulation and insulin sensitivity. *Diabetologia* 42: 21-28, 1991.

[58] P. Hildebrandt, K. Birch, B.M. Jensen, and C. Kuhl: Subcutaneous insulin infusion: Change in basal infusion rate has no immediate effect on insulin absorption rate. *Diabetes Care* 9: 561-564, 1986.

[59] J. Pickup, M. Mattock, and S. Kerry: Glycaemic control with continuous subcutaneous insulin infusion compared with intensive insulin injections in patients with type 1 diabetes: meta-analysis of randomised controlled trials. *BMJ* 324(705): 1-6, 2002

[60] J.L. Colquitt, C. Green, M.K. Sidhu, D. Hartwell, and N. Waugh: Clinical and cost-effectiveness of continuous subcutaneous insulin infusion for diabetes. *Health Technol Assess.* 8(43): 1-186, 2004.

[61] L. Heinemann, C. Weyer, M. Rauhaus, S. Heinrichs, and T. Heise: Variability of the metabolic effect of soluble insulin and the rapid-acting insulin analog insulin aspart. *Diabetes Care* 11: 1910-1914, 1998.

[62] B.A. Buckingham, J. Block, D. Wilson, K. Rebrin, G. Steiln: Novolog Pharmacodynamics in Toddlers. *Diabetes* 54 (Suppl 1): Abstract 1889-P, 2005.

[63] NovoLog® Physician Insert – Approved October 21, 2005

[64] J. Walsh, R. Roberts: **Pumping Insulin**, The Art Of Using An Insulin Pump, 1st ed., pages 70-73, 1989.

[65] A. Schiffrin and M. Belmonte: Multiple daily self-glucose monitoring: its essential role in long-term glucose control in insulin-dependent diabetic patients treated with pump and multiple subcutaneous injections. *Diabetes Care* 5: 479-484, 1982.

[66] N. Perrotti, D. Santoro, S. Genovese, et. al.: Effect of digestible carbohydrates on glucose control in insulin-dependent diabetic patients. *Diabetes Care* 7: 354-359, 1984.

[67] G. Boden and F. Jadali: Effects of lipid on basal carbohydrate metabolism in normal men. *Diabetes* 40: 686-692, 1991.

[68] F.Q. Nuttall, A.D. Mooradian, M.C. Gannon et al.: Effect of protein ingestion on the glucose and insulin response to a standardized oral glucose load. *Diabetes Care* 7: 465-470, 1984.

[69] D.J.A. Jenkins, T.M.S. Wolever and A.L. Jenkins: Starchy foods and glycemic index. *Diabetes Care* 11: 149-59, 1988.

[70] D.J.A. Jenkins, T.M.S. Wolever, et al.: Glycemic index of foods: a physiologic basis for carbohydrate exchange. *Amer J Clin Nutr* 34: 362-66, 1981.

[71] T.M.S. Wolever, L Katzman-Relle et al.: Glycemic index of 102 complex carbohydrate foods in patients with diabetes. *Nutr Res* 14: 651-69, 1994.

[72] Self reported data from pumpers at http://www.insulin-pumpers.org/about.shtml

[73] The earliest version of a "450 Rule" was developed by us for Regular insulin in 1992 in the *Insulin Pump Therapy Handbook*. This was also published in an insulin dose table on page 50 of the 1994 edition of **Pumping Insulin** and modified to a 500 Rule for rapid insulin in the 2000 edition of **Pumping Insulin.**

[74] E Bonora: Postprandial peaks as a risk factor for cardiovascular disease: epidemiological perspectives. *Int J Clin Pract* Suppl 129: 5-11, 2002.

[75] The original 1500 Rule was developed in 1988 for Regular insulin by Paul Davidson, M.D., in Atlanta, Georgia, and later modified by him to a 1716 Rule in 2003. We prefer a 2000 Rule for additional safety with rapid insulin when the basal is 50% of the TDD (or 1800 when the basal is 40% or 2200 when it is 60% of the TDD).

[76] B.W. Bode, et al: Continuous glucose monitoring facilitates sustainable improvements in glycemic control. *Diabetes* 49 (suppl. 1): 393, 2000.

[77] Bode et al, *Diabetes* 46: 143, 1997

[78] D. Cox, L. Gonder-Frederick, W. Polonsky, D. Schlundt, B. Kovatchev and W. Clark: Recent hypoglycemia influences the probability of subsequent hypoglycemia in Type I patients. *Diabetes* Abstract 399, ADA Conference 1993.

[79] E.W. ter Braak, et. al.: Clinical characteristics of type 1 patients with and without severe hypoglycemia. *Diabetes Care* 23(10): 1467-1471, 2000.

[80] H.M. Ramsli, S.P. Therkelsen, O. Sovik, and H. Thordarson: Unexpected and unexplained deaths among young patients with diabetes mellitus. *Tidsskr Nor Laegeforen* 124 (23): 3064-3065, 2004.

[81] O. Sovik and H. Thordarson: Death-in-bed syndrome in young diabetic patients. *Diabetes Care* 22 (Suppl 2): B40-42, 1999.

[82] S.N. Davis, S. Fowler, and F. Costa: Hypoglycemic Counterregulatory responses differ between men and women with Type 1 diabetes. *Diabetes* 49: 65-72, 2000.

[83] A. Avogaro, P. Beltramello, L. Gnudi, A. Maran, A. Valerio, M. Miola, N. Marin, C. Crepaldi, L. Confortin, F. Costa, I. MacDonald and A. Tiengo: Alcohol intake impairs glucose counterregulation during acute insulin-induced hypoglycemia in IDDM patients. *Diabetes* 42: 1626-1634, 1993.

[84] V. Bhatia and J.I. Wolfsdorf: Severe hypoglycemia in youth with insulin-dependent diabetes mellitus: frequency and causative factors. *Pediatrics* 88(6): 1187-1193, 1991.

[85] J. Anderson, S. Symanowski, and R. Brunelle: Safety of [Lys(B28), Pro(B29)] human insulin analog in long-term clinical trials. *Diabetes* 43(1): abstract 192, 1994.

[86] T. Veneman, A. Mitrakou, M. Mokan, P. Cryer and J. Gerich: Induction of hypoglycemia unawareness by asymptomatic nocturnal hypoglycemia. *Diabetes* 42: 1233-1237, 1993.

[87] C.G. Fanelli, L. Epifano, et al: Meticulous prevention of hypoglycemia normalizes the glycemic thresholds and magnitude of most of neuroendocrine responses to, symptoms of, and cognitive function during hypoglycemia in intensively treated patients with short-term IDDM. *Diabetes* 42: 1683-1688, 1993.

[88] D.D. Fredrickson, D.W. Guthrie, J.K. Nehrling, R. Guthrie: Effects of DKA and severe hypoglycemia in cognitive functioning: a prospective study. *Diabetes* 44 (suppl 1): abstract 97, 1995.

[89] M.H. Tanner et. al.: Toxic shock syndrome from staphylococcus areus infection at insulin pump infusion sites. *JAMA* 259: 394-395, 1988.

[90] A. Pietri and P. Raskin: Cutaneous complications of chronic continuous subcutaneous insulin infusion therapy. *Diabetes Care* 4: 624-627, 1981.

[91] K. E. Powell et al.: Physical activity and chronic disease. *Am J Clin Nutr* 49: 999-1006, 1989.

[92] M. Tanasescu et. al.: Physical activity in relation to cardiovascular disease and total mortality among men with Type 2 diabetes. *Circulation* 107(19): 2392-2394, 2003.

[93] G. Zoppini, M. Carlini, M. Muggeo: Self-reported exercise and quality of life in young type 1 diabetic subjects. *Diabetes Nutr Metab* 16(1): 77-80, 2003.

[94] A. Festa, C.H. Schnack, A.D. Assie, P. Haber and G. Schernthaner: Abnormal pulmonary function in Type I diabetes is related to metabolic long-term control, but not to urinary albumin excretion rate. *Diabetes* 43 (1): abstract 610, 1994.

[95] J. Wahren: Glucose turnover during exercise in healthy man and in patients with Diabetes Mellitus. *Diabetes* 28(1): 82-88, 1979.

[96] P. Felig and J. Wahren: Role of insulin and glucagon in the regulation of hepatic glucose production during exercise. *Diabetes* 28(1): 71-75, 1979.

[97] B.A. Perkins and M.C. Riddell: Diabetes and exercise: Using the insulin pump to maximum advantage. *Canadian J of Diabetes* 30(1): 72-79, 2006.

[98] E.B. Marliss and M. Vranic: Intense exercise has unique effects on both insulin release and its role in glucoregulation: implications for diabetes. *Diabetes* 51 (Suppl 1): S271-283, 2002.

[99] The PedPump Study: A Low Percentage of Basal Insulin and More Than Five Daily Boluses are Associated With Better Centralized A1C in 1041 Children on CSII in 17 Countries, *Diabetes* Abstract #1887-P, 2005.

[100] U.K Prospective Diabetes Study 16: Overview of 6 years of therapy of Type II diabetes – a progressive disease. *Diabetes* 44: 1249-1258, 1995.

[101] S. Fourlanos, C. Perry, et. al.: A clinical screening tool identifies autoimmune diabetes in adults. *Diabetes Care* 29: 970-975, 2006.

[102] P. Raskin, B.W. Bode, J.B. Marck, et al: Continuous subcutaneous insulin infusion and multiple daily injection therapy are equally effective in type 2 diabetes: a randomized, parallel-group, 24-week study. *Diabetes Car.* 26: 2598 -2603, 2003.

[103] Valensi P, Moura I, Le Magoarou M, Paries J, Perret G, Attali JR: Short-term effects of continuous subcutaneous insulin infusion treatment on insulin secretion in non-insulin-dependent overweight patients with poor glycaemic control despite maximal oral anti-diabetic treatment. *Diabetes Metab* 23: 51-57, 1997.

[104] Ilkova H, Glaser B, Tunckale A, Bagriacik N, and Cerasi E: Induction of long-term glycemic control in newly diagnosed type 2 diabetic patients by transient intensive insulin treatment. *Diabetes Care* 20: 1353-1356, 1997.

[105] Y. Ohkubo, H. Kishikawa, E. Araki, et al.: Intensive insulin therapy prevents the progression of diabetic microvascular complications in Japanese patients with non-insulin-dependent diabetes mellitus: a randomized prospective 6-year study. *Diabetes Res Clin Pract* 28: 103-117, 1995.

[106] A. Georgopoulos, S. Margolis, P. Bachorik, and P.O. Kwiterovich: Effect of improved glycemic control on the response of plasma triglycerides to ingestion of a saturated fat load in normotriglyceridemic and hypertriglyceridemic diabetic subjects. *Metabolism* 37: 866-871, 1988.

[107] G.B. Bolli, J.E. Gerich: The "dawn phenomenon"--a common occurrence in both non-insulin-dependent and insulin-dependent diabetes mellitus. *N Engl J Med* 310(12): 746-750, 1984.

[108] P. White: Pregnancy complicating diabetes. *Am J Med* 7: 609-616, 1949.

[109] J. Pedersen: Fetal mortality in diabetics in relation to management during the latter part of pregnancy. *Acta Endocrinol* 15: 282-294, 1954

[110] J. Pedersen and E. Brandstrup: Fetal mortality in pregnant diabetics: strict control of diabetes with conservative obstetric management. *Lancet* I: 607a-612, 1956.

[111] J. Pedersen, L. Molsted-Pedersen and B. Andersen: Assessors of fetal perinatal mortality in diabetic pregnancy. *Diabetes* 23: 302-305, 1974.

[112] K. Fuhrmann, H. Reiher, K. Semmler, F. Fischer, M. Fisher and E. Glockner: Prevention of congenital malformations in infants of insulin-dependent diabetic mothers. *Diabetes Care* 6: 219-223, 1983.

[113] J.L. Kitzmiller, L.A. Gavin, G.D. Gin, L. Jovanovic-Peterson, E.K. Main and W.D. Zigrang: Preconception care of diabetes: Glycemic control prevents congenital anomalies. *JAMA* 265: 731-736, 1991.

[114] B. Rosenn, M. Miodovnik, C.A. Combs, J. Khoury and T.A. Siddiqi: Preconception management of insulin-dependent diabetes: Improvement of pregnancy outcome. *Obstet Gynecol* 77: 846-849, 1991.

[115] J.M. Steel, F.D. Johnstone, D.A. Hepburn and A. Smith: Can prepregnancy care of diabetic women reduce the risk of abnormal babies? *Br Med J* 301: 1070-1074, 1990.

[116] M. Miodovnik, C. Skillman, J.C. Holroyde, J.B. Butler, J.S. Wendel and T. A. Siddiqi: Elevated maternal glycohemoglobin in early pregnancy and spontaneous abortion among insulin-dependent diabetic women. *Am J Obstet Gynecol* 153: 439-442.

[117] J.L. Mills, J.L. Simpson, S.G. Driscoll, L. Jovanovic-Peterson, M. Van Allen, J.H. Aarons, B. Metzger, et.al.: The National Institute of Child Health and Human Development: Diabetes in Early Pregnancy Study: Incidence of spontaneous abortion among normal women and insulin-dependent diabetic women whose pregnancies were identified within 21 days of conception. *NEJM* 319: 1617-1623, 1988.

[118] L. Jovanovic-Peterson, M. Druzin and C.M. Peterson: Effect of euglycemia on the outcome of pregnancy in insulin-dependent diabetic women as compared with normal control subjects. *Am J Med* 71: 921-927, 1981.

[119] C.A. Combs, B. Wheeler, E. Gunderson, L. Gavin, and J.L. Kitsmiller: Significance of microproteinuria in the first trimester of pregnancies complicated by diabetes. *Diabetes* 39: 36A, 1990.

[120] S. Bo et al: Clinical characteristics and outcome of pregnancy in women with gestational hyperglycaemia with or without antibodies to beta-cell antigens. *Diab Med* 20 (1): 64-68, 2003.

[121] I. Ostlund and U. Hanson: Occurrence of gestational diabetes mellitus and the value of different screening indicators for the oral glucose tolerance test. *Acta Obstet Gynecol Scand* 82 (2): 103-108, 2003.

[122] J.S. Sheffield, E.L. Butler-Koster, B.M. Casey, D.D. McIntire, K.J. Leveno: Maternal diabetes and infant malformations. *Obstet Gynecol* 100 (5 Pt 1): 925-930, 2002.

[123] L. Jovanovic-Peterson and C.M. Peterson: Dietary manipulation as a primary treatment strategy for pregnancies complicated by diabetes. *J Am Coll Nutr* 9: 320-325, 1990.

[124] B. Rosenn, M. Miodovnik, C.A. Combs, J. Khoury and T.A. Siddiqi: Preconception management of insulin-dependent diabetes: Improvement of pregnancy outcome. *Obstet Gynecol* 77: 846-849, 1991.

[125] L. Jovanovic, R.H. Knopp, Z. Brown, M.R. Conley, E. Park, J.L. Mills, B.E. Metzger, J.H. Aarons, L.B. Holmes, J.L. Simpson: Declining insulin requirement in the late first trimester of diabetic pregnancy. *Diabetes Care* 24(7): 1130-1136, 2001.

[126] E.A. Masson, J.E. Patmore, P.D. Brash, M. Baxter, G. Caldwell, I.W. Gallen, P.A. Price, P.A. Vice, J.D. Walker, S.W. Lindow: Pregnancy outcome in Type 1 diabetes mellitus treated with insulin lispro (Humalog). *Diabet Med* 20(1): 46-50, 2003.

[127] S.K. Garg, J.P. Frias, S. Anil, P.A. Gottlieb, T. MacKenzie, W.E Jackson: Insulin lispro therapy in pregnancies complicated by type 1 diabetes: glycemic control and maternal and fetal outcomes. *Endocr Pract* 9(3): 187-93, 2003.

[128] Bhattacharyya A, Brown S, Hughes S, Vice PA: Insulin lispro and regular insulin in pregnancy. *QJM* 94(5): 255-60, 2001.

[129] L. Jovanovic, S. Ilic, D.J. Pettitt, K. Hugo, M. Gutierrez, R.R. Bowsher, E.J. Bastyr 3rd: Metabolic and immunologic effects of insulin lispro in gestational diabetes. *Diabetes Care* 22(9): 1422-7, 1999.

[130] O. Langer, D.L. Conway, M.D. Berkus, E.M. Xenakis, O.N. Gonzales: A comparison of glyburide and insulin in women with gestational diabetes mellitus. *N Engl J Med* 343(16): 1134-1138, 2000.

[131] W.A. Bauman, S. Shaw, E. Jayatilleke, A.M. Spungen and V. Herbert: Increased intake of calcium reverses vitamin B12 malabsorption induced by metformin. *Diabetes Care* 23(9): 1227-1231, 2000.

[132] L. Jovanovic-Peterson, W. Bevier, and C.M. Peterson: The Santa Barbara County Health Care Services program: birth weight change concomitant with screening for and treatment of glucose-intolerance of pregnancy: a potential cost-effective intervention? *Amer J Perinatol* 14: 221-228, 1997.

Glossary

A1c

Glycosylated hemoglobin levels reflect blood glucose level during the previous two to three months. A1c is used to assess blood glucose control in people with diabetes. Normal A1c levels are generally 4% to 6%. Diabetes treatment typically aims for a target A1c of less than 6.5% or 7%.

Albuminuria

A condition in which high levels of a protein called albumin are found in the urine. Excess albumin in the urine is often a sign of early kidney disease.

Autoimmune antibodies

Antibodies in the blood stream of a person with an autoimmune disease. Type 1 and Type 1.5 are characterized by these.

Autoimmune disease

A disease caused by a defect in which the body's internal defense system attacks a part of the body itself. Type 1 diabetes is an autoimmune disease.

Basal/Bolus balance

Created by having the basal and bolus a balanced percentage of the Total Daily Dose (TDD), such as 50% basal/50% bolusl. Other balanced options are 60% basal/40% bolus and 40% basal/60% bolus. Assessing the basal/bolus balance is one way to troubleshoot poor control.

Basal insulin or rate

A continuous 24-hour delivery of insulin that matches background insulin need. When the basal rate is correctly set, the blood sugar does not rise or fall during periods in which the pump user is not eating. Basal rates are given as units/hour with typical rates between 0.4 u/hr and 1.6 u/hr for many pumpers.

Bolus

See Carb Bolus or High Blood Sugar Bolus.

Beta cells (b-cells)

Cells that make insulin and are found in the Islets of Langerhans within the pancreas.

Blood glucose level

The concentration of glucose in the blood (blood sugar). It is measured in milligrams per deciliter (mg/dl) in the U.S. or in millimoles (mmol) in other countries.

Body mass index (BMI)

A unit of measurement (kg/m^2) that describes weight in relation to height for people 20 to 65 years old.

C-peptide

Plasma C-peptide is a by-product of insulin production with a longer half-life than insulin. It measures how much insulin a person is able to make. A level below 0.3 is defined as type 1 diabetes.

Carbohydrate

One of the three main constituents (carbohydrates, fats, and proteins) of foods and the most important for blood sugar control. Carbohydrates (four calories per gram) are composed mainly of sugars and starches.

Carb bolus

A spurt of insulin delivered quickly to match carbohydrates in an upcoming meal or snack. Most pumpers use between 1 unit of rapid insulin for each 5 grams of carbohydrate and 1 unit for each 25 grams.

Carb counting

Counting the grams of carbohydrate in any food eaten. This is an effective way to determine the amount of insulin needed to maintain a normal blood sugar.

Carb factor

The number of grams of carbohydrate one unit of insulin covers for a person. This varies from person to person.

Catheter

The plastic tube through which insulin is delivered between the pump and the insertion set.

Classic insulin pump

An insulin pump available before late 2002 and early 2003. Does not have smart features.

Continuous monitor

A device often consisting of a sensor implanted under the skin sending blood sugar readings via radio waves to a transmitter. Often displays individual readings taken every 5 minutes, graphs of the readings over time and trend arrows. Often provides high and low blood sugar alarms.

Correction bolus

A spurt of insulin delivered quickly to bring a high blood sugar back within a person's target range for before a meal, after a meal, or a bedtime.

Correction factor

The distance a high blood sugar will drop for one unit of insulin for a person. Measured in mg/dl in the U.S. and mmol in other countries. This varies from person to person.

C-peptide

A byproduct of insulin production. Plasma C-peptide has a longer half-life than insulin and often is used to measure how much insulin a person is able to make. Generally, a level below 0.3 is defined as Type I diabetes.

CSII

Continuous subcutaneous insulin infusion, a fancy name for using an insulin pump.

DCCT

Diabetes Control and Complications Trial. The DCCT was a 9-year study of more than 1,400 people with Type I diabetes. Sponsored by the National Institute of Health, it showed that tight blood sugar control significantly reduces the risk of diabetic retinopathy, neuropathy, and nephropathy.

Dawn Phenomenon

An early morning rise in blood glucose levels, caused largely by the normal release of growth hormone that blocks insulin's effect during the early morning hours. It is more likely to raise blood sugar in Type I than Type II diabetes.

Diabetic coma

Loss of consciousness due to very high blood sugars. (See ketoacidosis)

Diabetic nephropathy

Kidney disease resulting from diabetes that usually has been poorly controlled for several years. There rarely are symptoms until very late in the disease.

Diabetic neuropathy

Damage to the nervous system most often resulting from poor control. Three different forms of neuropathy can be distinguished: peripheral neuropathy, sensory neuropathy, and autonomic neuropathy. Peripheral neuropathy affects the motor nerves, which can lead to problems with muscle movement and size. Sensory neuropathy impairs the nerves that control touch, sight, and pain perception. Autonomic neuropathy affects the nerves involved in such involuntary functions as digestion. Symptoms such as pain, loss of sensation, loss of reflexes, and/or weakness may occur.

Diabetic retinopathy

Damaged small blood vessels in the eye that can cause vision problems, including blindness.

Endogenous insulin

Insulin production within a person in the beta cells.

Fasting plasma glucose (FPG) test

The test is taken after fasting for 8 to 10 hours, typically overnight. FPG level less than 110 mg/dL is normal; one between 110 and 126 mg/dL indicates impaired glucose tolerance, and one greater than 126 mg/dL supports a provisional diagnosis of Type 2 diabetes.

Exogenous insulin

Insulin given by injection or pump; vital for Type 1 diabetes and needed by many with Type 2 diabetes.

Fat

One of the three main constituents (carbohydrate, fats, and protein) of foods. Fats occur alone as liquids or solids, such as oils and margarines, or they may be a component of other foods. Fats may be of animal or vegetable origin. They have a higher energy content than any other food (9 calories per gram).

Gestational diabetes

Elevated blood sugars usually diagnosed during the last half of pregnancy and triggered by insulin resistance. Gestational diabetes increases the risk of perinatal mortality and the development of diabetes in the mother years following the pregnancy.

Glucagon

A hormone made by the pancreas that raises blood sugar levels. It is injected during severe low blood sugars to raise the blood sugar quickly by releasing glucose stored in the liver.

Glucose

A simple sugar, also known as dextrose, that is found in the blood and is used by the body for energy.

Glycemic Index (GI)

A method to classify foods, especially carbohydrates, according to how they affect the blood glucose level.

Glycogen

Glycogen is the form in which the liver and muscles store glucose. It may be broken down to active blood glucose during a low blood sugar, fasting, or exercise.

Glycosylated hemoglobin

See A1c.

Gram

A small unit of weight in the metric system. Used in weighing food. One ounce equals 28 grams.

Hormone

A chemical substance produced by a gland or tissue and carried by the blood to other tissues or organs, where it stimulates action and causes a specific effect. Insulin and glucagon are hormones.

Hyperglycemia

A higher than normal level of glucose in the blood (high blood sugar).

Hypertension

High blood pressure (excess blood pressure in the blood vessels). Found to aggravate diabetes and diabetic complications.

Hypoglycemia

A lower than normal glucose level in the blood (low blood sugar), usually less than 60 mg/dl (3.3 mmol). Symptoms vary from confusion, nervousness, sweating, shakiness, headaches, and drowsiness to moodiness, or numbness in the arms and hands. Untreated, severe hypoglycemia can cause loss of consciousness or convulsions.

Infusion set

The hub, catheter, and insertion set used to transfer insulin from the pump through an infusion line under the skin.

Insertion set

The part of the infusion set inserted through the skin. It may be a fine metal needle or a larger metal needle, which is removed to leave a small teflon catheter under the skin.

Insulin

A hormone secreted by the beta cells of the Islets of Langerhans in the pancreas. Needed by many cells to use glucose for energy.

Insulin pump

A small, computerized, programmable device about the size of a beeper that can be programmed to deliver basal insulin and give a bolus of insulin for a meal or high blood sugar. It replaces insulin injections. A pump delivers fast-acting insulin via a plastic catheter to either a teflon infusion set or a small metal needle inserted through the skin for gradual absorption into the bloodstream. Doses as small as 0.025 unit can be delivered with accuracy.

Insulin resistance syndrome (IRS)

A basic metabolic abnormality underlying Type 2 diabetes. Insulin resistance describes reduced insulin sensitivity of cells to the action of insulin. AKA Metabolic Syndrome and Syndrome X.

Interstitial fluid

A relatively clear fluid between cells in which glucose measurements can be made without drawing blood by puncturing a blood vessel.

Islets of Langerhans

Special groups of pancreatic cells that produce insulin and glucagon.

Ketoacidosis

A very serious condition in which the body does not have enough insulin. An excess release of free fatty acids causes high levels of ketones in the blood and urine. This acidic state takes hours or days to develop, with symptoms of abdominal pain, nausea, and vomiting. It also causes dehydration, electrolyte imbalance, rapid breathing, coma, and possibly death.

Ketones

Acidic byproducts of fat metabolism.

Nephropathy

See Diabetic nephropathy

Neuropathy

See Diabetic neuropathy

Oral glucose tolerance test (OGTT)

A 2 or 3-hour test of plasma glucose with values over 200 mg/dL (> 11.1 mmol/L) used to confirm a suspected diagnosis of diabetes.

Pancreas

A gland positioned near the stomach that secretes insulin, glucagon, and many digestive enzymes.

Protein

One of the three main constituents (carbohydrate, fat, and protein) of foods. Proteins are made up of amino acids and are found in foods such as milk, meat, fish, and eggs. Proteins are essential constituents of all living cells and form important structures and enzymes. Proteins (four calories per gram) are burned at a slower rate than fats or carbohydrates.

Proteinuria

Protein in the urine. This may be a sign of kidney damage.

Reservoir/Syringe/Cartridge

A container which holds the fast-acting insulin inside a pump.

Retina

A very thin light-sensitive layer of nerves and blood vessels at the back of the inner surface of the eyeball.

Smart insulin pump

An insulin pump with smart features. Became available in late 2002.

Total Daily Dose (TDD)

The amount of insulin a person uses in a day. Calculations are made using the TDD to determine the basal rate, carb factor and correction factor.

Type 1 diabetes

In Type 1 diabetes the pancreas makes little or no insulin because the insulin-producing beta cells have been destroyed. It is an autoimmune disease caused by a defect in which the body's internal defense system attacks a part of the body itself. This type of diabetes usually appears suddenly and most commonly in people younger than 30. Treatment consists of daily insulin injections or use of an insulin pump, a planned diet, regular exercise, and daily self-monitoring of blood glucose through finger sticks or continuous monitoring.

Type 1.5 diabetes

Also called LADA. A slower form of Type 1 diabetes in adults in which only one or two types of autoimmune antibodies is present.

Type 2 diabetes

Type 2 diabetes is associated with insulin resistance and impaired beta cell function. It sometimes is controlled by diet, exercise, and daily monitoring of glucose levels, but at other times oral antihyperglycemic agents or insulin injections are needed. Type 2 diabetes accounts for 90% to 95% of diabetes cases.

School Care Plan For An Insulin Pump

Re: _____   Date: _____/_____/_____

To Whom It May Concern:

_____ is a patient in our Center with Type 1 Diabetes Mellitus (Insulin Dependent Diabetes Mellitus). To better control his/her diabetes, he/she is using insulin pump therapy.

An insulin pump is simply another way to deliver insulin. Through the pump, _____ _____ receives insulin around the clock via a small needle or plastic tube which is inserted in the abdomen. He/she has been taught how to program the pump to deliver insulin, as needed. This means he/she will program the pump before each meal to give insulin in a dose determined by his/her fingerstick blood glucose test.

To care for his/her diabetes at school, _____ will need to have the following items with him/her:

— The insulin infusion pump, which is worn
— Backup pump supplies (syringes, tubing, infusion sets, insulin), and regular syringe
— Glucagon injection kit for severe low blood sugar
— Blood glucose testing supplies (meter, strips, lancet device, and lancets)
— Snack foods and water (to handle extremes of blood glucose)
— Ketostix (to test urine ketones as needed)
— _____

There may be times when he/she will need to be excused to test a blood sugar or for ketones, or to use the bathroom.

In case of a low blood sugar emergency, the pump can be stopped for 30 to no more than 60 minutes, although it is usually more important to raise the blood sugar with a drink or food that contains sugar. _____ can show you how to detach the line ahead of time. If a severe low blood sugar occurs, the catheter can be temporaily detached from the infusion set near the skin site, but it is important to reattach within 30 to 60 minutes.

Pump therapy is a safe and effective way to manage diabetes. We are confident that this individual can handle this tool properly.

If you need further information, please contact his/her family or our office.

Sincerely,

_____   (   ) _____-_____

Index

10.1 Find Your Starting TDD From Your Weight, Current Doses, And Current Control

1. In A, find your weight on the left and circle the average TDD for this weight on the right.
2. In B, calculate your current TDD on injections.
3. In C, compare A and B to obtain a reduced starting TDD.
4. In D, adjust the result in C upward or downward as required based on your recent control.
   Consider a recent A1c, the average blood sugar on your meter, and the frequency of lows.

A. TDD By Weight

For this weight	an average TDD in	
in lbs(kg)	adults[1] is	children[2] is
40 (18)	-	5.0 u/day
60 (27)	-	7.5 u/day
80 (36)	20 u/day	10.0 u/day
100 (45)	25 u/day	12.5 u/day
120 (54)	30 u/day	-
140 (64)	35 u/day	-
160 (73)	40 u/day	-
180 (82)	45 u/day	-
200 (91)	50 u/day	-

B. Current TDD

1. Write down typical doses given at each time of day over the last week.
2. Add together to find your current average TDD.

Insulin	Rapid*	Long	*Rapid = carb + correction
Breakfast	_____ u	_____ u	
Lunch	_____ u	_____ u	
Dinner	_____ u	_____ u	Total = Current TDD
Bedtime	_____ u	_____ u	
Totals	_____ u +	_____ u =	_____ u/day

C. Is the TDD in A less than or greater than B?

A is greater than B:

Suggests excess insulin or some insulin resistance. Add A and B and multiply by 0.45 to obtain 90% of the average as your starting TDD:

TDD from A = _____ u/day

TDD from B = _____ u/day

A + B = _____ u/day

x 0.45

TDD = _____ u/day

A is less than B:

Suggests you are sensitive to insulin. Multiply A times 0.9 to obtain 90% of A as your starting TDD:

TDD from A = _____ u/day

x 0.9

TDD = _____ u/day

D. Your Starting TDD

Consider raising the TDD found in C for a recent high A1c or a high average blood sugar on your meter or lowering it if lows have been frequent or you plan to start a diet or exercise program.

TDD from C of _____ u/day modified to Starting TDD of _____ u/day

[1] An average adult dose ranges from 0.23 to 0.32 unit/lb/day (0.5 to 0.7 unit/kg/day). We use 0.25 u/lb/day.
[2] The average pediatric dose ranges from 0.09 to 0.23 unit/lb/day (0.2 to 0.5 unit/kg/day). We use 0.125 u/lb/day here.

Steps To Take For Optimum Control

You need to perform certain core steps to achieve optimum control on your pump. Workspace 10.1 on the previous page shows how to determine an optimum TDD. Table 10.4 below shows how to distribute this TDD into basal rates and carb and correction factors that should work. (Look also at Tables 10.6 and 10.7 in the book if you require a lower or higher percentage of your TDD for basal delivery.)

Workspace 11.2 on the next page, along with Workspace 12.2 for your carb factor and Workspace 13.3 for your correction factor, show how to test these numbers to ensure that they are the best ones for you to stay in control. Check also that your duration of insulin action is set for the best time for you, as shown on page 154.

10.4 50% Basal And 50% Bolus

Once a starting TDD is determined, find your value in column one and look across that row for close estimates of your starting basal rate, carb factor, and correction factor.

Starting TDD[1] =	Day's Basal[2]	Average Basal[3]	Carb Factor[4] 1u covers:	Corr. Factor[5] 1u lowers BG:
18 units	9 units	0.38 u/hr	28 grams	111 mg/dl (6.1 mmol)
22 units	11 units	0.46 u/hr	23 grams	91 mg/dl (5.0 mmol)
26 units	13 units	0.54 u/hr	19 grams	77 mg/dl (4.2 mmol)
30 units	15 units	0.63 u/hr	17 grams	67 mg/dl (3.7 mmol)
35 units	18 units	0.75 u/hr	14 grams	56 mg/dl (3.1 mmol)
40 units	20 units	0.83 u/hr	12 grams	50 mg/dl (2.8 mmol)
45 units	23 units	0.96 u/hr	11 grams	45 mg/dl (2.4 mmol)
50 units	25 units	1.04 u/hr	10 grams	38 mg/dl (2.2 mmol)
60 units	30 units	1.25 u/hr	8 grams	33 mg/dl (1.8 mmol)
70 units	35 units	1.46 u/hr	7 grams	29 mg/dl (1.5 mmol)
80 units	40 units	1.67 u/hr	6 grams	25 mg/dl (1.3 mmol)
90 units	45 units	1.88 u/hr	6 grams	22 mg/dl (1.2 mmol)
100 units	50 units	2.08 u/hr	5 grams	20 mg/dl (1.1 mmol)

[1] Calculate the starting TDD on page 117.
[2] Day's basal is 50% of the TDD
[3] Avg Basal = day's basal/24 hrs

[4] Carb Factor = 500/TDD
[5] Correction Factor = 2000/TDD in mg/dl or 110/TDD in mmol

11.2 Test Your Basal Rates

1. Start your basal test:
   - at least 5 hours after your last bolus and at least 3 hours after your last carb intake
   - when your starting BG is reasonable, such as between 100 and 150 (5.6 to 8.3 mmol)
   - on a day when there has been no unusual strenuous activity, moderate or severe hypoglycemia, or stress.
2. Monitor your glucose every 1-2 hours (or at 0, 4, and 8 hours for an overnight basal test).
3. Record times, BGs, and change from starting BG in mg/dl or mmol.
4. Plot the change in your BG.
5. If your glucose level rises or falls more than 30 mg/dl (1.7 mmol), refer to Table 11.4 for how much to change your basal.

Basal Test

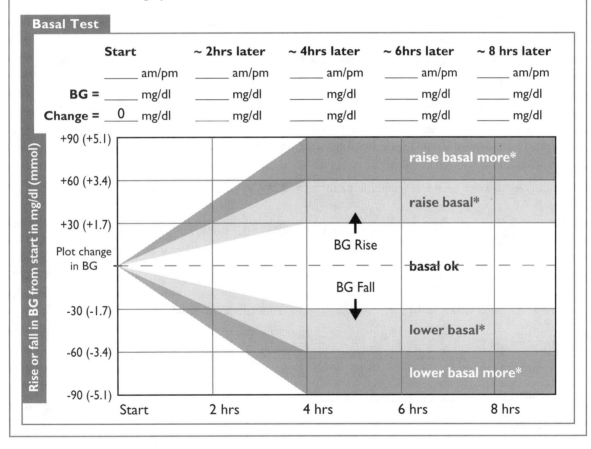

	Start	~ 2hrs later	~ 4hrs later	~ 6hrs later	~ 8 hrs later
	_____ am/pm	_____ am/pm	_____ am/pm	_____ am/pm	_____ am/pm
BG =	_____ mg/dl	_____ mg/dl	_____ mg/dl	_____ mg/dl	_____ mg/dl
Change =	0 mg/dl	_____ mg/dl	_____ mg/dl	_____ mg/dl	_____ mg/dl

Order Pumping Insulin And Other Helpful Diabetes Books

Send me _____ copy(ies) of **Pumping Insulin** 4th edition at $23.95 each, plus shipping. (California residents add 7.75% sales tax.) This and many other diabetes books and products are available at www.diabetesnet.com/ishop/ Call for discounts on quantity orders.

Name _____

Address _____

City _____ State _____ Zip _____

Phone ( ) _____ – _____ Email _____@_____

_____ **Pumping Insulin** 4th edition at $23.95 each ($25.81 in Calif.) $ _____

_____ **Using Insulin** at $23.95 each ($25.81 in Calif.) $ _____

_____ **Smart Charts** (refill for 4 mos.) at $8.95 ($9.64 in Calif.) $ _____

_____ **Smart Charts** (refill for 12 mos.) at $21.45 ($23.11 in Calif.) $ _____

Shipping: ❑ Priority Mail $4.50 ❑ Bookrate $3.25 $ _____
(+ $1.25 for each add.) (+ $0.50 for each add. item)
Total $ _____

Payment: ❑ Check ❑ Visa ❑ MC ❑ Amer Express ❑ Discover

Card #: _____ Expires: _____ /_____

Signature: _____

Mail to:

Torrey Pines Press /
Diabetes Mall
1030 West Upas St.
San Diego, CA 92103

Call: (800) 988-4772
Fax: (619) 497-0900
Online: www.diabetesnet.com/ishop/